Textbook of
Forensic Pharmacy

Textbook of Forensic Pharmacy

Dr. Reema Dheer
Ph.D., FISHE
Associate Professor,
LBS College of Pharmacy, Jaipur

Manoj Dheer
Assistant Drugs Controller,
Govt. of Rajasthan

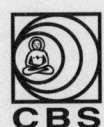

CBS Publishers & Distributors Pvt. Ltd.
New Delhi • Bengaluru • Chennai • Kochi • Kolkata • Mumbai • Pune
Hyderabad • Nagpur • Patna • Vijayawada

Textbook of Forensic Pharmacy

> **Disclaimer**
> Science and technology are constantly changing fields. New research and experience broaden the scope of information and knowledge. The authors have tried their best in giving information available to them while preparing the material for this book. Although, all efforts have been made to ensure optimum accuracy of the material, yet it is quite possible some errors might have been left uncorrected. The publisher, the printer and the authors will not be held responsible for any inadvertent errors or inaccuracies.

ISBN: 978-81-239-2803-6

Copyright © Authors and Publisher

First Edition: 2016
Reprint: 2018, 2023

All rights reserved. No part of this book may be reproduced or transmitted in any form or by any means, electronic or mechanical, including photocopying, recording, or any information storage and retrieval system without permission, in written, from the author and the publisher.

Published by Satish Kumar Jain and produced by Varun Jain for
CBS Publishers & Distributors Pvt Ltd
4819/XI Prahlad Street, 24 Ansari Road, Daryaganj, New Delhi 110 002, India
Ph: 011-23289259, 23266861   Website: www.cbspd.com
                                 e-mail: delhi@cbspd.com
Corporate Office: 204 FIE, Industrial Area, Patparganj, Delhi 110 092, India
Ph: 011-4934 4934   Fax: 011-4934 4935   e-mail: publishing@cbspd.com; publicity@cbspd.com

Branches

- **Bengaluru:** Seema House 2975, 17th Cross, KR Road, Banasankari 2nd Stage, Bengaluru 560 070, Karnataka, India
  Ph: +91-80-26771678/79   Fax: +91-80-26771680   e-mail: bangalore@cbspd.com
- **Chennai:** 7, Subbaraya Street, Shenoy Nagar, Chennai 600 030, Tamil Nadu, India
  Ph: +91-44-26680620, 26681266   Fax: +91-44-42032115   e-mail: chennai@cbspd.com
- **Kochi:** 42/1325, 1326, Power House Road, Opp KSEB, Power House, Ernakulam, Kochi 682 018, India
  Ph: +91-484-4059061-65   Fax: +91-484-4059065   e-mail: kochi@cbspd.com
- **Kolkata:** 147, Hind Ceramics Compound, 1st Floor, Nilgunj Road, Belghoria, Kolkata 700 056, West Bengal, India
  Ph: +91-33-25633055-56   e-mail: kolkata@cbspd.com
- **Lucknow:** Basement, Khushnuma Complex, 7-Meerabai Marg (behind Jawahar Bhawan), Lucknow 226 001, India
  Ph: +91-522-4000032   e-mail: tiwari.lucknow@cbspd.com
- **Mumbai:** PWD Shed. Gala no. 25/26, Ramchandra Bhatt Marg, Next to JJ Hospital Gate no. 2, Opp. Union Bank of India, Noorbaug Mumbai 400 009, Maharashtra, India
  Ph: +91-22-66661880/89   e-mail: mumbai@cbspd.com

Representatives

- **Hyderabad** 0-9885175004 • **Jharkhand** 0-9811541605 • **Nagpur** 0-9421945513
- **Patna** 0-9334159340 • **Pune** 0-9923910676 • **Uttarakhand** 0-9716462459

Printed at Nikunj Print Process, Sonipat, Haryana

DEDICATION

We admit with all humbleness that this book would not have seen the light of the day without the untiring support, guidance and motivation which we received from our associates, friends and family.

Without naming people and their individual contributions, we dedicate this book to all of them with profound regards, heartfelt gratitude and thanks.

We take this opportunity to convey thanks to our Parents and Teacher, Prof. V.N. Sharma for showing us the way and leading us on the path in our endeavour to impart knowledge to our students.

As Teachers at heart, we pray to God to be with all students and help them to do well in life.

Reema Dheer
Manoj Dheer

Dr. V.N. Sharma
M.B.B.S., M.Sc. (Med),
Ph.D. (Pharmacology), F.A.M.S.

A-9/1, Vijay Path, Tilak Nagar
Jaipur – 302 004
Phone: 141 2620692
Mobile: 98290 85788
E-mail: silveron_c@yahoo.co.in

Emeritus Prof. Pharmacology, SMS Medical College, Jaipur
Technical Advisor, LBS College of Pharmacy, Jaipur
Chairman, Ethics Committee, SMS Medical College & Hospital,
Fortis Hospital and Monilek Hospital, Jaipur
Former Prof. & Head, Deptt. of Pharmacology &
Principal and Controller, Associated Group of Hospitals
Medical Colleges, Jodhpur and Bikaner

FOREWORD

As the Technical Advisor in LBSCOP, Jaipur, I was associated with Dr. Reema Dheer for nearly two decades. I always appreciated her knowledge and analytical approach amalgamated with dedication and excellent teaching skills.

During my frequent and extensive academic interactions, I realized the strength of Manoj Dheer as a teacher since he was combining his knowledge of the subject with the practical experience gained by him as an ADC, Rajasthan.

In my opinion, both Dr. Reema Dheer and Manoj Dheer belong to the category of exceptional teachers who inspire the students to understand the subject while studying and their method of presentation makes the subject interesting.

The authors have prepared an updated book in simple language, keeping the syllabus in view. I feel happy for the students and professionals who stand to gain a lot from this effort of Reema and Manoj Dheer.

I have gone through the manuscript of the book, prepared for publication. Each chapter has an introduction and contains essential information of the topic. I am sure that, in the coming times, this will become a 'must possess' book not only for the students of pharmacy but also for the pharmacy professionals who are employed in private or public sector.

This book will always be a useful tool to consult in matters related to regulations, regulatory requirements, ethical practices and legal aspects.

I wish all success to this much needed effort in Forensic Pharmacy.

Dr. V.N. SHARMA

Preface

The profession of pharmacy has shown a rapid growth in the recent years. In terms of volume, the Indian pharmaceutical industry is not just the world's third largest but is also very vibrant and hence it is transforming and undergoing continuous changes. It is the need of the day and also the requirement of the regulating authorities that the pharmacy student should be equipped with updated knowledge of the Acts and the Rules & Regulations specified therein.

Forensic pharmacy has become an important subject for the students of pharmacy as it deals with the application of scientific knowledge to legal problems and legal proceedings considering the changing scenario.

This book provides a systematic coverage of the theory as well as the application thereof in the field of forensic pharmacy. Efforts have been made to incorporate all the latest changes made by the Government from time to time in the Acts.

Every chapter gives the definitions, objectives, administrative agencies, procedures, offences and other related aspects, under the respective Act.

The systematic structure of the book is assigned to cover the major syllabi of Forensic Pharmacy in 20 chapters and includes all topics of syllabus proposed by AICTE while broadly covering the syllabi of diploma, undergraduate and postgraduate courses in pharmacy.

The main objective of the book is to provide updated and comprehensive knowledge of the subject and fulfill the requirements of the students as per the curriculum of the various universities and competitive and entrance examinations held for jobs and postgraduate courses. At the end of each chapter, questions for revision have also been added for the benefit of students.

The chapters covered in the book are: Pharmaceutical Legislation in India; Code of Pharmaceutical Ethics; The Pharmacy Act, 1948; The Drugs and Cosmetics Act, 1940 and Rules, 1945; The Medicinal and Toilet Preparations (Excise Duties) Act, 1955 and Rules, 1956; The Narcotic Drugs and Psychotropic Substances Act, 1985 and Rules; The Drug Price Control Order (DPCO), 2013; New Drug Policy; The Drugs and Magic Remedies (Objectionable Advertisements) Act, 1954; The Poisons Act, 1919; The Medical Termination of Pregnancy Act, 1971; The Insecticides Act, 1968; The Prevention of Cruelty to Animals Act, 1960; The Shops and Establishment Act, 1954; The All India Council for Technical Education Act, 1987; The Factories Act, 1948; The Minimum Wages Act, 1948; Intellectual Property Rights; The Legal Meterology Act, 2009; The Patents Act, 1970; Right to Information Act, 2005.

The List of Drugs Prohibited for Manufacture and Sale as per the Drugs and Cosmetics Act, 1940, List of Essential Drugs, Psychotropic Substances and the Prescribed Standards for Disinfectant Fluids, has been included in the Appendices.

For any requirement of legal interpretations, the readers are advised to refer the latest Gazette Notifications issued by the Ministry of Health, Government of India, New Delhi.

We are thankful to Mr. Satish Kumar Jain, CMD, CBS Publishers & Distributors Pvt. Ltd., and Mr. B.M. Singh for excellent arrangement of the text, editorial support, and publication of the book on priority basis.

Comments/suggestions from readers are welcome and the same may be incorporated in subsequent edition.

Reema Dheer
Manoj Dheer

Contents

Foreword vii
Preface ix

1. Pharmaceutical Legislation in India 1
2. Code of Pharmaceutical Ethics 6
3. The Pharmacy Act 12
4. The Drugs and Cosmetics Act, 1940 and Rules, 1945 29
    (a) Administration of the Act *33*
    (b) Schedules *44*
    (c) Import of Drugs and Cosmetics *64*
    (d) Manufacture of Drugs and Cosmetics *72*
    (e) Sale of Drugs *90*
    (f) Labelling and Packing of Drugs *102*
    (g) Provisions Applicable to Ayurvedic, Siddha and Unani Drugs *109*
    (h) Provisions Applicable to Homeopathic Medicines *116*
    (i) Provisions Applicable to Cosmetics *120*
    (j) General Provisions About Offences *125*
    (k) Miscellaneous – List of colours permitted to be used in drugs *126*
5. Medicinal and Toilet Preparations (Excise Duties) Act, 1955 and Rules, 1956 130
6. The Narcotic Drugs and Psychotropic Substances Act, 1985 149

7. The Drugs and Magic Remedies
   (Objectionable Advertisements) Act, 1954 168
8. Drugs (Price Control) Order, 2013 174
9. The Poisons Act, 1919 184
10. Medical Termination of Pregnancy Act, 1971 187
11. Prevention of Cruelty to Animals Act 192
12. The Insecticides Act, 1968 198
13. Shops and Establishment Act 208
14. The AICTE Act, 1987 215
15. The Factories Act, 1948 222
16. The Legal Metrology Act, 2009 235
17. Minimum Wages Act, 1948 245
18. Intellectual Property Rights 253
19. The Patents Act, 1970 263
20. Right to Information Act, 2005 275

Appendices 283
Appendix A   Banned Drugs   *283*
Appendix B   Scheme of Testing and Inspection for Certification
             of Disinfectant Fluid, Phenolic Type According to
             IS 1061:1997 (With Amendment No. 1)   *288*
Appendix C   The Schedule – List of Psychotropic Substances   *292*
Appendix D   List of Essential Medicines   *295*

List of Abbreviations 313
Index 315

Chapter 1

Pharmaceutical Legislation in India

The pharmaceutical legislation is related with legal system which regulates the conduct of pharmacy business and practice of profession of pharmacy. The in-depth knowledge of pharmaceutical legislation helps the pharmacists to understand their legal and ethical responsibility and can prevent the undesirable legal proceedings. The pharmaceutical legislation safeguards the health of the people by making the right medication available to the general public as well as protects the rights of the pharmacist practising the profession of pharmacy.

Objectives of pharmaceutical legislation

1. To facilitate and promote healthcare by regulating the manufacture, sale, import, etc. and hence quality of the drugs.
2. To make the drugs available to the public at a reasonable price and through a qualified person.
3. To exercise control over the false and misleading advertisements related to drugs and magic remedies.
4. To promote research and development indigenously.

History of pharmacy legislation in India

In the early part of the 20th century, there was practically no legislative control on drugs as well as on the profession of pharmacy. Although, the Opium Act, 1878, the Poisons Act, 1919 and the Dangerous Drugs Act, 1930 were in force, these were specific in nature and grossly inadequate in controlling the chaotic conditions prevailing at that time.

In 1927, a resolution was passed by the council of states to recommend to the Governor General in Council to urge provincial governments to take immediate steps to control indiscriminate use of drugs and to legislate for the standardization of the preparation and sale of drugs. The government of India in pursuance to the resolution appointed a committee known as the Drugs Enquiry Committee (DEC) in 1928. Government of India on 11th August 1930, appointed a committee under the chairmanship of *Late Col. R.N. Chopra*, known as Chopra Committee, to see into the problems of Pharmacy in India and recommend the measures to be taken. This committee published its report in 1931 and it was reported that there was no recognized specialized profession of Pharmacy. A set of people known as compounders were filling the gap.

Recommendations of Chopra Committee

The DEC recommended the following:

1. Central legislation to control drugs and pharmacy.
2. Setting up testing laboratories in all the states to control and ensure the quality of manufactured and imported drugs.
3. To set up Advisory Board to advise the Government in making rules.
4. Start courses for training in pharmacy and prescribing minimum qualification for pharmacist.
5. Development of pharmaceutical industry.

Just after the publication of the report *Prof. M.L. Schroff* (Prof. Mahadeva Lal Schroff) initiated pharmaceutical education at the university level in the Banaras Hindu University. In 1935, United Province Pharmaceutical Association was established which was later converted into Indian Pharmaceutical Association. The Indian Journal of Pharmacy was started by Prof. M.L. Schroff in 1939. All India Pharmaceutical Congress Association was established in 1940.

Government of India brought 'Import of Drugs Bill' which was later withdrawn. Subsequently, in 1940, Government brought 'Drugs Bill' to regulate the import, manufacture, sale and distribution of drugs in British India. This Bill was finally adopted as 'Drugs Act of 1940'. In 1941, the first Drugs Technical Advisory Board (DTAB) under this Act was constituted and Central Drugs Laboratory was established in Calcutta.

In 1945, 'Drugs Rule under the Drugs Act of 1940' was notified. Since then, the Drugs Act has been modified from time to time and at present the provisions of the Act cover cosmetics and Ayurvedic, Unani and Homeopathic medicines in some respects. The present Drugs and Cosmetics Act is an improved version of the Drug Act 1940. In 1945, the Government brought the Pharmacy Bill to standardize the Pharmacy Education in India and in 1946, The Indian Pharmacopoeial List was published under the chairmanship of *Late Col. R.N. Chopra*. It consisted of lists of drugs in use in India at that time, which were not included in British Pharmacopoeia. In 1948, Pharmacy Act 1948 was published and a Indian Pharmacopoeial Committee was constituted under the chairmanship of late *Dr. B.N. Ghosh* in the same year.

After independence, the **Indian Pharmacopoeial Committee** was constituted in 1948 which compiled The Pharmacopoeia of India (I.P.), an official book of Government of India, in 1955. Its first edition was published in the year 1955 followed by a supplement to it in 1960. The next edition was published in 1966, which contained Western as well as traditional drugs. The supplement to 1966 edition was published in 1975. In the next edition of 1985 and its addendum in 1989 and 1991, traditional drugs were not included. The fourth edition of I.P. was published in 1996 and its addendum/supplement 2000 and 2002, the fifth edition in 2007, sixth edition of I.P. in 2010 and seventh in 2014. The seventh edition of 2014-2015 includes indigenous herbs, herbal products, veterinary vaccines, products of biotechnology, additional anti-cancer and anteroviral drugs. Standards of new drugs and drugs used under National Health Programme are added and the drugs as well as their formulations not in use now-a-days are omitted from this edition. 19 new radiopharmaceutical monographs and one general chapter are first time being included in this edition. All pharmaceutical manufacturers and persons dealing with drugs shall comply with the standards of monographs in Indian Pharmacopoeia.

In the year 1949, Pharmacy Council of India (P.C.I.) was established under Pharmacy Act. After that, in 1954, the Education Regulations came in force in some states but other states lagged behind. *Drugs and Magic Remedies (Objectionable Advertisements) Act 1954* was passed in the same year to stop misleading advertisements (e.g. Cure all pills). In 1955, *Medicinal and Toilet Preparations (Excise Duties) Act 1955* was introduced to enforce uniform duty for all states for alcohol products.

To have efficient control and vigilance, "*Prevention of Food Adulteration Act 1954*", "*Factory Act 1948*", The "*Indian Patent and Design Act 1970*", "*Medicinal and Toilet Preparations Act 1955*", "*Medical Termination of Pregnancy Act 1971*", etc. were enforced and amended from time to time.

Further, in 1985, *Narcotic and Psychotropic Substances Act* was enacted to protect society from the dangers of addictive drugs. Similarly, to control the price of drugs in India by Drugs Price Order was enforced by the Government, which changed as and when required.

Several other committees were constituted like the **Bhore Committee** under the chairmanship of *Sir Joseph Bhore* in 1948, **Bhatia Committee** under the chairmanship of *Major General S.L. Bhatia* in 1953, **Mudaliyar Committee** under the chairmanship of *Dr. A. Lakshmanswamy Mudaliyar* in 1961 and **Hathi Committee** under the chairmanship of *Jaisukh Lal Hathi*.

The Hathi Committee took a comprehensive look into the various facets of the drug industry in India. The report covered all aspects of the import, licensing, price control, role of foreign sector, quality control, etc. It encouraged the development of indigenous industry vis-à-vis the foreign dominated multinational drug companies. The prices of large number of drugs in the interest of the consumers was also taken care of.

To attract foreign capital and technology, a new drug policy was announced in September 1994 in the form of "*Modifications in Drug Policy, 1986*". The globalization of economy is expected to provide greater momentum to production, improved quality, easy flow of goods and services including pharmaceutical across national frontiers.

"**Pharmacy Practice Regulations 2015**" have been released on 16th January 2015 and is expected, that, they will largely benefit the patients in coming days. The comprehensive changes in the regulations will lead to improved quality of health care and will ensure that pharmacists maintain high standards in their duty, to reduce cost of health care and to inhibit criminal abuse of medicines. As per the clauses in the regulations, a registered pharmacist will now allow review the patient record and each prescription presented for supply for the purpose of promoting therapeutic appropriateness.

Another important aspect of the "Pharmacy Practice Regulations, 2015" is that the pharmacist is authorised (as a healthcare professional) to undertake process and outcome research, health promotion and education and provide health information. It also allows the registered pharmacists to undertake the pharmacoepidemiological studies.

Evolution of pharmacist as an integral part of the healthcare system

The pharmacist now plays a major role in the healthcare system and is no longer considered as a mere compounder or a small manufacturer. He is the most important link between patient and a Registered Medical Practitioner (RMP).

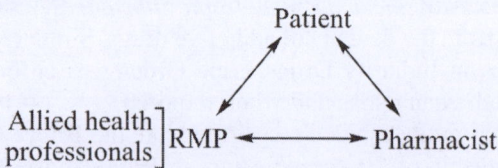

QUESTIONS FOR REVISION

1. Give an account of Pharmaceutical legislation in India.
2. Write notes on:
   (a) Chopra Committee,
   (b) Development of Pharmacy as a profession.

Chapter 2

Code of Pharmaceutical Ethics

The word "Ethics" originated from a Greek word "Ethikos" meaning custom or character and ethics may be defined as *"the code of moral principles"* or as *"the science of morals"*. The conduct of individuals in any society is governed by governmental controls as well as social customs and duties.

Professionals' ethics play an important role in smooth functioning of the society. The law of the land may prevent a person from causing injury to another but cannot force him to help his neighbours in hours of need, for example, the Drugs and Cosmetics Rules can stop a pharmacist from selling adulterated, misbranded drugs, etc. but cannot prevent him from practices performed for meagre material gains and indulging in cut throat competition. However, morality can be taught through codes or lessons.

Profession of Pharmacy is a noble profession as it is indirectly helping the persons to get well with the help of medical practitioners and other co-professionals. Government has restricted the practice of Pharmacy to only Professional Pharmacists i.e. registered Pharmacist under the Pharmacy Act 1948. Standards of professional conduct for pharmacy are necessary in the public interest to ensure an efficient pharmaceutical service and safeguard the people's health. Therefore, *Pharmacy Council of India (PCI) has framed the following ethics for Indian Pharmacists, which may be categorized under the following headings:*

1. Pharmacist in relation to his job
2. Pharmacist in relation to his trade
3. Pharmacist in relation to medical profession
4. Pharmacist in relation to his profession.

OBJECTIVES

The code of ethics framed by the Pharmacy Council of India is meant to guide the Indian Pharmacist as to how he should conduct himself in relation to himself, his patrons and the general public, co-professionals, and members of the medical and other health professions.

1. Pharmacist in relation to his job

The salient features of code of pharmaceutical ethics in relation to his job are:

(i) **Scope of Pharmaceutical services:** Pharmacy premises (medicine shops) should be registered and it should provide reasonable comprehensive pharmaceutical services like supply of commonly required medicines to the patients as per the requirement and provide emergency supplies at all times without delay.

(ii) **Conduct of the Pharmacy:** A qualified pharmacist should have control over the pharmacy. Error of accidental contamination in the preparation, dispensing and supply of medicines should be checked and professionalism should reflect in the appearance of the premises. It should be clearly evident that Practice of Pharmacy is being carried out in the premises.

A Pharmacist should always be there in every pharmacy. At the premises a notice, indicating and stating that dispensing is carried out under Employees State Insurance Scheme (E.S.I.S.) or any other similar scheme sponsored by the government, should be exhibited.

(iii) **Handling of prescription:** A pharmacist should receive a prescription without any comment on it that may cause anxiety to the patient and may even shake the faith in his physician. Question on a prescription should be answered carefully so as not to disclose any information and should neither disclose the secrecy of the prescription to the patient.

The pharmacist should neither add, omit or substitute any ingredient nor alter the composition of a prescription, without the consent of the prescriber. In case of any obvious error, due to any omission, incompatibility or overdose, the prescription should be referred back to the prescriber for correction or approval of the change suggested.

The pharmacist should guide and advice the patient about any special instructions to be followed while using the medicine.

(iv) **Handling of drugs:** A prescription should always be dispensed correctly and carefully with standard quality drug or excipients.

Drugs that have abusive potential should not be supplied to any one. All ingredients should be weighed and measured properly.

(v) **Apprentice Pharmacist:** Experienced pharmacists should provide all the facilities for practical training of the apprentice pharmacists. Until and unless the apprentice proves himself or herself, certificate should not be granted to him/her.

2. Pharmacist in relation to his trade

Following are the provisions which pharmacist should keep in mind while dealing with his trade:

(i) **Price structure:** The prices charged should be fair, keeping with the quality, quantity and labour or skill required in making it ready for use, so that adequate remuneration is ensured to the pharmacist, taking into consideration his knowledge, skill, and the time consumed, but at the same time without unduly overcharging the purchaser.

(ii) **Fair trade practice:** Fair practice should be adopted by a pharmacist in the trade without any attempt to capture other pharmacist's business. If a customer brings a prescription (by mistake) to him which was to be dispensed by some other pharmacy, the pharmacist should refuse to accept the prescription and should direct him to the right place. Imitation of copying of the labels, trade marks and other signs or symbols of other pharmacy should not be done.

He should not offer any sort of prizes or gifts or any kind of allurements to patronize or by deliberately charging less price than those charged by fellow pharmacists.

(iii) **Purchase of drugs:** Pharmacists should buy drugs from genuine and reputable sources. The pharmacist should always be careful not to aid or help directly or indirectly the manufacture, possession, distribution and sale of spurious or sub-standard drugs.

(iv) **Hawking of drugs:** Hawking of drugs and medicinals should not be encouraged and neither should an attempt be made to solicit orders for such substance from door to door.

Distribution of therapeutic substances without an expert supervision is highly undesirable, so "self-service" method of operating pharmacies and medical stores should be discouraged.

(iv) **Advertising and displays:** The sale of medicines or medical appliances or display of materials in undignified style on the premises, in the press or elsewhere, which contains the following are prohibited:

- Any warnings, design or illustration, reflecting unfavorably on a pharmacist, collectively or upon any group or individuals.

- A disparaging reference, direct or by implication to other supplier, products, remedies, or treatments.
- Misleading or exaggerated statements or claims.
- The word 'cure' or reference to an ailment or symptoms of ill health.
- A guarantee of therapeutic efficacy.
- An appeal to fear.
- An offer to refund money paid.
- A prize, competition or similar scheme.
- Any reference to medical practitioner or a hospital or the use of terms "Doctor" or "Dr" or "Nurse", as connection with the name of a preparation not already established.
- A reference to sexual weakness, premature ageing or loss of virility.
- A reference to complaints of sexual nature in terms which lack the reticence proper to the subject.
- Contraceptive preparations and appliances or their illustrations, except a notice approved by regulations or bearing the words "Family Planning Requisites", should not be exhibited.
- *Under no circumstance should lustful, obscene and indecent publications of any kind or description be sold or distributed, as this practice may prove highly detrimental to the moral welfare of the nation.*

3. Pharmacist in relation to medical profession.

Following are the code of ethics of a pharmacist in relation to medical profession:

(i) **Limitation of professional activity:** The professional activity of the pharmacists should be confined to their own field only and under no circumstances indulge into medical practice and should not diagnose diseases and prescribe medicines. A pharmacist may, however, deliver first aid to the victim in case of accident or emergency.

Pharmacist should never recommend a medical practitioner unless specifically asked to do so.

(ii) **Clandestine arrangements:** A pharmacist should not enter into a secret arrangement or contract with a physician by offering him any commission or any advantages.

(iii) **Liaison with public:** A pharmacist should always maintain proper link between physicians and people. He should advise the physicians on pharmaceutical matters and should educate the people regarding health and hygiene. The pharmacist should always keep himself/herself up-to-date with pharmaceutical knowledge from various journals or publications. Any information acquired by a pharmacist during his professional activities should not be disclosed to any third party until and unless required to do so by law.

4. Pharmacist in relation to his profession

Regarding the profession, the following code of ethics should be fulfilled:

(i) **Professional vigilance:** A pharmacist must abide by the pharmaceutical laws and he/she should see that other pharmacists are abiding it. He should not be afraid of bringing or causing a miscreant to be brought to book, even if he is a member of his own profession.

The pharmacist should extend help and cooperation to a fellow member in his legitimate needs, scientific, technical or otherwise, but at the same time should be vigilant to weed the undesirable out of the profession and thus help to maintain its fair name and traditions.

He should be prepared to serve any time of the day in case of emergencies and above all should be a good and responsible citizen.

(ii) **Law-abiding citizens:** The pharmacists should have a fair knowledge of the laws of the country pertaining to food, drug, pharmacy, health, sanitation, etc.

(iii) **Relationship with professional organizations:** A pharmacist should be actively involved in professional organizations, should advance the cause of such organizations.

(iv) **Decorum and propriety:** A pharmacist should not indulge in doing anything that goes against the decorum and propriety of Pharmacy Profession.

PHARMACIST'S OATH

A young prospective pharmacist should feel no hesitation in assuming the following pharmacist's oath:

"I promise to do all I can to protect and improve the physical and moral well-being of society, holding the health and safety of my community above other considerations. I shall uphold the laws and standards governing my profession, avoiding all forms of misinterpretation, and I shall safeguard the distribution of medical and potent substances.

Knowledge gained about patients, I shall hold in confidence and never divulge unless compelled to do so by law.

I shall strive to perfect and enlarge my knowledge to contribute to the advancements of pharmacy and the public health.

    I furthermore promise to maintain my honour in all transactions and by my conduct never bring discredit to myself or to my profession nor to do anything to diminish the trust reposed in my professional brethren.

   May I prosper and live long in favour as I keep and hold to this, my Oath, but if violated these sacred promises, may the reverse be my lot."

QUESTIONS FOR REVISION

1. Describe briefly the essential features of code of ethics related to his job framed by Pharmacy Council of India.
2. Write notes on:
   (a) Pharmacist in relation to his trade.
   (b) Pharmacist in relation to his profession.
   (c) Pharmacist in relation to medical profession
   (d) Pharmacist's Oath.

Chapter 3

The Pharmacy Act

Medicines have an important role to play in safeguarding the public health and so does the pharmacist, as he has the key role in handling, compounding, dispensing and storage, etc. of these medicines or drugs.

Earlier there was no restriction at the entry level and hence any person without having any knowledge of pharmacy or pharmacology or pharmaceutical chemistry was engaged in the practice of pharmacy. The pharmaceutical profession was represented only by the so-called 'compounders' who were almost at par with the lowest cadre worker in the health profession and were not required to undergo any formal education. Anyone who could read a prescription and do some mixings in a dispensary could harbour ambition of becoming a compounder.

There were no regulations for the education to be imparted or the practical training necessary for the pharmacist, but now the scenario has changed and there are provisions for control, starting from procurement, preparation, handling, dispensing, etc. of drugs. Every country now has number of laws to provide for the education and training of persons entering the profession of pharmacy.

In India, "The Pharmacy Act, 1948" was passed with the broad objective of regulating the practice of pharmacy, formalizing education and training of would be pharmaceutical professionals and exercise control to uplift the almost non-existent profession.

The Act extends to entire India (except, Jammu & Kashmir) and has been amended thrice in 1959, 1976 and 1982 to cater to the changed social needs.

Objectives of the Act

As indicated above, the Act was passed with the following objectives in view:

(a) To frame a programme of education and practical training for persons willing to enter and practice the profession of pharmacy. This objective is achieved through Pharmacy Council of India (PCI).

(b) To limit the practice of profession to such qualified and trained professionals, who are registered with the State Pharmacy Council or Joint Pharmacy Councils only and to monitor their professional work.

The above objectives can be achieved by entrusting responsibilities on Pharmacy Council of India (Central Council) and State Pharmacy Councils. The constitution, procedures, etc. of these are discussed in the following sections:

(i) Central Council means the Pharmacy Council of India.
(ii) State Council means the State Council of Pharmacy constituted under the Act and includes the Joint State Council of Pharmacy.
(iii) Central Register means the register of Pharmacists maintained by the Central Council.
(iv) Medical Practitioner means a person holding medical qualification as provided in the Indian Medical Degree's Act or Indian Medical Council Act or a person registered or eligible for registration in the medical register of the State or a Dentist or a Veterinarian.
(v) Registered Pharmacist means a person whose name for the time being is entered in the Register of Pharmacists of the state in which he is for the time being residing or engaged in the profession or business of Pharmacy.

THE PHARMACY COUNCIL OF INDIA

To ensure and fulfill quality and uniform education and training, the Act has provided for the constitution of the Pharmacy Council of India (PCI). The Pharmacy Council of India is constituted by the Central Government every five years. It has the power and responsibility to frame courses of study for pharmacists and for approving institutions which conduct the courses. The first Pharmacy Council of India was constituted in 1949, soon after the enactment of the Pharmacy Act. The present constitution of the Pharmacy Council of India and its functions, etc. are discussed below.

Constitution of Pharmacy Council of India

The Pharmacy Council of India (PCI) constituted by the Central Government has the following composition:

A. Elected members

(i) Six members, at least one teacher each of Pharmacy, Pharmaceutical Chemistry, Pharmacology and Pharmacognosy elected by UGC from the teaching staff of an Indian University or an affiliated college granting a degree or diploma in Pharmacy.
(ii) One member, elected by the Medical Council of India from amongst its members.
(iii) One member elected by each State Pharmacy Council who shall be a Registered Pharmacist.

B. Nominated members

(i) Six members, nominated by the Central Government, including at least four persons possessing degree or diploma in Pharmacy and engaged in the practice of Pharmacy or Pharmaceutical Chemistry.
(ii) One representative each of University Grants Commission and the All India Council for Technical Education.
(iii) One Registered Pharmacist to represent each State nominated by the State Government/Union Territory Administration.

C. Ex-officio members

(i) The Director General of Health Services.
(ii) The Director of Central Drugs Laboratory.
(iii) The Drugs Controller of India.

The President and Vice-President of the Pharmacy Council are elected by its members from amongst themselves for a term of five years. The elected and the nominated members of the Council hold office for a term of five years, but they can resign from their membership at any time by writing to the President of PCI. Any member remaining absent, for three consecutive meetings, without sufficient reasons, deemed to have vacated his seat from the Council. A casual vacancy in the PCI is usually filled by fresh nomination or election and the person so nominated or elected holds the office only for the remaining term. All members of the Council are eligible for re-election or re-nomination. The members nominated by U.G.C. or Medical Council of India or State Pharmacy Councils shall no longer remain members of PCI as soon as they cease to be a staff in university or a college, or a member of MCI or a registered pharmacist in the state.

The Council has the authority to fix the rate of allowances payable to its members, lay down rules for its procedures, decide the mode of elections and conduct elections. The Council may constitute, amongst its members, such committees which can be helpful in the functioning of council and for the same, may coopt persons who are not a member of the council for a period not exceeding 5 years.

Copies of the minutes of the meetings, summary of the annual activities, the accounts, etc. are required to be submitted to the Central Government. The accounts should be maintained as per the directions of the Controller and Auditor-General of India and are subject to audit by him or his nominee. The reports or abstracts may be published by the government, in the manner it may think proper.

For effective working, the Council may appoint:
(i) A Secretary who may acts as its Registrar and, if necessary, its treasurer as well.
(ii) Other officers and servants for carrying out its statutory functions.
(iii) The Executive Committee of the PCI consisting of the President (Chairman of the Committee) and the Vice-President and five other members elected by the Central Council from amongst its members.

Functions of Pharmacy Council of India

The Pharmacy Council of India has been entrusted with the following functions:

1. Design of Educational Pattern

The main important task of PCI is to frame the educational structure for the would be pharmacist and to keep it tuned to the changing needs with passage of time. The standards of education for pharmacists framed by the Council are known as the Education Regulations and its main features are:

(i) Minimum qualification for admission to the course;
(ii) Duration of the course of study to be covered, training to be undertaken;
(iii) Nature and period of practical training to be undertaken after the completion of the regular course. (Not less than 500 hours covered in a minimum of 3 months in a recognized institution, hospital, pharmacy or dispensary; or licensed chemist and druggist shop);
(iv) The subjects of examinations and the standards to be attained therein for qualification;
(v) Minimum equipments and facilities to be provided by the institutions running approved courses of study;
(vi) Conditions to be fulfilled by institutions giving practical training and the authorities holding approved examinations.

The Education Regulations have to be framed with the approval of the Government of India and after circulating the draft to each State Government and taking into consideration their comments, if any. The Regulations have to be monitored from time to time by the Executive Committee of the Council and may recommend to the Council amendments considered essential. Whenever any amendment is sought to be done in the Regulations, the Council has to follow the procedure presented for their initial drafting namely circulation to the State Governments and approval of the Central Government.

After the formation of the State councils the State Governments were supposed to promulgate the Education Regulations in the States in consultation with the respective State Pharmacy Councils. In case if any State Government takes no action on this behalf, the Act provides that the Education Regulations shall be deemed to have taken effect in that State automatically, on the expiry of three years from the date of the constitution of the State Council.

2. Approval of Institutions/Withdrawal of Approvals

An institution or authority, which conducts a course of study or holds an examination for the pharmacists, has to apply to the Pharmacy Council of India for approval of the course or the examination. The procedure involves:

(a) Application by the institute to PCI.

(b) Inspection by PCI: Whenever PCI receives any application from an institution or authority seeking approval of the course conducted by it, the Council may depute its Inspectors to visit the institution to check whether the prescribed facilities for imparting training or holding examinations are in accordance with the Education Regulations or not. The Inspectors then report to the Council of the facts and facilities available in the institution and on the conduct and standards of the examinations held.

(c) Approval: If on the report of the Inspectors, PCI is satisfied that the course or the examination under consideration is in conformity with the Education Regulations, it may accord approval to it and then the said course or examination shall be deemed to be approved for qualifying for registration as a pharmacist under the Act.

(d) Declaration of approval is published in the Official Gazette by passing a resolution at a meeting of the Council.

If it comes to the notice of the Pharmacy Council of India, that any approved institute does not continue to be in conformity with the Education Regulations, the Council may give notice to the institution or authority concerned, of its intention to withdraw the approval. After looking into any representation that may be made by the institution or authority (through the respective State Governments within three months of the notice), the Council may decide whether the approval is to be withdrawn or is to be continued conditionally, subject to fulfillment of specified conditions by the authority or the institution concerned.

3. Recognition of Foreign Qualifications

PCI may recognize any qualification, granted by an authority outside India, which affords guarantee of requisite skill and knowledge to be a sufficient qualification for registration as a pharmacist under the Act. The Council may further specify that such qualification shall be deemed to be sufficient only when granted before or after a particular date, subject to such additional conditions as may be specified by the Council. In normal cases, only citizens of India possessing such qualifications shall be eligible for registration. Citizens of other countries, holding qualifications granted there, shall be registrable in this country when an Indian national, holding the same qualification, is by law, allowed to enter and practice the profession of pharmacy in that country.

4. Maintenance of Central Register of Pharmacists

Under the provisions of the Pharmacy (Amendment) Act 1976, the Pharmacy Council of India is required to maintain a Register containing names of all persons registered as pharmacists in different States. This Register has to be maintained by the Registrar of the Council in accordance with the directions of the Pharmacy Council of India and has to be revised suitably from time to time and published in the Gazette of India. This Register would be deemed to be a public document within the meaning of the Indian Evidence Act 1872.

The State Pharmacy Councils are required to supply to the Pharmacy Council of India, five copies of their Registers as soon as possible, after 1st April each year and inform it about any amendments made in the Registers from time to time.

Constitution of State and Joint State Pharmacy Council

The Pharmacy Act, 1948 provides for the constitution of a State Pharmacy Council in each State. Two or more States can also enter into an agreement to form a Joint State Pharmacy Council or otherwise the State Pharmacy Council of one State may serve the needs of the other participating States.

Constitution of State Pharmacy Council

Elected Members

1. Six members elected amongst themselves by Registered Pharmacists of the State.
2. One member elected by the Medical Council of the State from amongst its members.

Nominated Members

Five members nominated by the State Government, of whom at least three should possess a degree or diploma in pharmacy or pharmaceutical chemistry or be Registered Pharmacists.

Ex-officio Members
1. Chief Administrative Medical Officer of the State.
2. Officer-in-charge of Drugs Control Administration of the State.
3. Government Analyst of the State or where there is more than one analyst, such one as may be appointed by the State Government.

Constitution of Joint State Pharmacy Council

Elected Members
1. Six members elected amongst themselves by Registered Pharmacists of each participating State.
2. One member elected by the Medical Council of each State from amongst its members.

Nominated Members
Two to four members nominated by each participating State Government of whom more than half should possess a degree or diploma in pharmacy or pharmaceutical chemistry or be Registered Pharmacists.

Ex-officio Members
1. Chief administrative medical officer of each of the participating States.
2. Officer-in-charge of Drugs Control Administration of each participating State.
3. Government Analyst of each participating State or where there is more than one Analyst, such one as may be appointed by the State Government.

Every State Council shall have a President and Vice-President, elected by the members from amongst themselves for tenure of five years from the first constitution of the council. The State Government may nominate the President. If he is not already a member of the council, he becomes a member of the council in addition.

The nominated and elected members of the council hold office for a period of five years. They may, however, resign from their membership by writing to the President. Any member who remains absent for three consecutive meetings, without sufficient excuse, is deemed to have vacated his seat from the council. A casual vacancy in the council is usually filled by fresh nomination or election as the case may be. All members of the council are eligible for re-election or re-nomination. The members, who are elected by the State Pharmacy Council or State Medical Council, shall no longer remain members of Councils as soon as they cease to be a member of State Medical Council or a Registered Pharmacist in the state.

The Council usually appoints a registrar (who may also act as its Secretary and Treasurer) and other necessary officers and staff as may be required to carry out its functions under the Pharmacy Act. The State Council is also required to constitute an Executive Committee similar to that of the Central Council. It should furnish necessary information and annual report to the State Government and to the Pharmacy Council of India.

Functions of State Pharmacy Councils and Joint State Pharmacy Councils

Functions of State Pharmacy Councils and Joint State Pharmacy Councils are as follows:

(a) Inspection by State Councils:

The State Pharmacy Councils or Joint State Pharmacy Councils, with permission from the respective State Governments, may appoint sufficient number of Inspectors having prescribed qualification to:

(i) Inspect any premises where drugs are compounded or dispensed.
(ii) Inquire regarding the registration of the person engaged in compounding and dispensing.
(iii) Investigate any complaint made in writing regarding contravention of the Act.
(iv) Institute prosecution under the direction of the executive committee of the State.
(v) Exercise such other powers as may be deemed necessary in order to give effect to certain provisions of the Act.

(b) Maintenance of the first and subsequent Registers of Pharmacists

Registration of Pharmacists

The Pharmacy Act, 1948 provides for the registration of pharmacists in all the States of India. The State Government prepares the First Register of Pharmacists in a State. After the constitution of the State Pharmacy Councils, the maintenance of the first and subsequent Registers becomes the responsibility of the State Councils. Before the end of June each year, the State Councils are required to pay to the Pharmacy Council of India, a sum equivalent to one-fourth of the fees realized by them during the period of 12 months, ending on the 31st day of March in that year.

The **Register of Pharmacists** includes the following particulars:
(i) Full name and residential address of the registered person.
(ii) Date of his first entry in the register.
(iii) Qualification of the person for registration.
(iv) Professional address of the person and, in case of employed persons, the name of the employer.
(v) Such other particulars as may be prescribed.

First Register

For preparing the First Register, the State Government constitutes a Registration Tribunal consisting of three persons and a Registrar who also acts as its secretary. A date is appointed by the State Government before which all applications for registration, accompanied by the prescribed fee, should reach the registration tribunal. All the applications are examined by the tribunal received upto the appointed date and when satisfied that an applicant is duly qualified, directs his or her name to be entered into the Register.

Conditions required for the entry into first register

(i) Should have attained the age of 18 years.
(ii) Should pay the prescribed fee.
(iii) Should be a resident of the State or should carry out his business or profession of pharmacy in the State.
(iv) Should have the following qualifications:
  (a) A degree or diploma in pharmacy or pharmaceutical chemistry or a chemist and druggist diploma of an Indian university or a State Government or possess any other qualification granted outside India which is recognized as adequate for registration, or
  (b) A degree of an Indian university other than a degree or diploma in pharmacy or pharmaceutical chemistry along with an experience of not less than three years in dispensing and compounding of drugs in a hospital or dispensary or any other place where drugs are regularly dispensed on the prescription of a Registered Medical Practitioner, or
  (c) Should have passed an examination recognized by the State Government as adequate for compounders and dispensers, or
  (d) Should have an experience of not less than five years in dispensing and compounding of drugs in a hospital or dispensary or any other place where drugs are dispensed regularly on the prescription of a Registered Medical Practitioner, prior to the date notified by the State Government for receipt of applications, for entry of names on the First Register.

The First Register may be published as directed by the State Government. Any person, who is dissatisfied with the decision of the tribunal, has a right to appeal to the authority, appointed by the Government in this behalf, within 60 days of the publication of the Register. The decision of the State Government is considered to be final and the tribunal has to amend the Register in accordance with the directions of the Government. Upon the constitution of the State Council the register is handed over into its custody.

Subsequent Registers

After the preparation of the First Register and before the Education Regulations have taken effect in a State, a person who wants his name to be registered in the subsequent Register:
 (i) Should be at least 18 years of age.
 (ii) Should have paid the prescribed fee.
 (iii) Should be a resident of the State or should carry out his business or profession of pharmacy in the State.
 (iv) Should fulfill the following requirements:
   (a) Requirements as prescribed for registration and where no such requirements have been prescribed, possess the qualifications which would have entitled him to have his name registered on the first Register and is at least matriculate, or
   (b) Is a Registered Pharmacist in another State, or
   (c) Possess a qualification granted outside India which is recognized as adequate for registration and is at least matriculate.

(c) Entry and Removal of Names

After an appointed date, all applications for registration should be addressed to the Registrar of the State Pharmacy Council. On receipt of the application, if the Registrar is of the opinion that the applicant has the requisite qualifications for registration, he may give directions to enter his or her name in the Register. Persons whose names have been removed from the Registers of other States shall not be entitled to registration, unless the State Council gives its consent thereto. Any person, whose application for registration has been rejected by the Registrar, may appeal to the State Council, within three months of the rejection of application. The decision of the State Council shall be final.

Once the name of a person is entered in the Register, the Registrar is required to issue to him a certificate of registration in the prescribed form. The retention of the name on the Register shall be subject to payment of the prescribed fee annually to the State Council by due date, as specified in this behalf. If the renewal fee is not paid by the due date, the Registrar shall remove the name of the defaulter from the Register. The name so removed may, however, be restored to the Register on the prescribed conditions being satisfied. On payment of the fees, the Registrar is required to issue a receipt thereof and such receipts are deemed to be proofs of renewal of registration. Any professional qualifications attained by the registered pharmacist (which he may have obtained after his first registration) is entered against his name in the Register, subject to the payment of fees prescribed on that behalf.

(d) Removal of Names from the Register

The name of a pharmacist may be removed from the Register on following reasons:

(i) If his name has been entered in the Register due to error, mis-representation or suppression of facts, or

(ii) If he has been convicted of an offence in any professional respect, which, in the opinion of the Executive Committee, renders him unfit to be on the Register of Pharmacists, or

(iii) If a person, employed to work under him in connection with any business of pharmacy, has been convicted of an offence or held guilty of an infamous conduct, such that if he was a registered pharmacist himself, his name would have been removed from the Register. Action against the pharmacist can be taken only if it is proved that:

1. The objectionable conduct was instigated or connived at by the pharmacist himself, or
2. The registered pharmacist, during the period of 12 months preceding the offence, has been guilty of a similar offence or conduct, or
3. Any person, employed by the pharmacist for purposes of business of pharmacy, has been guilty of similar offence during the preceding 12 months and the pharmacist had the knowledge of the offence, or
4. The offence or conduct had continued over a long period and the pharmacist had or should have had the knowledge of the continuing offence, or
5. The act is an offence under the Drugs and Cosmetics Act, 1940 and the pharmacist did not use his intelligence to see that the provisions of this Act were being observed at his place of business by persons under his control.

Names can be removed only by an order of the Executive Committee of the State Pharmacy Council, after it has made due enquiries and given opportunity to the person concerned to explain his conduct. The removal of names from the Register may either be permanent or only for specified periods of time. The order of Executive Committee directing removal of a name from the Register should be confirmed by the State Pharmacy Council and it takes effect only after three months of the date of the order. This rule implies that any pharmacist, who is held guilty and whose name has been removed from the Register, shall continue to remain a registered pharmacist for the next three months and only after the expiry of that period he shall cease to be a registered pharmacist. This period of grace is probably given to allow the person to find an alternative means of livelihood. A person, aggrieved by the order directing the removal of his name, may appeal to the State Government, within 80 days, whose decision shall be final. A person, whose name has been removed from the Register, is required to surrender his certificate of registration to the Registrar of the Pharmacy Council concerned. The State Pharmacy Council may, at any time, for reasons appearing sufficient to it, order that the name of a person shall be restored to the Register. Where an appeal against the removal was made and rejected by the State Government, the name cannot be restored, unless confirmed by the State Government.

(e) Printing of Registers

The Registrars of the State Pharmacy Councils were required to publish the Registers on the 1st April following the commencement of the Pharmacy (Amendment) Act, 1959 as they stood on that date. Later on, each year after the first of April, they were required to publish supplements to the Registers showing all additions or amendments. All Registers should be updated three months before ordinary elections of the State Pharmacy Council and printed. Copies of printed registers, and all their supplements, should be supplied to persons applying for them, on payment of the prescribed costs. These Registers and supplements are deemed to be proofs that the persons, whose names are contained therein, are registered pharmacists.

THE EDUCATION REGULATIONS

The Education Regulations are framed under Section 10 of the Act and prescribe:

(i) Qualification for pharmacists.

(ii) Minimum qualification for admissions to Diploma Course in Pharmacy, Duration of the course, No. of hours to be covered for theory and practical, mode of examinations, eligibility for appearing in the examinations, minimum pass marks for passing examination, etc.

(iii) Period and other conditions for practical training, etc.
(iv) Detailed syllabus of Diploma in Pharmacy.
(v) Conditions to be fulfilled by the institutions for approval of course of study under Section 12 of the Act. These conditions include details of infrastructural facilities which an institution seeking approval of the course of study has to create i.e. accommodation area, qualification, experience and No. of teaching staff, staff-student ratio, non-teaching staff, equipments, museum, library, etc.
(vi) Conditions to be fulfilled by the examining authority conducting examinations of the students.
(vii) Conditions to be fulfilled by the institutions to be recognised for giving practical training.
(viii) Practical training contract form for pharmacists.

Presently, the "Education Regulations 1991 for the Diploma Course in Pharmacy" (E.R. 91) are in vogue. The Education Regulations for B.Pharm, **Bachelor of Pharmacy (Practice) Regulations, 2014** have been notified on 18th December by the Pharmacy Council of India, with the approval of the Central Government.

The **Master of Pharmacy (M.Pharm) Course Regulations, 2014** have been notified on 10th December 2014 by the Pharmacy Council of India, with the approval of the Central Government. Master of Pharmacy (M.Pharm) shall consist of a certificate, of having passed the course of study and examination as prescribed in these regulations, for the purpose of registration/addition of qualification as a pharmacist for practising the profession under the Pharmacy Act, 1948.

A pharmaceutical service requires constant interaction with patients and other professionals to monitor, advise and follow-up on drug efficacy, any side effects and complications. The profession also requires constant interaction with different health professionals at various levels to provide the best patient care.

On 15th January, 2015, **Pharmacy Practice Regulations, 2015** have been issued by the Pharmacy Council of India, with the approval of the Central Government.

Objectives for making Practice Regulations

Professions exist to serve society. The mission of the pharmacy profession is to render service to humanity with full respect for the dignity of profession and man, besides addressing the needs of society and of individual patients. The public places great trust in the knowledge, skills and professional judgments of pharmacists. This trust requires the pharmacists to ensure and maintain throughout their career high standards of personal and professional conduct, up-to-date knowledge and professional competence relevant to their domain of practice.

The registered pharmacist should merit the confidence of patients entrusted to their care, rendering to each a full measure of service and devotion for which the registered pharmacist should try continuously to improve his knowledge and skills and should make available to their patients and colleagues the benefits of their professional attainments.

The registered pharmacist should practice methods of practice founded on scientific basis and should not associate professionally with anyone who violates this principle. The honoured ideals of the pharmacy profession imply that the responsibilities of the registered pharmacist extend not only to individuals but also to society.

This calls for framing of the regulations for practice of pharmacy, laying down responsibilities of pharmacist towards patient, another registered pharmacist and the public in general. Primary reasons to regulate pharmacy profession are:

(i) To improve quality of health care.
(ii) To ensure that Pharmacists maintain high standards in their duty.
(iii) To reduce cost of health care.
(iv) To inhibit criminal abuse of medicines.

It is also a call for laying down the activities which may be construed as misconduct and provision for taking disciplinary action.

Qualification for registration as a pharmacist as per Education Regulations

(i) The minimum qualification for registration as a pharmacist is a pass in "Diploma course in Pharmacy" (D.Pharm) from an institution approved u/s 12 of the Act. D.Pharm is a two years course after 10+2 (science academic stream) followed by 500 hours of practical training spread over a period of 3 months.
(ii) "Degree course in Pharmacy" (B.Pharm) from an institution approved by the PCI u/s 12 of the Act. B.Pharm is a 4 years course after 10+2 (science academic stream).
(iii) Master of Pharmacy (M.Pharm), a two year course, studied and passed the examination as prescribed in these regulations, is qualified for the purpose of registration/addition of qualification as a pharmacist for practicing the profession under the Pharmacy Act, 1948.

Regulation of Pharmacy Education under the Pharmacy Act

(i) By prescribing minimum qualification for registration as a pharmacist.

(ii) By prescribing norms to be fulfilled by the pharmacy institutions seeking approval for the purpose of registration as a pharmacist.
(iii) Uniform implementation of prescribed norms all over the country.
(iv) Verification of the prescribed norms by inspecting pharmacy institutions.
(v) Granting approval or otherwise (withdrawal of approval/rejection of application) depending on the merits of the case.

Regulation of Pharmacy Profession under the Pharmacy Act

(i) Registration as a pharmacist is done by the State Pharmacy Council constituted under Section 19 of the Pharmacy Act.
(ii) Minimum Statutory requirements for registration as a pharmacist under the Pharmacy Act (Ref. Section 32(2) of the Pharmacy Act):
   (a) Applicant should have attained the age of 18 years and should pay the prescribed fee.
   (b) Applicant should reside or carry on the business, or profession of Pharmacy, in the State.
   (c) Applicant should have passed an approved examination. Or should possess a qualification approved under Section 14 of the Pharmacy Act. Or is a registered pharmacist in another state.
(iii) An approved examination is "Diploma in Pharmacy" or "Degree in Pharmacy" from an institution approved under Section 12 of the Pharmacy Act.
(iv) Pharmacy Act states that no person other than a Registered Pharmacist shall compound, prepare, mix, or dispense any medicine on the prescription of a medical practitioner and whosoever contravenes it, shall be punishable with imprisonment for a term which may extend to six months, or with fine not exceeding one thousand rupees or with both.
(v) Pharmacy Act empowers the State Pharmacy Council, with the previous sanction of the State Govt., to appoint inspectors, who may:
   (a) Inspect any premises where drugs are compounded or dispensed;
   (b) Enquire whether a person who is engaged in compounding or dispensing of drugs is registered pharmacist;
   (c) Investigate any complaint made in writing in respect of any contravention of this Act;
   (d) Institute prosecution under the order of the Executive Committee of the State Council;
   (e) Exercise such other powers as may be necessary for carrying out the purposes of Chapters III, IV and V of this Act, or any rules made thereunder.

Offences and Penalties

(a) Falsely claiming to be a Registered Pharmacist
A person who falsely claims to be a Registered Pharmacist, or uses in connection with his name or title, any words or letters, to show that his name is entered in the Register of Pharmacists, is liable to a fine of up to Rs. 500 on first conviction and to a fine of up to Rs. 1000 and/or imprisonment for up to 6 months on second or subsequent conviction. The use of the words Pharmacist, Chemist, Druggist, Pharmaceutist, Dispenser, Dispensing Chemist or any of their combinations with any other words shall be deemed to suggest that the person is a Registered Pharmacist. If, however, a person is a Registered Pharmacist in another State and, at the time of making such a claim, has filed an application for registration in the State, he shall not be deemed to be guilty of the offence. The onus of proving that his name is on the Register of Pharmacists shall be on the person claiming to be a Registered Pharmacist. Cognizance of the offence on this account can be taken only on the complaints by the State Government or by an officer authorized in this behalf or by the order of the Executive Committee of the State Pharmacy Council.

(b) Dispensing by Unregistered Persons
After the date notified in this behalf by the State Government, no person other than a Registered Pharmacist can compound, mix or dispense drugs on the prescription of a Registered Medical Practitioner. This, however, does not apply to dispensing of medicine by a Medical Practitioner to his own patients, or with the permission of the State Government to the patients of other medical practitioner.

Dispensing by unregistered persons is a punishable offence with imprisonment of up to six months or a fine of up to Rs. 1000 or both. Cognizance of this offence can be taken only on the complaints by the State Government or by an officer authorised in this behalf or by the order of the Executive Committee of the State Pharmacy Council.

(c) Failing to Surrender Certificate of Registration
If a person whose name has been removed for the time being from the Register, fails without sufficient reason to surrender his certificate of registration, is liable to a fine of up to Rs. 50. Cognizance of this offence shall not be taken except by an order of the Executive Committee of the State Pharmacy Council.

(d) Penalty for Obstructing State Pharmacy Council Inspectors
Any person willfully obstructing an Inspector of the State Pharmacy Council shall be liable to imprisonment of up to 6 months or a fine of up to Rs. 1000 or both.

QUESTIONS FOR REVISION
1. What are the main objectives of Pharmacy Act.
2. Describe the constitution and functions of Pharmacy Council of India.
3. Discuss the main features of Education Regulations (ER).
4. Mention the procedures for approval or withdrawal of approval of Institution imparting Pharmacy Education.
5. Write a note on constitution and functions of State/Joint Pharmacy Councils.
6. Describe the conditions required for entry into the first register and subsequent register.
7. Write a note on offences and penalties prescribed under Pharmacy Act 1948.

Chapter 4

The Drugs and Cosmetics Act, 1940 and Rules, 1945

Drugs are of paramount importance for the prevention and cure of disease and ailments and hence are classified as "essential commodity" under the Essential Commodities Act, 1955. Although the drugs have a dubious past and had their origins in superstitions and magic but now have established themselves on scientific basis. Therefore, manufacture, sale, stock and distribution, etc. of drugs warrant the specialized knowledge, skill and expertise and hence are required to be regulated under a legal framework.

Cosmetics are although luxury item, they may contain some ingredients, the constant use of which might prove to be harmful and hence their manufacturing needs to be controlled.

All countries in the world have enforced effective laws and rules which ensure the availability of safe, effective and standard drugs to the public without any difficulty.

In India, the first Act in this behalf was enacted in 1940 under the title of Drug Act which sought to exercise some control over operations related to allopathic drugs only. However, since then this act has been amended a number of times to include under its purview Ayurvedic, Unani, Siddha and Homeopathic drugs as well as cosmetics, contraceptives, mosquito repellents, creams, lotions and medical devices, etc. used for internal and external use for diagnosis.

Objectives

The Drugs and Cosmetics Act, 1940 was enacted with the following objectives:

1. Control over the manufacture of drugs and cosmetics in the country so as to prevent the production of sub-standard, adulterated, misbranded or spurious drugs or cosmetics.
2. Regulation of import of drugs and cosmetics into the country, to prevent entry of sub-standard or harmful drugs and cosmetics.
3. Regulation of sale and distribution of drugs and cosmetics.
4. Regulation of manufacture and sale of Ayurvedic, Unani, Siddha drugs and manufacture and sale of Homeopathic drugs, wherever applicable.
5. Regular inspections of establishments engaged in manufacture of drugs (including AYUSH drugs) and cosmetics, by taking samples and getting them tested in drug testing control laboratories of State and Centre.

This Act also provides for constitution of two "Boards", namely the Drug Technical Advisory Board and Ayurvedic & Unani Drug Technical Advisory Board to advise the Central and State Governments on technical matters and to carry out other function assigned to it by this Act. It also provides the establishment of consultative committees, one for the Allopathic and other for Ayurvedic, Siddha and Unani to advice various governments and boards on matters tending to secure uniformity throughout the country in the administration of the Act.

There are two Schedules to the Drugs and Cosmetics Act and more than thirty Schedules to the Rules.

The Drugs and Cosmetics Act, 1940 has been divided into V chapters. The Drugs and Cosmetics Rules, 1945 has been divided into XIX parts, each part dealing with a particular object.

The Central Drugs Standard Control Organization (CDSCO), headed by the Drugs Controller General (India) (DCGI), discharges the function allocated by central government and similarly Drugs Controller is responsible at the state level.

Definitions

(i) **Drug** includes:
   (a) All medicines for internal or external use of human beings or animals and all substances intended to be used for or in the diagnosis, treatment, mitigation or prevention of any disease or disorder in human beings or animals, including preparations applied on human body for the purpose of repelling insects like mosquitoes.
   (b) Such substances other than food intended to affect the structure/function of the human body or intended to be used for the destruction of vermin or insects, which cause disease in human beings or animals as may be specified from time to time by the Central Government by notification in the official gazette.

(c) All substances intended for use as components of a drug including empty gelatin capsules.
  (d) Such devices intended for internal or external use in the diagnosis, treatment, mitigation or prevention of disease or disorder in human beings or animals, as may be specified from time to time by the Central Government by notification in the official gazette.
(ii) **Misbranded drug:** A drug is termed as misbranded:
  (a) If it is so coloured, coated, powdered or polished that damage is concealed or if it is made to appear of better or greater therapeutic value than it really is.
  (b) If it is not labelled in the prescribed manner.
  (c) If its label or container or anything accompanying the drug bears any statement, design or device which makes any false claim for the drug or which is false or misleading in any particular way.
(iii) **Adulterated drug:** A drug is termed as adulterated:
  (a) If it consists, in whole or in part, of any filthy, putrid or decomposed substance.
  (b) If it has been prepared, packed or stored under insanitary conditions whereby it may have been contaminated with filth or whereby it may have been rendered injurious to health.
  (c) If its container is composed, in whole or in part, of any poisonous or deleterious substance, which may render the contents injurious to health.
  (d) If it bears or contains, for purposes of colouring only, a colour other than one which is prescribed.
  (e) If it contains any harmful or toxic substance which may render it injurious to health.
  (f) If any substance has been mixed therewith so as to reduce its quality or strength.
(iv) **Spurious drug:** A drug is termed as spurious:
  (a) If it is imported under a name which belongs to another drug.
  (b) If it is an imitation of, or is a substitute for, another drug or resembles another drug in a manner likely to deceive or bears upon its label or container the name of another drug unless it is plainly and conspicuously marked so as to reveal its true character and its lack of identity with such other drug.
  (c) If the label or container bears the name of an individual or company purporting to be the manufacturer of the drug, which individual or company is fictitious or does not exist.
  (d) If it has been substituted, wholly or in part, by another drug or substance.
  (e) If it purports to be the product of a manufacturer of whom it is not truly a product.

(v) **Cosmetic** means any article intended to be rubbed, poured, sprinkled or sprayed on, or introduced into, or otherwise applied to, the human body or any part thereof for cleansing, beautifying, promoting attractiveness, or altering the appearance and includes any article intended for use as a component of cosmetic.

(vi) **Misbranded cosmetics:** A cosmetic is deemed to be misbranded:
1. if it contains a colour which is not prescribed; or
2. if it is not labelled in the prescribed manner; or
3. if the label or container or anything accompanying the cosmetic bears any statement which is false or misleading in any particular way.

(vii) **Spurious cosmetics:** A cosmetic is deemed to be spurious:
1. if it is manufactured under a name which belongs to another cosmetic; or
2. if it is an imitation of, or is a substitute for, or resembles another cosmetic in a manner likely to deceive or bears upon it or upon its label or container the name of another cosmetic, unless it is plainly and conspicuously marked so as to reveal its true character and its lack of identity with such other cosmetic; or
3. if the label or container bears the name of an individual or a company purporting to be the manufacturer of the cosmetic, which individual or company is fictitious or does not exist; or
4. if it purports to be the product of a manufacturer of whom it is not truly a product.

(viii) **Patent or proprietary medicines:**
(a) In relation to Ayurvedic, Siddha or Unani-Tibb systems of medicine all formulations containing only such ingredients mentioned in the formulae described in the authoritative books of Ayurveda, Siddha or Unani-Tibb systems of medicine specified in the first schedule, but does not include a medicine which is administered by parenteral route and also a formulation included in the authoritative books as specified in clause (a).
(b) In relation to any other systems of medicine, a drug which is a remedy or prescription presented in a form ready for internal or external administration of human beings or animals and which is not included in the edition of the Indian Pharmacopoeia for the time being or any other Pharmacopoeia authorised in this behalf by the Central Government after consultation with the Drugs Technical Advisory Board constituted under Section 5.

(ix) **Ayurvedic, Siddha or Unani drugs** include all medicines intended for internal or external use for or in the diagnosis, treatment, mitigation or prevention of disease or disorder in human beings or animals and manufactured exclusively in accordance with the formulae described in the authoritative books of Ayurvedic, Siddha and Unani-Tibb systems of medicine specified in the first schedule.

(x) **Homeopathic medicine** includes any drug which is recorded in homeopathic proving, therapeutic efficacy of which has been established through long clinical experience as recorded in authoritative homeopathic literature of India and abroad and which is prepared according to the techniques of homeopathic medicines, but, not a medicine which is administered by parenteral route.

(xi) **Manufacture** in relation to any drug or cosmetic includes any process or part of a process for making, altering, ornamenting, finishing, packing, labelling, breaking up or otherwise treating or adopting any drug or cosmetic with a view to its sale or distribution but does not include the compounding or dispensing of any drug, or the packing of any drug or cosmetic, in the ordinary course of retail business.

ADMINISTRATION OF THE ACT

For the efficient administration of the Act and Rules, the Drugs and Cosmetics Act provides for the establishment of following agencies (Table 4.1).

I. ADVISORY

(a) Drugs Technical Advisory Board (DTAB)

DTAB is constituted by the Central Government to advise the Central and State Governments on technical matters arising out of the administration of this Act. It consists of 18 members, of whom 8 are ex-officio, 5 nominated and 5 elected members, as follows:

Constitution and Composition

Ex-officio Members

(i) Director General of Health Services as Chairman
(ii) Drugs Controller of India
(iii) Director, Central Drugs Laboratory, Calcutta
(iv) Director, Central Research Institute, Kasauli
(v) Director, Indian Veterinary Research Institute, Izatnagar
(vi) President, Pharmacy Council of India
(vii) President, Medical Council of India
(viii) Director, Central Drugs Research Institute, Lucknow

Table 4.1

Agency	Function

I. Advisory
  (a) Drugs Technical Advisory Board (DTAB)
  (b) Drugs Consultative Committee (DCC)
	1. To advise Central & State Govts. on technical matters arising out of the operation of the Act.
	2. To advise governments and DTAB on issues related to uniform operation of the Act throughout country.

II. Analytical
  (a) Central Drugs Laboratory (CDL)
  (b) State Drug Control Laboratories
  (c) Government Analyst
	1. To analyze and report on samples of drugs/cosmetics sent by customs collectors/courts/consumers.
	2. To analyze and report on samples of drugs/cosmetics sent by Drug Inspectors (Drugs Control Officers).
	3. Can analyze samples of private agencies on prescribed payment.

III. Executive
  (a) Controlling and Licensing Authority
  (b) Drug Inspectors
  (c) Customs Collectors
	1. Incharge of Drugs Control issues approval of licences and implementation of Act.
	2. To inspect manufacturing and sale establishments and assist Licensing Authorities in implementation of the Act.
	3. Implementation of the Act to certain extent with respect to imported drugs/cosmetics.

Nominated Members

(i) Two persons from amongst persons who are in charge of the drug control agencies in the States, to be nominated by the Central Government.

(ii) One person from pharmaceutical industry to be nominated by the Central Government.

(iii) Two persons holding the appointment of Government Analyst under this Act, to be maintained by Central Government.

Elected Members

(i) A teacher in pharmacy, pharmaceutical chemistry or pharmacognosy on the staff of a university or affiliated college elected by the Executive Committee of Pharmacy Council of India.

(ii) A teacher in medicine or therapeutics on the staff of a university or affiliated college elected by the Executive Committee of the Medical Council of India.

(iii) One person to be elected by the Central Council of the Indian Pharmaceutical Association.
(iv) One person elected by the Council of the Indian Medical Association.
(v) One pharmacologist, elected by the Governing Body of the Indian Council of Medical Research.

The nominated and elected members hold the office for three years but are eligible for re-nomination or re-election. A Secretary of the board is appointed by the Central Government and the board is provided with clerical and other staff as necessary.

(b) Drugs Consultative Committee (DCC)

Consists of two representatives nominated by the Central Government and one nominee of each of the State Governments and has power to regulate its own procedure. The DCC shall meet as and when required to do so by Central Government. The committee may constitute sub-committees to examine the technical issues referred by Drugs Consultative Committee.

II. ANALYTICAL

(a) Central Drugs Laboratory (CDL)

The Central Drugs Laboratory (established in Calcutta under the control of a Director) is entrusted with the following functions:

(i) Analysis or test of samples of drugs or cosmetics sent to it by customs collectors or courts;
(ii) To carry out such duties, as may be entrusted to it by the Central Government or by the State Governments with the permission of the Central Government and in consultation with DTAB.

Biological and other special product, analysis, tests are not carried out in the Central Drugs Laboratory at Calcutta and hence samples of sera, vaccines, toxins, antigens, antitoxins, sterilized surgical ligature and suture, bacteriophages and solutions of serum proteins for injection are required to be sent to the Director of the Central Research Institute, Kasauli and antisera, vaccines, toxoids and diagnostic antigens for veterinary use to the Director, Indian Veterinary Research Institute, Izatnagar, who exercise all the functions of the Director of Central Drugs Laboratory, in respect of such classes of drugs.

Tests on condoms are carried out at the Central Testing Laboratory, Mumbai and Director of this laboratory exercises functions of Director, Central Drugs Laboratory in this respect. Tests on oral polio vaccine, human blood and its products including test for freedom from HIV antibodies, testing of diagnostic reagents and kits are to be carried out at the National Institute of Biologicals, NOIDA. Director of this institute exercises the functions of the Director of the Central Drugs Laboratory in respect of these drugs.

The Homeopathic medicines should be sent to the Homeopathic Pharmacopoeial Lab., Ghaziabad, whose Director exercises the functions of the Central Drugs Laboratory in respect of homeopathic medicines.

The functions of the Laboratory in respect of intrauterine devices and falope rings shall be carried out by the Central Drug Testing Laboratory, Thane and the functions of the Director in respect of the said devices shall be exercised by the Head of the said department.

All samples of drugs or cosmetics, sent to the Central Drugs Laboratory for analysis by courts, should be sent under registered and sealed covers together with a memorandum to the Director. A copy of the memorandum and a specimen impression of the seal used to seal the packet should also be sent to him separately by registered post. The Director or other officer, authorized by him, should record the condition of the seals, on receipt of the packet.

On completion of the test or analysis, the Director is required to supply a report of the analysis with full protocols of the test applied. The report should be signed by the Director or other officer so authorized by the Central Government by notification in the Official Gazette.

(b) State Drug Control Laboratories

Each state of India is required to establish a laboratory for the analysis and testing of drugs and cosmetics, manufactured or sold within their respective areas. Samples of drugs and cosmetics, taken by drug inspectors during the course of inspection of the licensed manufacturing houses, wholesale and retail establishments, are required to be analyzed in these laboratories, in order to ascertain whether they meet the prescribed standards or not. Drug Control Laboratories may also undertake analysis and testing of drugs on behalf of private persons or concerns, who do not possess such facilities of analysis in their respective establishments, on payment of the prescribed fees (see Schedule B) and furnish them with a report of the analysis in writing.

(c) Government Analysts

A. Qualifications of Government Analyst

A person appointed as a Government Analyst under the Act shall be a person who:

(a) is a graduate in medicine or science or pharmacy or Pharmaceutical Chemistry [University established in India by law or has an equivalent qualification recognized and notified by the Central Government for such purpose], and has had not less than five years' postgraduate experience in the testing of drugs in a laboratory under control of:
  (i) a Government Analyst appointed under the Act, or
  (ii) the head of an institution or testing laboratory approved for the purpose by the appointing authority [or has completed two years' training on testing of drugs, including items stated in Schedule C, in Central Drugs Laboratory], or
(b) possesses a postgraduate degree in medicine or science or pharmacy or Pharmaceutical Chemistry [University established in India by law or has an equivalent qualification recognized and notified by the Central Government for such purpose], or possesses the Associateship Diploma of the Institution of Chemists (India) obtained by passing the said examination with 'Analysis of Drugs and Pharmaceuticals' as one of the subjects and has had after obtaining the said postgraduate degree or diploma not less than three years' experience in the testing of drugs in a laboratory under the control of:
  (i) a Government Analyst appointed under the Act, or
  (ii) the head of an institution or testing laboratory approved for the purpose by the appointing authority [or has completed training on testing of drugs, including items stated in Schedule C, in Central Drugs Laboratory]:

Provided that
  [(i) for purpose of examination of items in Schedule C,
    (ia) the persons appointed under clause (a) or (b) and having degree in Medicine, Physiology, Pharmacology, Microbiology, Pharmacy should have experience or training in testing of said items in an institution or laboratory approved by the appointing authority for a period of not less than six months;
    (ib) the person appointed under clause (a) or (b) but not having degree in the above subjects should have experience or training in testing of said Schedule C drugs for a period of not less than three years in an institution or laboratory approved by the appointing authority or have completed two years training on testing of drugs including items stated in Schedule C in Central Drugs Laboratory;
  (ii) for a period of four years from the date on which Chapter IV of the Act takes effect in the States, persons whose training and experience are regarded by the appointing authority as affording, subject to such

further training, if any, as may be considered necessary, a reasonable guarantee of adequate knowledge and competence, may be appointed as Government Analysts. The persons so appointed may, if the appointing authority so desires, continue in service after the expiry of the said period of four years;

(iii) no person who is engaged directly or indirectly in any trade or business connected with the manufacture of drugs shall be appointed as a Government Analyst for any area:

Provided further that for the purpose of examination of antisera, toxoid and vaccines and diagnostic antigens for veterinary use, the person appointed shall be a person who is a graduate in veterinary science, or general science, or medicine or pharmacy and has had not less than five years' experience in the standardization of biological products or person holding a postgraduate degree in veterinary science, or general science, or medicine or pharmacy or pharmaceutical chemistry with an experience of not less than three years in the standardization of biological products: Provided also that persons, already appointed as Government Analysts may continue to remain in service, if the appointing authority so desires, notwithstanding the fact that they do not fulfil the qualifications as laid down in clause (a), clause (b) or the preceding proviso.

B. Duties of Government Analysts

(i) To analyse and test samples of drugs and cosmetics sent by drug inspectors or other persons, and furnish reports of test or analysis according to the Rules.

(ii) To engage in any research work possible and forward to the Government from time to time, results of analytical and research work with a view to publication at the discretion of the Government.

C. Procedure on receipt of sample

On receipt of samples of drugs and cosmetics from drug inspectors, the analysts should record the condition of the seal on the package and compare it with the impression of the seal received separately. On completion of the analysis, a report in triplicate, together with full details of the tests protocol applied, should be supplied.

Reports signed by government analyst are taken to be evidences of the facts stated therein unless they are challenged within 28 days to either inspector or in court. In case of a challenge, the samples may be sent for test or analysis to the Central Drugs Laboratory (Appellate Laboratory), whose report shall be deemed to be conclusive.

III. EXECUTIVE

(a) Licensing Authorities

The Central Government notifies such person holding appointment under its control to work as Licensing Authority for issue of licences for the import of drugs, issue of NOC for test licence, issue/approval of New Drugs meant for export and as Licence Approving Authority for approval of such licences under dual licensing system. The State Governments appoint Licensing Authorities for their respective territories to issue licences for the manufacture and sale of drugs and for the manufacture of cosmetics.

Qualification of a Licensing Authority

No person shall be qualified to be a Licensing Authority under the Act unless:

(i) he is a graduate in Pharmacy or Pharmaceutical Chemistry or in Medicine with specialisation in Clinical Pharmacology or Microbiology from a University established in India by law; and

(ii) he has experience in the manufacture or testing of drugs or enforcement of the provisions of the Act for a minimum period of five years.

The Licensing Authorities have the discretion to issue or refuse to issue licences to the prospective applicants, depending on whether they satisfy the prescribed rules or not. The Licensing Authorities are also empowered to cancel or suspend the licences issued by them if the licensees fail to observe any of the conditions of licences, after giving them reasonable opportunity of explaining their case. The decision of the Licensing Authorities is, however, subject to challenge in the courts of law as discussed earlier.

Such authorities are designated differently in different states; mostly they are given the designation of 'Drug Controller' but in some states they are called 'Director, Drug Control Administration' and yet in some `Officer-in-charge, Drug Control'. The Licensing Authority is assisted by Deputy Drugs Controller and Assistant Drugs Controller to work under them.

(b) Drugs Inspector (Drugs Control Officer)

The Central Government or the State Governments are required to appoint a suitable number of drugs inspectors (DCO's) for their respective areas who are public servants within the meaning of Section 21 of Indian Penal Code. The Inspectors may be appointed either to inspect the premises licensed for the sale of drugs or to inspect the establishments licensed for the manufacture of drugs and cosmetics. No person having any financial interest in the import, manufacture or sale of drugs and cosmetics can be appointed as a drugs inspector kunder the Act. Inspectors are required to keep all information acquired by them, in the course of their duty, confidential and not to disclose it except for official business or when required to do so before a court of law. Inspectors held guilty of any vexatious searches, seizures, etc. are liable to fine up to Rs. 1,000.

A. Qualifications for the appointment of Inspectors

A person who is appointed an Inspector under the Act shall be a person who has a degree in Pharmacy or Pharmaceutical Sciences or Medicine with specialization in Clinical Pharmacology or Microbiology from a University established in India by law: Provided that only those Inspectors:

(i) who have not less than 18 months' experience in the manufacture of at least one of the substances specified in Schedule C, or
(ii) who have not less than 18 months' experience in testing of at least one of the substances in Schedule C in a laboratory approved for this purpose by the Licensing Authority, or
(iii) who have gained experiences of not less than three years in the inspection of firms manufacturing any of the substances specified in Schedule C during the tenure of their services as Drugs Inspectors; shall be authorised to inspect the manufacture of the substances mentioned in Schedule C:

[Provided further that the requirement as to the academic qualification shall not apply to persons appointed as Inspectors on or before the 18th day of October, 1993.]

B. Duties of Inspectors

The duties of drug inspectors may be classified under the following two headings:
1. Inspection of premises licensed for the sale of drugs.
2. Inspection of premises licensed for the manufacture of drugs and cosmetics.

Inspection of premises licensed for the sale of drugs

Subject to the instructions of the controlling authority, the following are the duties of a drugs inspector:

(i) To inspect, not less than twice a year, all premises licensed for the sale of drugs in his area, and to satisfy himself that the conditions of the licence are being observed.
(ii) To obtain and send samples of drugs for analysis. The samples may also be taken from dealers or from persons who are conveying, delivering or preparing to deliver any drug to a purchaser.

(iii) To investigate any complaints, made to him in writing, and to make such inspections and enquiries as may be necessary to detect the sale of drugs in contravention of the Act and the Rules.
(iv) To enter and search, at all reasonable times, with such assistants, as may be necessary, all places, vessels, vehicles or persons where or by whom an offence under the Act is believed to be committed, to order any person in possession of contraband drugs to not to dispose of such drugs for a specified period not exceeding 20 days, or if the defect is such that it cannot be remedied by the possessor, to seize the stock of the drugs.
(v) To institute legal proceedings in case of any breach of the Act and the Rules.
(vi) When authorized by the State Government to do so, to detain packages of imported drugs as are prohibited to be imported.
(vii) To exercise such other powers, as may be necessary, to give effect to the provisions of the Act and Rules.
(viii) To maintain records of all inspections and of actions taken, including the taking of samples and seizure of stocks, and to submit copies of such records to the licensing or the controlling authority.

Inspection of the premises licensed for the manufacture of drugs

Subject to the instructions of the controlling authority the following are the duties of the drug inspectors, specially authorized to inspect the manufacture of drugs and cosmetics:

(i) To inspect, not less than twice a year, all premises licensed for the manufacture of drugs (in the case of establishments licensed for the manufacture of Schedule C and C1 drugs to inspect the plant, the process of manufacture, the means employed for standardizing and testing of drugs or cosmetics), the methods and places of storage, details of location, construction and administration of the establishment and enquire into the technical qualifications of the staff employed, in order to satisfy himself that the provisions of the Act and the Rules are being observed.
(ii) To take samples of drugs or cosmetics manufactured on the premises and send them for test or analysis.
(iii) To check all records and registers, required to be maintained under the Rules, in order to satisfy himself that the provisions are being observed.
(iv) To send detailed report of each inspection to the controlling authorities indicating how far the provisions of the Act and the Rules are being observed.
(v) To institute prosecutions in respect of breaches of the Act and Rules thereunder.

C. Procedure of Inspection

(a) For taking samples of drugs and their dispatches to the government analysts

Whenever any inspector takes sample of a drug or cosmetic, he should intimate the purpose to the person from whom he takes the sample in prescribed form 17, in writing.

Tender a fair price thereof in cash or on credit and obtain receipt for the same. If, however, the price is not accepted, he should tender a receipt for the quantity of drug taken by him in the prescribed form 17A.

The samples should then be divided in four parts in the presence of the person from whom the samples have been taken unless he willfully absents himself, and seal each part, suitably mark the same and allow the person to add his mark or seal to such parts if he so desires.

When the samples are taken from the premises licensed for the manufacture of drugs, samples may, however, be divided into three parts only. If the drug is made up in containers of small volume or if the drug is such that it may deteriorate on exposure, the Inspector may take 3 to 4 such containers and mark and seal them in the usual manner.

One portion of the sample should then be sent to the government analyst, one reserved for production before the court if the proceedings are instituted in respect of such sample, the third sent to the vendor from whom purchase has been disclosed of the impugned drug, if any, and the fourth returned to the person from whom the sample was taken.

The portion of the sample sent to the government analyst should be sent by registered post or delivered personally in a sealed packet along with a specimen seal impression separately used to seal the sample portion. After the report of analysis or test has been received from the government analyst, the inspector will decide whether any further action is necessary in the matter or not, depending on results of such test/analysis.

(b) For entry and search, etc. of places, persons, vehicles, vessels, etc.

An Inspector, if he has reason to believe that some drugs in contravention of the Act are stocked in any place, he may enter such place at all reasonable times with a view to search them or any vessels or persons, either alone or with such assistants as may be necessary.

The inspectors can stop and search any vehicle suspected to be carrying any drug in contravention of the Act. The provisions of the Code of Criminal Procedure 1898, apply to any search or seizure, made under Chapter IV of the Act, as they apply to any search or seizure made under the authority of a warrant issued under Section 98 of the Code. Any wilful obstruction may be removed by the inspectors. The inspectors may also examine any records, registers, documents or material objects, if they have reasons to believe that they may be evidences of the commission of an offence under the Act or the Rules.

(c) For seizure of stocks

Whenever any stocks, records, registers, documents, material objects, etc. are believed to be evidences of the commission of an offence under the Act, the same may be seized by the Inspectors. An inspector should inform a magistrate as soon as possible and take his orders for the custody of such seized articles. Records should be returned to the owner within 20 days after making copies, extracts etc., if necessary.

(d) Prohibition of manufacture and sale of certain drugs and cosmetics

The Inspector ensures that no person shall himself or by any other person on his behalf—

(a) manufacture for sale (or for distribution), or sell, or stock or exhibit (or offer) for sale or distribute—
  (i) any drug which is not of a standard quality, or is misbranded, adulterated or spurious;
  (ii) any cosmetic which is not of a standard quality or is misbranded or spurious;
  (iii) any patent or proprietary medicine, unless there is displayed in the prescribed manner on the label or container thereof, [the true formula or list of active ingredients contained in it together with the quantities thereof];
  (iv) any drug which by means of any statement, design or device accompanying it or by any other means, purports or claims [to prevent, cure or mitigate] any such disease or ailment, or to have any such other effect as may be prescribed;
  (v) any cosmetic containing any ingredient which may render it unsafe or harmful for use under the directions indicated or recommended;
  (vi) any drug or cosmetic in contravention of any of the provisions of this Chapter or any rule made thereunder;
(b) sell, or stock or exhibit (or offer) for sale, or distribute any drug [or cosmetic] which has been imported or manufactured in contravention of any of the provisions of this Act or any rule made thereunder;
(c) manufacture for sale (or for distribution) or sell, or stock or exhibit or offer for sale, or distribute any drug [or cosmetic], except under, and in accordance with the conditions of, a licence issued for such purpose.

Provided that nothing in this section shall apply to the manufacture, subject to prescribed conditions, of small quantities of any drug for the purpose of examination, test or analysis.

QUESTIONS FOR REVISION

1. Write the main objectives of the Drugs and Cosmetics Act, 1940.
2. Define
   (i) Drug
   (ii) Cosmetics
   (iii) Patent or Proprietary medicines
   (iv) Adulterated drugs
   (v) Spurious drugs
   (vi) Misbranded drugs.
3. Write notes on:
   (i) Drug Technical Advisory Board
   (ii) Drug Consultative Committee
   (iii) Central Drugs Laboratory
   (iv) Government Analyst
   (v) Drugs Inspector (Drugs Control Officer).
4. Write the qualifications and duties of a Government Analyst.
5. Write the qualifications and duties of a Drug Inspector (Drugs Control Officer). Describe the procedures followed by the drug inspector in drawing a sample.

SCHEDULES

There are two Schedules to the Drugs and Cosmetics Act, 1940, and more than thirty Schedules to the Rules, 1945.

A. SCHEDULES TO THE DRUGS AND COSMETICS ACT, 1940

- First Schedule of the Act: List of authoritative books of Ayurvedic, Siddha and Unani-Tibb systems of medicine.
- Second Schedule of the Act: Standards to be compiled with imported drugs manufactured for sale, stocked or exhibited for sale or distributed.

B. SCHEDULES TO THE RULES, 1945

Schedule A	Specimens of the prescribed forms for making application for licences, issue and renewal of licences, forms for taking samples test/analysis reports, etc.
Schedule B	Rates of fee for test or analysis by the CDL or state drug laboratories, e.g. pyrogen test - INR 500/-, bioassay of antibiotic - INR 400/-, etc.
Schedule C	List of biological and special products (like ophthalmic preparations, parenteral preparations and sterile disposable devices, etc.) whose import, manufacture, sale and distribution are governed by special provisions.

Schedule C1	List of other special products not meant to be injected like digitalis, adrenaline, liver extract, vitamins, antibiotics, hormones, in vitro blood grouping sera, etc., whose import, manufacture, sale and distribution are governed by special provisions.
Schedule D	List of drugs that are exempted from certain provisions that are applicable to the import of drugs and cosmetics.
Schedule D-I	Registration of the manufacturer or his authorized agent for import of drugs.
Schedule D-II	Registration of bulk drugs/formulations/special products for its import in India.
Schedule E	(Omitted in June 1982) List of poisonous substances.
Schedule E-I	List of poisonous substances under Ayurvedic, Siddha and Unani systems.
Schedule F	Space, equipment, supply, GMP/SOP, sterile air classification, Master formula, Quality assurance for Blood Banks, Blood donation camps and manufacture of blood products.
Schedule F(I)	Requirement of operating blood banks and manufacture of blood products and cord blood derived stem cells. Special provisions applicable to manufacture and testing of vaccines, antiserums and diagnostic antigens.
Schedule F(II)	Standards for surgical dressing.
Schedule F(III)	Standards for umbilical tapes.
Schedule FF	Standards for ophthalmic preparations.
Schedule G	List of substances that are required to be taken under medical supervision and therefore are to be labelled with word caution accordingly, e.g. bleomycin, ethosuximide, antihistaminics like pheniramine, etc.
Schedule H	List of substances which are required to be sold by retail on the prescription of a registered medical practitioner only (list of prescription drugs), e.g., Cetrizine hydrochloride, Diclofenac, Ciprofloxacin, Ranitidine, etc.
Schedule H-1	List of drugs and their salts which are required to be labelled with words: Warning: "It is dangerous to take this preparation except in accordance with the medical advice and are not to be sold by retail without prescription of RMP", e.g., Alprazolam, Codeine, Pentazocine, Rifampicin, etc.

Schedule I	(Omitted in June 1982) Particulars regarding calculation of proportions of poisons in certain cases.
Schedule J	Diseases and ailments which a drug may not purport to prevent or cure or make claims to prevent or cure, e.g. AIDS, cancer, obesity, paralysis, etc.
Schedule K	Class of drugs that are exempted from certain provisions related to the manufacture, sale and distribution of certain drugs and cosmetics.
Schedule L	(Omitted in June 1982) List of certain prescription drugs.
Schedule L-1	Good Laboratory Practices and Requirement of premises and equipments.
Schedule M	GMP and requirements of factory premises, plants and equipments for pharmaceutical products.
Schedule M_1	GMP and requirements of factory premises, plants and equipments for manufacture of homeopathic drugs.
Schedule M_2	GMP and requirements of factory premises, plants and equipments for manufacture of cosmetics.
Schedule M_3	GMP and requirements of factory premises, plants and equipments for manufacture of medical devices.
Schedule N	List of minimum equipments (apparatus) and books for the efficient running of a Pharmacy.
Schedule O	Classification and standards for disinfectant fluids. Standard for disinfectants shall conform to Indian Standard Specification (IS:1061:1997) laid down from time to time by Bureau of Indian Standards.
Schedule P	Life periods and storage conditions for certain drugs.
Schedule P-I	Pack sizes of drugs for marketing.
Schedule Q	List of coal tar dyes, coloring agents and pigments permitted to be used in cosmetics and soaps.
Schedule R	Sampling, testing and standards for condoms and other mechanical contraceptives.
Schedule R-I	Standards for medical devices.
Schedule S	Standards for cosmetics.
Schedule T	GMP for Ayurvedic, Siddha and Unani medicines.
Schedule T-A	Forms of records of raw materials by Ayurvedic, Siddha and Unani manufacturers.
Schedule U	Particulars to be shown in manufacturing raw materials and analytical records of drugs.

Schedule U-I	Particulars to be shown in manufacturing and raw materials of cosmetics.
Schedule V	Standards for patent and proprietary medicines.
Schedule W	(Omitted in Feb 2000) List of drugs which shall be marketed under generic names only.
Schedule X	List of drugs whose import, manufacture and sale, labelling and packaging are governed by special provisions.
Schedule Y	Requirements and guidelines for permissions to import and/or manufacture of new drugs for sale or to undertake clinical trials.

Rule 127 gives the list of colours permitted to be used in drugs.

DETAILS OF IMPORTANT SCHEDULES

SCHEDULE D

Class of drugs that are exempted from certain provisions applicable to import of drugs and cosmetics:

1. Substances not intended for medicinal use.
2. The following substances, which are used both as articles of food as well as drugs:
   (i) All condensed or powdered milk whether pure, skimmed or malted, fortified with vitamins and minerals.
   (ii) Farex, Oats, Lactose and all other similar cereal preparations whether fortified with vitamins or otherwise excepting those for parenteral use.
   (iii) Virol, Bovril, Chicken essence and all other similar predigested foods.
   (iv) Ginger, Pepper, Cumin, Cinnamon and all other similar spices and condiments unless they are specifically labelled.
3. Drugs and cosmetics imported for manufacture and export by units situated in "Special Economic Zones" as notified by the Government of India from time to time.

The extent of exemption for above is with respect to requirement of import licence, import registration and import through notified port of entry.

SCHEDULE J

Diseases and ailments (by whatever name described) which a drug may not purport to prevent or cure or make claims to prevent or cure:

- AIDS
- Angina pectoris
- Appendicitis
- Arteriosclerosis
- Baldness
- Blindness
- Bronchial asthma
- Cancer and benign tumour
- Cataract
- Change in colour of the hair and growth of new hair
- Change of foetal sex by drugs
- Congenital malformations
- Deafness
- Diabetes
- Diseases and disorders of uterus
- Epileptic fits and psychiatric disorders
- Encephalitis
- Fairness of the skin
- Form, structure of breast
- Gangrene
- Genetic disorders
- Glaucoma
- Goitre
- Hernia
- High/low blood pressure
- Hydrocele
- Insanity
- Increase in brain capacity and improvement of memory
- Improvement in height of children/adults
- Improvement in size and shape of the sexual organ and in duration of sexual performance
- Improvement in the strength of the natural teeth
- Improvement in vision
- Jaundice/hepatitis/liver disorders
- Leukaemia
- Leucoderma
- Maintenance or improvement of the capacity of the human being for sexual pleasure
- Mental retardation, subnormalities and growth
- Myocardial infarction
- Obesity

- Paralysis
- Parkinsonism
- Piles and fistulae
- Power to rejuvenate
- Premature ageing
- Premature greying of hair
- Rheumatic heart diseases
- Sexual impotence, premature ejaculation and spermatorrhoea
- Spondylitis
- Stammering
- Stones in gall bladder, kidney, bladder
- Varicose veins

SCHEDULE K

Exemptions: The following classes of drugs are exempted from the provisions of Chapter IV of the Act relating to the manufacture, sale and distribution of drugs (Table 4.2):

SCHEDULE M

Good Manufacturing Practices: Maintaining the quality of drugs is basically the responsibility of manufacturer and the Good Manufacturing Practices (GMP) guidelines are a means to assure this very quality. The GMP regulations were prepared in 2001 which could be finalized and implemented in 2005, in the form of amended Schedule M.

To achieve the objectives of GMP, the licensee shall comply with the requirements of GMP as laid down in Schedule M. The licensee shall evolve methodology and procedures which should be documented and kept for reference and inspection.

Part I deals with Good Manufacturing Practices relating to factory premises, and Part II deals with the Plant and Equipment for manufacture of drugs.

Part I – Factory Premises

1. General requirements

A. **Location and surroundings:** The location of the factory, and its surrounding, shall ensure freedom from contamination due to sewage, drain, etc. and obnoxious odour or fumes, or large quantity of soot, dust or smoke.

B. **Buildings:** The factory building shall be so constructed as to ensure production of drugs under hygienic conditions. It shall conform to conditions laid down in the Factories Act, 1948.

Table 4.2

No.	Classes of Drugs	Extent and Conditions of Exemption
1.	Drugs not intended for medicinal use	Exempted from all provisions relating to manufacture, sale and distribution of drugs, provided the drugs are not sold for medicinal use or for use in the manufacture of drugs and do not claim to come up to the prescribed standards.
2.	Quinine and other antimalarial drugs	No licence required for sale when sold by retail under arrangements made by the State Governments.
3.	Drugs supplied by a registered medical practitioner to his own patients or to the patients of another practitioner at latter's request and drugs supplied by a hospital or dispensary maintained or supported by a Government or local body or by charity or voluntary subscription	No licence required to effect their supply provided the registered medical practitioner is not keeping an open shop or is not engaged in the manufacture, importation, sale or distribution of drugs. Drugs should be purchased from a licensed dealer or manufacturer.
4.	Drugs supplied by a hospital or dispensary, maintained or supported by Government or local body	Exempt from all provisions applicable to the sale of medicines except that dispensing and supply shall be carried out by or under supervision of a qualified person.
5.	Quinine sulphate	Would not be considered substandard if it is coloured pink with an edible coloring matter or contains not more than 06% of other cinchona alkaloids or leaves a residue not exceeding 0.14% on incineration, and in the B.P. test for readily carbonisable substances, produces a yellow colour of an intensity four times the colour produced by B.P. quinine sulphate.
6.	Magnesium sulphate	Exempted from being treated as not of standard quality to the extent in chloride present in the salt shall not exceed 0.12% in case of product prepared from sea water.

(Contd.)

No.	Classes of Drugs	Extent and Conditions of Exemption
7.	Substances which are used both as drugs as well as foods such as all condensed and powdered milks, lactose, farex, oats or similar cereal preparations, whether fortified with vitamins or not, excepting those intended for parenteral use. Virol, Bovril, chicken essence and other similar spices and condiments unless they are labelled to be of pharmacopoeial quality	No restrictions on their manufacture, sale or distribution.
8.	Household remedies such as aspirin tablets, paracetamol tablets, analgesic balms, antacid preparations, gripe water for infants, inhalers containing drugs for treatment of cold and nasal congestion, syrups, lozenges, pills and tablets for cough, liniments, skin ointments, burn ointments, absorbent cotton wool, castor oil, liquid paraffin, epsom salts, eucalyptus oil, Tr. iodine, Tr. Benz. Co., mercurochrome solution, quinine sulph. tablets I.P., tablets of iodochlorohydroquinoline (250 mg)	Sale licence is not subject to the following conditions: (i) The drugs are sold only in a village having population of not more than one thousand persons and where there is no licensed dealer under the Drugs and Cosmetics Act; (ii) The drugs do not contain any substance specified in Schedules G, H or X; (iii) The drugs are sold in the original unopened containers of the licensed manufacturers.
9.	Substances intended to be used for destruction of vermin or insects, which cause disease in human beings or animals viz. insecticides and disinfectants	Sale licence is not necessary, provided the person selling such substances complies with the requirement of not selling it after the expiry date or not violating any statement or direction recorded on the label of such container.
10.	Mechanical contraceptives	Sale licence is not necessary, provided the person selling such substances complies with the requirement of not selling it after the expiry date or not violating any statement or direction recorded on the label of such container.
11.	Chemical contraceptives	Sale licence is not required for sale or distribution of chemical contraceptives (tablets of specified composition).

(Contd.)

No.	Classes of Drugs	Extent and Conditions of Exemption
12.	Cosmetics	Sale licence is not required, provided that the cosmetics sold, if of Indian origin, are manufactured by licensed manufacturers.
13.	Oral rehydration salts (manufactured as per the following formula): Sodium chloride 3.5 g/litre, Trisodium citrate dihydrate 2.9 g/litre, Potassium chloride 1.5 g/litre. May be replaced by Sodium bicarbonate (Sodium hydrogen carbonate) 2.5 g/litre, when citrate salt is not available	Sale licence is not required, subject to the condition that such a product has been manufactured under a valid drug manufacturing licence.
14.	White or yellow petroleum jelly I.P. (non-perfumed)	Sale licence is not required, subject to the conditions that such a product has been manufactured under a valid drug manufacturing licence.
15.	Medicated dressing and bandages for first aid	Sale licence is not required, subject to the conditions that such a product has been manufactured under a valid drug manufacturing licence.
16.	Preparations applied to human body for the purpose of repelling insets like mosquitoes	Sale licence is not required, subject to the condition that such a product has been manufactured under a valid drug manufacturing licence.
17.	Radiopharmaceuticals	All provisions relating to manufacture, sale and distribution.
18.	Hair fixers used by men for fixing beard	All provisions relating to manufacture, sale and distribution.
19.	Tablets of chloroquine salts	Sale licence not required, provided the drug in strip pack is sold under the Commercial Distribution Scheme of the National Malaria Eradication Programme and duly labelled as "National Malaria Eradication Programme".

(*Contd.*)

No.	Classes of Drugs	Extent and Conditions of Exemption
20.	Sales from restaurant cars of trains and from coastal ships of household remedies, which do not require the supervision of a registered pharmacist for their sale	Sale licence not required, but the records of purchase and sale of drugs shall be maintained by the person in charge of sale of such drugs, which shall be available for inspection and drawing of sample for test by an Inspector appointed under the Act.
21.	Drugs supplied by: (i) Multipurpose Workers attached to Primary Health Centers/Sub-Centers; (ii) Community Health Volunteers under the Rural Health Scheme; (iii) Nurses, Auxiliary Nurse, Midwives and Lady Health Visitors attached to Urban Family Welfare Centers/Primary Health Centers/Sub-Centers; and (iv) Anganwadi Workers	Sale licence not necessary, provided the drugs are supplied under the Health or Family Welfare Programme of the Central or State Government.
22.	Morphine tablets	Sale licence is not required, subject to the following conditions, namely: (i) The drug shall be supplied by the Palliative Care Centres approved by the State Government to terminally-ill cancer patients; (ii) The drug shall be kept under the custody of the Medical Officer in-charge of the said centre; (iii) The drug shall be purchased from a dealer or a manufacturer who holds licence under these rules, and records maintained as per Act and such records shall be open to inspection by an Inspector appointed under the Act, who may also take samples for test.
23.	Nicotine gum and lozenges containing upto 2 mg of nicotine	No sale licence required, provided it has been manufactured under a valid manufacturing licence.

C. **Water supply:** The water used in the manufacture shall be pure and of a drinkable quality, free from pathogenic microorganisms.
D. **Disposal of waste:** Waste water and other residues from the laboratory shall be suitably treated before disposal to render it harmless.

2. Sterile products manufacturing area

A. **Sterile products:** For the manufacture of sterile drugs separate enclosed areas specifically designed for the purpose shall be provided. These areas shall be provided with air locks for entry and ventilated with air supply through HEPA filters. All surfaces in the manufacturing areas shall be designed to facilitate cleaning and disinfection. During manufacturing operation, routine microbial counts of area is necessary. Access to the manufacturing areas shall be restricted to authorised personnel. The design of area must preclude the possibility of mix up between sterile and non-sterile products.
B. **Working space:** Adequate working space and adequate room for orderly placement of equipment and materials shall be provided to eliminate any risk of mix up between different drugs, and cross contamination. In storage area separate space shall be provided for "under test", "approved" and "rejected" materials, including space for returned and recalled goods.
C. **Health, clothing and sanitation of workers:** All the personnel, including temporary staff, coming in direct contact with the products including raw materials shall be free from contagious or obnoxious diseases and shall undergo periodic health check up.
D. **Medical services:** The manufacturer shall provide:
   (i) Adequate facilities for the first aid.
   (ii) Medical examination of workers at the time of employment and periodic check up thereafter once in a year.
   (iii) Facility for vaccination or other exigencies. Services of a qualified physician for assessing the health status of personnel involved in the manufacturing and quality control of drugs shall also be made available.
E. **Sanitation in the manufacturing premises:** The manufacturing area shall not be utilised for any other purpose and shall be maintained clean and in an orderly manner, free from accumulated waste, dust, debris, etc. A routine sanitation programme shall be drawn up and observed.
F. **Equipment:** Equipment used for the manufacture of drugs shall be constructed, designed, installed and maintained so as to:
   (i) Achieve operational efficiency to attain the desired quality.
   (ii) Prevent physical, chemical and physicochemical change through surface contact.

(iii) Prevent contact of any substance required for the operation of the equipments like lubricants, etc.
(iv) Facilitate thorough cleaning wherever necessary.
(v) Minimise any contamination of drugs and their containers during manufacture.

G. **Raw materials:** The licensee shall keep an inventory of all raw materials to be used at any stage of manufacture of drugs and maintain records as per Schedule U. All such materials shall be:
   (i) Identified and their containers examined for damage and assigned control number.
   (ii) Stored at optimum temperature and relative humidity.
   (iii) Conspicuously labelled indicating the name of the materials; control number, name of the manufacturer and be specifically labelled "under test" or "approved" or "rejected".
   (iv) Systematically sampled by quality controlled personnel.
   (v) Tested for compliance with required standards of quality.
   (vi) Released from quarantine by quality control personnel through written instructions.
   (vii) So organised that stock rotation is on the basis of first in first out principle in the storage area.
   (viii) So arranged that all rejected materials are conspicuously identified and are destroyed or returned to the suppliers as soon as possible and records maintained thereof.

H. **Master formula records:** The licensee shall maintain master formula records relating to all manufacturing procedures for each product, which shall be prepared and endorsed by the competent technical staff. The master formula records shall give:
   (i) The patent or proprietary name of the product along with the generic name, if any, strength and the dosage form.
   (ii) A description or identification of the final containers, packaging materials, labels and closures to be used.
   (iii) The identity, quantity and quality of each raw material to be used, irrespective of whether or not it appears in the finished product. The permissible overages that may be included in a formulated batch shall be indicated.
   (iv) A description of all vessels and equipments and the size used in the process.
   (v) Manufacturing and control instructions along with parameters for critical steps such as mixing, drying, blending, sieving, sterilizing the product, etc.
   (vi) The theoretical yield to be expected from the formulation at different stage of manufacture and permissible yield limits.

(vii) Detailed instructions on precautions to be taken in manufacture and storage of drugs and of semi-finished products.
(viii) The requirements of in-process quality control test and analysis to be carried out during each stage of manufacture including the designation of persons or departments responsible for the execution of such tests and analysis.

I. **Batch manufacturing records:** The licensee shall maintain batch manufacturing record as per Schedule U for each batch of the drug product. Manufacturing records are required to provide a complete account of the manufacturing history of each batch of a drug, showing that it has been manufactured, tested and analysed in accordance with the manufacturing procedures and written instructions as per the master formula.

J. **Manufacturing operations and controls:** All manufacturing operations and controls shall be carried out under the supervision of approved competent technical staff. Critical steps in the process relating to selection, weighing and measuring of raw materials; addition during the process and weighing and measuring during the various stages shall be performed under the direct personal supervision of a competent technical staff. Even the non-sterile products are required to be free from pathogens like *Salmonella*, *E. coli*, *Pyocyanea*, etc. All vessels, containers and mechanical manufacturing equipment shall be conspicuously labelled with the name of the product and batch number, batch size and stage of manufacture. Labels shall also be attached to all mechanical manufacturing equipment during their operation.

K. **Reprocessing and recovery:** If a product batch has to be reprocessed, reprocessing procedure shall be authorised and recorded. An investigation shall be carried out into the causes necessitating reprocessing and appropriate corrective measures shall be taken for prevention of recurrence. Recovery of product residue may be carried out by incorporating in subsequent batches of the product, if permitted in the master formula.

L. **Product containers and closures:** All containers and closures shall comply with the pharmacopoeial requirements. Suitable specifications, test methods, cleaning procedures and sterilization procedures, when indicated, shall be used to assure that containers, closures and other component parts of drug packages are suitable and they are not reactive, additive, adsorptive, absorptive or leach to an extent that significantly affects the quality or purity of the drug. Wherever bottles are being used, the written schedule of cleaning shall be laid down and followed. Where bottles are not dried after washing, they shall be rinsed with deionised water or distilled water.

M. **Labels and other printed materials:** Printed and packaging materials including leaflets shall be stored, handled and accounted in such a way as to ensure that batch packaging materials and leaflets relating to different products do not become intermixed. Prior to issue, all labels for containers, cartons and boxes and all circulars, inserts and leaflets shall be examined and released as satisfactory, for use by the quality control personnel. Records shall be maintained for each shipment received of each packaging materials indicating receipt, control reference number and whether accepted or rejected.

N. **Distribution records:** Records for distribution of drug shall be maintained for distribution of finished batch in order to facilitate prompt and complete recall of the batch, if necessary.

O. **Records of complaints and adverse reactions:** Reports of serious adverse reactions resulting from the use of drug along with the comments shall be maintained and informed to the concerned Licensing Authority as early as possible.

P. **Quality control system:** Every manufacturing establishment shall have a quality control department supervised by approved expert staff directly responsible to the management but independent of other departments. The quality control department shall control all raw materials, monitor all in-process quality checks and control the quality and stability of finished products.

Part II – Plant and Equipment

Part II of Schedule M recommends the requirements of plant and equipment for the manufacture of drugs under the following sections:

  (i) Ointments, Emulsions, Lotions, Solutions, Pastes, Creams for external use.
 (ii) Syrups, Elixirs and Solutions, Emulsions, Suspensions for internal/oral use.
(iii) Pills, Compressed Tablets and Hypodermic Tablets.
(iv) Powders.
 (v) Hard Gelatin Capsules.
(vi) Surgical Dressings other than Absorbent Cotton Wool.
(vii) Eye Ointments, Eye Lotions and other preparations for external use (manufactured under aseptic conditions).
(viii) Pessaries and Suppositories.
(ix) Inhalers and Vitrallae.
 (x) Repacking of Drugs, Pharmaceuticals and Chemicals.
(xi) Parenteral preparations.

For most of the sections, an area of minimum 30 sq. metres (150 sq. metres for parenteral section and 90 sq. metres for tablets) is recommended for the basic installation. Recommended requirements do not include requirement of machinery, equipment and premises required for preparation of containers and closures for different categories of drugs. However, the Licensing Authority shall have the discretion to relax or alter the requirements of the Schedule in the circumstances of a particular case. In respect of other categories of drugs, not included above, such as chemicals and pharmaceutical aids, gauze and bandages, medicinal gases, empty gelatin capsules, mechanical contraceptives, new dosage forms, etc., the Licensing Authority shall have the discretion to examine the factory premises, space, plant and machinery, etc. and direct the manufacturer to carry out necessary modifications. Areas for formulations meant for external use and areas for formulations meant for internal use shall be separately provided to avoid mix-up even though they are from the same category of formulations.

Grant of licence to testing institutions

Manufacturers which may not be having testing facilities of their own for sophisticated tests, may get their raw materials and finished goods tested from any approved institution. Application for approval of such institution should be made to the Licensing Authority in Form 36. The Licensing Authority may, after making any enquiry as it deems fit and after satisfying himself that the institution has necessary facilities for analysis, grant approval for analysis of specified substances on Form 37.

Conditions for the grant of Licence

Before approval is granted, the following conditions must be complied with by the applicant:

(i) The premises where the tests are being carried out shall be well lighted and properly ventilated except where the nature of tests of any drug or cosmetic warrants otherwise.

(ii) The applicant shall provide adequate space having regard to the nature and number of samples of drugs or cosmetics proposed to be tested.

(iii) If it is intended to carry out tests requiring the use of animals, adequate facilities for the proper care of animals should be available.

(iv) The applicant shall provide and maintain suitable equipment with regard to the nature and number of samples of drugs or cosmetics proposed to be tested.

(v) The testing of drugs and cosmetics, as the case may be, shall be under the active direction of a person whose qualifications and experience are considered adequate by the Licensing Authority.

(vi) The testing of drugs and cosmetics, as the case may be, shall be carried out by persons whose qualifications and experience are considered adequate by the Licensing Authority.

(vii) The applicant shall provide books of standards recognised under the provisions of the act and rules thereunder and such other reference books as may be required.

Conditions of Approval

(i) The approved institution shall provide and maintain adequate staff and adequate premises and equipment.

(ii) The approved institution shall provide proper facilities for storage so as to preserve the properties of the samples to be tested by it.

(iii) The approved institution shall maintain all records related to testing and such records shall be retained for a period of two years beyond the expiry date and for a period of six years in case of other substances.

(iv) The approved institution shall allow any inspector to inspect the premises and records.

(v) The approved institution shall notify to the Licensing Authority any change in person-in-charge of testing or in the expert staff responsible for testing, as the case may be, and any material alterations in the premises or changes in the equipment used for the purpose of testing.

(vi) Analytical reports shall be furnished in the prescribed form and in case any sample is determined to be substandard, a copy of the report shall be sent to the Licensing Authority.

(vii) The institution shall maintain an inspection book and comply with further requirements which may be prescribed. Approval can be suspended or cancelled by the approving authority, but the institution may appeal to the State Government within three months of the date of such order.

SCHEDULE N

Pharmacy and the minimum requirements for running a Pharmacy

The term Pharmacy means and includes every store or shop or other place:

(i) Where drugs are dispensed,

(ii) Where drugs are prepared,

(iii) Where prescriptions are compounded,

(iv) Which by sign, symbol or indication gives the impression that the operations mentioned above are carried out in the premises,
(v) Which has upon it or displayed within it or affixed to or used in connection with it a sign bearing the word(s) 'Pharmacy', 'Pharmacist', 'Dispensing Chemist' or 'Pharmaceutical Chemist',
(vi) Which is advertised in these terms.

Before granting a licence for a Pharmacy, the Licensing Authority may consider:

(a) The average number of licences issued during the period of 3 years immediately preceding.
(b) The occupation, trade or business ordinarily carried out by such applicant during the preceding 3 years.

Schedule N specifies the list of minimum requirements for running a Pharmacy. These include the following:

1. **Entrance:** The front of a Pharmacy shall bear an inscription "Pharmacy".
2. **Premises:** The premises of Pharmacy shall be separated from rooms for private use. The premises shall be well-built, dry, well-lit and ventilated and, of sufficient dimensions so that all goods, especially medicaments and poisons, can be kept in a clearly visible and appropriate manner. The area of dispensing department shall be not less than 6 sq. metres for one pharmacist with additional 2 sq. metres for each additional pharmacist. The height of the premises shall be at least 2.5 metres. The floor of the Pharmacy shall be smooth and washable. The walls shall be plastered or tiled or oil painted. A pharmacy department shall also be provided with ample quantity of good quality water. The dispensing department shall be separated by a barrier to prevent the admission of the public.
3. **Furniture:** Drugs, chemicals and medicaments shall be kept in a room appropriate to their properties and in such special containers as will prevent any deterioration of the contents. Drawers, glasses and other containers used for keeping medicaments shall be of suitable size and capable of being closed tightly to prevent the entry of dust. Every container shall bear a label of appropriate size, easily readable with names of medicaments as given in the Pharmacopoeias. A Pharmacy shall be provided with a dispensing bench, the top of which shall be covered with washable and impervious material like stainless steel, laminated plastic, etc. A Pharmacy shall be provided with a cupboard with lock and key for the storage of poisons and shall be clearly marked with the word POISON in red letters on a white background.

4. **Apparatus:** A Pharmacy shall be provided with the appropriate apparatus – balance, bottles, corks, measuring cylinder, etc. and books necessary for making official preparations and prescriptions.
5. **Books:** The Drugs and Cosmetics Act, 1940, The Drugs and Cosmetics Rules, 1945, The Pharmacopoeia of India (Current Edition), National Formulary of India (Current Edition), The Pharmacy Act, 1948 and The Narcotic Drugs and Psychotropic Substances Act, 1985.
6. **General:** A Pharmacy shall be run under the continuous personal supervision of a Registered Pharmacist, whose name shall be displayed conspicuously in the premises. The Pharmacist shall always put on clean white overalls. The premises and fittings of the Pharmacy shall be properly kept and everything shall be in good order and clean. All records and registers shall be maintained as required by the laws in force. Any container taken from the poison cupboard shall be replaced therein immediately after use in the personal custody of the responsible person. Medicaments, when supplied, shall have the labels conforming to the provisions of the laws in force.

Particulars to be recorded during dispensing and compounding of Drugs

The compounding and dispensing of all the drugs should be carried out by a registered pharmacist himself or under his direct and personal supervision. Supply of drugs should be recorded at the time of supply in a prescribed register maintained for the purpose and the serial number of the entry in a register shall be entered on the prescription. Following particulars shall be entered in the register:

(i) Serial number of the entry,
(ii) Date of supply,
(iii) Name and address of the prescriber,
(iv) Name and address of the patient or the name and address of the owner of the animal, if the drug is supplied for the veterinary use,
(v) Names of ingredients along with the quantities thereof of preparation supplied,
(vi) Signature of the registered pharmacist under whose supervision the medicine was made or supplied. If the drugs are not compounded in the premises and supplied in the original container, then particulars specified above may be entered in a cash or credit memo book.

In case of refill prescriptions, the entry shall include a serial number, the date of supply, the quantity supplied and a reference to the entry when the drug was dispensed in the previous occasion. However, it is not

necessary to record the particulars in the register or cash or credit memo in case:
(a) The drugs are supplied against prescriptions under the Employees's State Insurance Scheme, if all the particulars are given in that prescriptions; and
(b) If drugs, other than those specified in Schedule C and H or H1, are supplied in their original unopened containers.

SCHEDULE O

Standard for Disinfectants shall conform to Indian Standard Specification (IS:1061:1997) laid down from time to time by Bureau of Indian Standards. See Appendix C for details.

SCHEDULE P

Schedule P gives the list of drugs, their life period in months and applicable storage conditions (temperature centigrade).

For all other drugs not specified under this Schedule, the maximum life period can be upto sixty months.

For the purpose of storage, the condition shall be

- Cold place – Not exceeding 8 degree centigrade.
- Cool place – Temperature between 10 degree centigrade to 25 degree centigrade.

All capsules shall be stored at a temperature not exceeding 30 degree centigrade.

Schedule P-I: Specifies pack sizes of certain drugs, while indicating the dosage forms, e.g. Pack size of Albendazole Suspension shall be 10 ml, Atenolol tablets in pack size of 14 tablets, Oral Rehydration Salts (ORS) powder in pouches to be reconstituted to one litre pack or in 5 unit dose sachets in one pack, etc.

SCHEDULE U

The method or format of keeping the manufacturing record of all batches manufactured are given in this Schedule U of the D & C Rules. A complete history and details of each batch are to be maintained, including the details of raw materials and packing materials, like container and closures used, in producing the batch. This shall conform to the GMP. These include the analytical and test report references of the raw materials used, the in-process reports, the finished product report, the yield, the quantity transferred to warehouse, the signatures of the approved competent technical staff responsible for the manufacture and that of testing head who released the batch for sale.

This schedule also gives format for the analytical reports of raw materials and the finished products.

These details are to be kept for two years from the expiry of such date and in the case of other substances for a period of five years from the date of manufacture. From this records, one can get all the information connected with the batch.

SCHEDULE V

Schedule V lays down the standards for Patent or Proprietary Medicines.

1. General Standards: In case of pharmaceutical products containing several active ingredients, the selection shall be such that the ingredients do not interact with one another, and do not affect the safety and therapeutic efficacy of the product. The combination shall not also lead to analytical difficulties for the purpose of assaying the content of such ingredients separately. The substances added as additives shall be innocuous, shall not affect the safety or therapeutic efficacy of the active ingredients, and shall not affect the assays and identity tests in the quantity present.
2. Patent or proprietary medicines shall comply with the general requirements of the dosage form under which it falls as given in the Indian Pharmacopoeia. If the dosage form, is not included in I.P., but is included in any other Pharmacopoeia, it shall comply with the general requirements of the dosage of such Pharmacopoeia.
3. Patent or proprietary medicines containing vitamins for prophylactic, therapeutic or pediatric use shall contain the vitamins in quantities, not less than and not more than those specified in the table given under this Schedule.
4. The content of active ingredients shall be as follows:

Ingredients	Percentage of label claim
(a) Other than vitamins, enzymes and antibiotics	90 to 110
(b) Enzymes and vitamins	Lower limit of 90 and no upper limit
(c) Dry formulations containing antibiotics	90 to 130
(d) Liquid formulation antibiotics	90 to 140

QUESTIONS FOR REVISION

1. Write short notes on Schedules C, C1, D, F(II), FF, G, H, H1, J, K, M, N, O, P and V.

2. Discuss the standards applicable to Patent and Proprietary medicines.
3. What is GMP? Why it is essential for a drug industry?
4. Discuss as to how following GMP in the manufacture of drugs helps in maintaining the quality of drugs produced.
5. Write short note on Total Quality Management (TQM) in drug production.
6. Write notes on Schedules M, N, U of Drugs and Cosmetics Rules.

IMPORT OF DRUGS AND COSMETICS

The term "import" is derived from the conceptual meaning as to bring in the goods and services into the part of a country. The buyer of such goods and services is referred to an importer and the overseas based seller is called as exporter.

The Drugs and Cosmetics Act and the Rules thereunder, provide for the import of drugs and cosmetics. Generally, drugs or cosmetics may be imported into India under the authority of a licence except those whose import is prohibited. Some drugs or cosmetics can be imported without any permit, provided they are of standard quality and statement that they comply with the provisions relating to import has been given to the custom collector by the manufacturer or importer.

Standard quality in relation to a drug means that the drug complies with the standard set out in the Second Schedule, and in relation to a cosmetic, that the cosmetic complies with such standard as may be prescribed.

Categories of drugs and cosmetics that are prohibited to be imported in India

The import of following categories of drugs are prohibited into India:
  i. Any drug or cosmetic which does not conforms to prescribed standard.
  ii. Any misbranded, adulterated or spurious drug.
  iii. Any misbranded or spurious cosmetic.
  iv. Any drug or cosmetic for import of which a licence is prescribed.
  v. Any patent or proprietary medicine, unless displayed in the prescribed manner on the label or container thereof, the true formula or list of active ingredients contained in it, together with the quantities thereof.
  vi. Any drug which, by means of any statement, design or device accompanying it or by any other means, claims to cure or mitigate any such disease or ailment, or to have any such other effect, as may be prescribed.

vii. Any cosmetic containing any ingredients which may render it unsafe or harmful for use under the direction indicated or recommended.
viii. Drugs which claim to prevent or cure any of the diseases or ailments specified in Schedule J to the rules.
ix. Drugs which have not been labelled and packed in the prescribed manner.
x. Any drugs whose manufacture, sale and distribution is prohibited in the country of origin, except when required for the purpose of examination, test or analysis.
xi. Biological and other special products specified in Schedule C and C1 after the date of their expiry as marked on the label or those not complying with the standards of strength, quality and purity as may be specified.
xii. Any new drug except with the permission of the Licensing Authority.
xiii. Any drug or cosmetic the import of which is prohibited under the Rules.

The Central Government may after consultation with the Drugs Technical Advisory Board, permit import of any drug or class of drugs not being of standard quality. And, if the Central Government is satisfied that the use of any drug or cosmetic is likely to involve any risk to human beings or animals or that any drug does not have the therapeutic value claimed; it may by notification in the official gazette, prohibit the import of such drug or cosmetic.

Categories of drugs which can be imported under licence or permit

Following are the classes of drugs that can be imported under the licence or permit:

i. All drugs specified in Schedule C and C1
ii. Drugs specified in Schedule X.
iii. Small quantities of drugs imported for the purpose of examination, test or analysis.
iv. Drugs imported for personal use covered by a prescription of registered medical practitioner.
v. Any new drug.

An application for import licence should be made to the proper authority in the prescribed form. A licence remains valid up to three years from the date of issue, unless earlier suspended or cancelled. Any person who is not satisfied by a suspension or cancellation order, passed by the Licensing Authority, may appeal within 30 days to the Central Government.

A separate licence is necessary in respect of import of drugs from each manufacturer. If a single manufacturer abroad has more than one factory situated in different places, manufacturing the same or different drugs, a separate import licence is required in respect of drug manufactured at each such factory. A single licence on one application form may be issued in respect of the import of more than one drug or class of drugs manufactured by the same manufacturer provided that the drugs or classes of drugs are manufactured at one factory or more than one factory, functioning conjointly as a single manufacturing unit. Any change in the constitution of a licensed firm should be informed to the Licensing Authority.

Conditions for getting Import Licence

An import licence is subjected to the following conditions:

i. The manufacturer shall comply with the conditions at all times given by him or on his behalf in undertaking.
ii. The licensee shall allow any Inspector authorized by the Licensing Authority to enter any premises where the imported substance is stocked, to inspect the means, if any, employed for testing the substances, and to take samples for test/analysis.
iii. The licensee shall furnish a sample adequate for examination as required by the Licensing Authority, together with full protocols of the tests, if any, which have been applied; from all batches or from such batch as directed by the Licensing Authority.
iv. If directed by the Licensing Authority, the licensee shall not sell or offer for sale any batch in respect of which a sample or protocols are furnished as indicated above, until a certificate is issued to him by or on behalf of the Licensing Authority.
v. In case the licensee is informed by the Licensing Authority that any drug does not comply with the prescribed standard of strength, quality and purity; he should withdraw the remainder of that batch from the market. The licensee shall maintain a record of all sales of imported substances showing particulars of the substance and of person to whom sold and such other particulars as specified by the Licensing Authority. Such records should be open to the inspection of any authorized Inspector.
vi. In respect of the sale or distribution of drugs specified in Schedule X, the licensee shall maintain a separate record or register showing the following particulars:
   (a) Name of the drug.
   (b) Batch number.
   (c) Name and address of the manufacturer.

- (d) Date of transaction.
- (e) Opening stock on the business day.
- (f) Quantity of drug received, if any, and the source from which received.
- (g) Name of the purchaser, his address and licence number.
- (h) Balance quantity of drug at the end of the business day.
- (i) Signature of the person under whose supervision the drugs have been supplied.

vii. The licensee shall comply with such further requirements as may be prescribed by the Licensing Authority and of which he has been given not less than four months notice.

(i) Import of Schedule C, C1 and X Drugs

Separate import licences are granted for the import of biological or other special products specified in Schedule C and C1 excluding X, and for drugs specified in Schedule X. Application for import in Form 8 or 8A is to be submitted to the Licensing Authority. An undertaking is given in Form 9 and prescribed fee is to be paid. In addition to the general conditions for the import licence, the Licensing Authority takes into consideration the following factors before granting the licence:

- (a) The premises where the imported substances will be stocked by the importer should be equipped with proper storage accommodation for preserving the properties of imported drugs.
- (b) Must have proper drug selling/manufacturing licence.
- (c) The licensee must maintain records, showing the particulars of the name of drugs and of the persons to whom they have been sold or the details of the usage in the manufacturing of other drugs.
- (d) The licensee shall allow authorized Inspector to inspect the premises and records.
- (e) Samples shall be provided for test and analysis, as and when asked for.
- (f) The licensee must comply with the undertaking given in Form 9 and the conditions stipulated in Licence Form 10 or 10A.
- (g) The licensee shall comply with any further requirements as may be specified by the Licensing Authority.

(ii) Import of Drugs for Examination, Test or Analysis

Small quantities of drugs can be imported for the purpose of examination, test or analysis subject to the following conditions:

i. Drugs shall be imported only under a licence in Form 11 from the Licensing Authority.

ii. The imported substances shall be used exclusively for the purpose of examination, test or analysis in the place specified in the licence or in any other place authorised by the Licensing Authority.
iii. The licensee shall allow any authorised Inspector to enter, inspect the premises, and to investigate the manner in which the substances are being used and to take samples thereof.
iv. The licensee shall keep a record of, and shall report to the Licensing Authority, the substances imported under the licence together with their quantities, the date of importation and the name of manufacturer.
v. The licensee shall comply with any further requirements as may be specified.

A licence for import for examination, test or analysis may be cancelled by the Licensing Authority for breach of any of the conditions of the licence. However, the licensee, whose licence has been cancelled, may appeal to the Central Government within 3 months of the date of such order.

(iii) Import of Drugs for Personal Use

Small quantities of drugs, whose import is otherwise prohibited, can be imported for personal use subject to the following conditions:

i. The drugs shall form part of the passenger's bonafide baggage and shall be the property of, and be intended for, the exclusive personal use of the passenger.
ii. The drugs must be declared to the Customs Authorities, if so directed.
iii. The quantity of any single drug, so imported, shall not exceed one hundred average doses.

The Licensing Authority may, in an exceptional case, sanction the import of a large quantity.

Any drug, imported for personal use but not forming the part of the bonafide personal baggage of the passenger, may be allowed to be imported subject to the following conditions:

(a) The Licensing Authority, on an application made to it in the specified form is satisfied that the drug is for bonafide personal use.
(b) The quantity is reasonable in the opinion of the Licensing Authority and covered by a prescription from a registered medical practitioner.

A permit is granted in respect of the said drug by the Licensing Authority in the specified form.

(iv) Import of New Drugs

A 'New drug' can be defined as a drug, the composition of which is not generally recognised as safe for use and includes any drug which has not been used to any large extent and for any appreciable length of time, after investigation study. Any patent or proprietary medicine containing any new drug is also to be considered as new drug.

No new drug can be imported except with the written permission of the Licensing Authority. While applying for such a permission, all documentary and other evidence relating to the standards of quality, purity and strength, etc. should be supplied to the Licensing Authority as provided in Schedule Y.

(v) Import of drugs by Govt. hospital/autonomous medical institution for treatment of patients

Small quantities of a new drug, otherwise prohibited for import, may be imported for treatment of patients suffering from life-threatening diseases or diseases causing serious permanent disability, or such diseases requiring therapies for unmet medical needs, by a Medical Officer of Govt. Hospital or an Autonomous Medical Institution providing tertiary care. Application for such import is to be made in Form 12AA.

PROCEDURE FOR IMPORT OF DRUGS

Any drug cannot be imported unless it is packed and labelled in conformity with the prescribed rules. Each consignment of drugs to be imported should be accompanied by an invoice or other statement showing the name and address of the manufacturer and the names and quantities of the drugs. Before importing drugs, for which a licence is not required, a declaration signed by the manufacturer on behalf of the importer, that the drugs comply with the provisions of the Act and Rules, should be supplied to the Customs Collector.

If he has reason to doubt whether any of the drugs complies with the provisions of the Act and the Rules, or if requested by an officer appointed for this purpose by the Central Government, the Customs Collector shall take samples of any drug in the consignment. The samples are sent to the director of the laboratory notified for this purpose by the Central Government. He may detain the consignments of drugs, of which samples have been taken, till the report of analysis of such samples is received. If the importer gives an undertaking in writing not to dispose of the drugs without the consent of the Customs Collector, and, to return the consignment to him within 10 days of the receipt of the notice, the Customs Collector may make over the consignment to the importer.

If the report indicates that a drug in the consignment is not of standard quality or contravenes any of the provisions of Chapter III of the Act or the Rules thereunder, and the contravention cannot be remedied by the importer, the Customs Collector may direct the importer to export the consignment back to the manufacturer abroad within two months, or forfeit it to the Central Government for destruction.

If aggrieved by the report, the importer may make representation to the Customs Collector who shall forward the samples together with representation to the Licensing Authority, whose decision shall be final. If the contravention is such that it can be remedied by the importer, the Customs Collector can permit the importer to import the drug, after taking a written undertaking not to dispose of the drug without the permission of the officer authorized in this behalf by the Central Government.

Places through which drugs may be imported into India

Drugs may be imported into India only through one of the following places:

(i) Ferozpur Cantonment and Amritsar Railway Stations: In respect of drugs imported by rail across the frontier with Pakistan.
(ii) Ranaghat, Bongaon and Mohiassan Railway Stations: In respect of drugs imported by rail across the frontier with Bangladesh.
(iii) Petraplole Road in West Bengal, Sutarkandi in Assam, Old Raghna Bazar and Agartala in Tripura: In respect of drugs imported by road from Bangladesh.
(iv) Raxaul in respect of drugs imported by road and railway lines connecting Raxaul in India and Birganj in Nepal.
(v) Chennai, Kolkata, Mumbai, Cochin, Nhava Sheva Kandla, Inland container Depot at Tuglakabad and Patparganj in Delhi, Tuticorin and Marmagaon port in Goa: In respect of drugs imported by sea into India.
(vi) Chennai, Kolkata, Mumbai, Delhi and Ahmedabad, Hyderabad, Goa and Bengaluru: In respect of drugs imported by air into India.

Consignments of drugs in transit through India to foreign countries, and which are not intended to be sold or distributed in India, are exempted from the provisions regulating the import of drugs. However, if such consignments are covered by import licences granted by countries of destination, the importer has to produce such licences at the time of import.

The substances exempted from provisions relating to import of drugs

The substances specified in Schedule D exempted from the provisions regulating import of drugs are as follows:

1. Substances not intended for medicinal use, provided these are imported in bulk and the importer certifies that these have been imported for

non-medicinal uses. If imported otherwise than in bulk, each container bears a label indicating that the substance is not intended for medicinal use.
2. The following substances, which are used both as articles of food as well as drugs:
   (i) All condensed or powdered milk whether pure, skimmed or malted, fortified with vitamins and minerals.
   (ii) Farex, Cerelac, Lactose and all other similar cereal preparations whether fortified with vitamins or otherwise except those for parenteral use.
   (iii) Virol, Bovril, chicken essence and all other similar predigested foods.

Ginger, pepper, cumin, cinnamon and all other similar spices and condiments unless they are specifically labelled as conforming to the standards in the Indian Pharmacopoeia or the official Pharmacopoeias and the official compendia of drug standards prescribed under the Act and Rules.

Power of Central Government to prohibit import in public interest

Where it is satisfied that the use of any drug or cosmetic is likely to involve any risk to human beings or animals or that any drug does not have the claimed therapeutic value or contains ingredients in such quantity for which there is no therapeutic justification, the Central Government may, in public interest, prohibit the import of such drug or cosmetic.

Application of laws relating to sea customs

The Customs Collector and other officers authorized in this behalf by the Central Government may detain any imported packages which he suspects to contain any drug or cosmetic, the import of which is prohibited under this Act, and report such detention to the Drugs Controller, India and if necessary, forward any package or sample of any suspected drug or cosmetic to the Central Drugs Laboratory for analysis.

Offences and Penalties related to import of drug

Any person, himself or by any other person on his behalf, imports consignment of the drugs or cosmetics in respect of which the offence has been committed are liable to confiscation. Offences cannot be tried by any court inferior to that of a Metropolitan Magistrate or of a Judicial Magistrate of the first class (Table 4.3).

Table 4.3. Offences and Penalties relating to import of drugs

Offence	Penalty	
	First Conviction	Subsequent Conviction
1. Import of adulterated or spurious drugs or spurious cosmetic or any cosmetic containing any ingredient which may render it unsafe or harmful for use under the directions recommended.	Imprisonment upto three years and fine upto Rs 5,000	Imprisonment upto five years or fine upto Rs 10,000 or both
2. Import of any drugs or cosmetics other than referred above, the import of which is prohibited.	Imprisonment upto six months or fine upto Rs 500 or both	Imprisonment upto one year or fine upto Rs 1,000 or both
3. Import of any drug or cosmetic in contravention of any notification issued by Central Government whereby prohibiting import of any drug or cosmetic in public interest.	Imprisonment upto three years or fine upto Rs 5,000 or both	Imprisonment upto 5 years or fine upto Rs 10,000 or both

Note: Penalties under 1, 2 or 3 above are in addition to any penalty awarded under the provisions of Sea Customs Act.

QUESTIONS FOR REVISION

1. Give an account on import of different classes of drugs and state the classes of drugs which are prohibited to be imported.
2. Write the conditions for getting import licence for import of drugs.
3. Write short notes on:
    (a) Import of Schedules C and C1 drugs.
    (b) Import of drugs for personal use.
    (c) Drugs which are prohibited to be imported.
    (d) Places of drugs where import can be made by air and sea.
    (e) Offences and penalties relating to import of drugs.
    (f) Import of new drugs.
    (g) Import of drugs without licence.
    (h) Import of drugs for examination, test or analysis.

MANUFACTURE OF DRUGS AND COSMETICS

Manufacture is a process or a part of a process for making, altering, ornamenting, finishing, packing, labelling, breaking up or otherwise treating or adopting any drug or cosmetic with a view to its sale or distribution, but does not include the compounding or dispensing of any drug, or the packing of any drug or cosmetic, in the ordinary course of retail business. The following licences are granted for the manufacture of drugs under the Drugs and Cosmetics Act and Rules.

1. Drugs other than those specified in Schedules C, C1, X and LVP.
2. Drugs specified in Schedules C, C1 but not specified in Schedule X.
3. Drugs specified in Schedules C, C1 and X.
4. Drugs specified in Schedule X but not in Schedules C and C1.
5. Manufacture of large volume of parenterals (LVP), sera and vaccine and recombinant DNA derived drugs specified in Schedules C and C1 and excluding those specified in Schedule X.
6. Drugs for the purpose of examination, test or analysis.
7. Loan licences.
8. Repacking licences.
9. Blood products.
10. Any new drugs.

Table 4.4 gives Application Form No. and Licence and Inspection Fee for manufacturing of drugs and cosmetics.

General Procedure for Getting the Manufacturing Licences

1. Application to be made in the prescribed form along with the prescribed application fee and inspection fee.
2. The premises should comply with the plan of premises Schedules M, M1, M2, M3 or T requirements, as the case may be.
3. An analytical and testing section, headed by a competent person, should be there.
4. The name of the company, constitution, products to be manufactured and all other required details should be furnished by the applicant to the Licensing Authority.

The Licensing Authorities appointed by the State Government issue the licences for the manufacture of drugs for which so authorized. A licence is valid only for a set of premises and if the drugs are manufactured on more than one set of premises, separate licences are required in respect of each such set of premises. The licence issued by the Licensing Authority is valid for a period of five years, on and from the date on which it was granted. Subsequently, it is renewed on renewal application, accompanied with prescribed renewal fee for a period of five years.

In the event of any change in the constitution of a licensed firm, the licensee should inform the Licensing Authority accordingly. Licence of such firms are deemed to be valid for a maximum period of 3 months from the date of change, unless in the meantime a fresh licence has been obtained from the Licensing Authority.

Table 4.4. Application Form No. and Licence and Inspection Fee for manufacturing of Drugs and Cosmetics

S. No.	Type of Licence	Application Form No.	Licence Form No.	Licence & Inspection Fee (as on date)
1.	Drugs other than those specified in Schedule C, C1 and Schedule X	Form 24	Form 25	Rs 6000 + Rs 1500
2.	Loan manufacturing for other than those specified in Schedule C and C1 and Schedule X	Form 24-A	Form 25-A	Rs 6000 + Rs 1500
3.	Repacking of drugs of Drugs other than those specified in Schedule C & C1 & X	Form 24B	Form 25B	Rs 500
4.	Drugs specified in Schedule X	Form 24F	Form 25F	Rs 6000 + Rs 1500
5.	Drugs those are specified in Schedules C and C1 excluding Part X-B and Schedule X (X-B: LVP and Blood Products)	Form 27	Form 28	Rs 6000 + Rs 1500
6.	Loan manufacturing for those specified in Schedule C and C1 excluding Part X-B and Schedule X (X-B: LVP and Blood Products)	Form 27A	Form 28-A	Rs 6000 + Rs 1500
7.	Drugs those are specified in Schedules C, C1 and X	Form 27-B	Form 28-B	Rs 6000 + Rs 1500
8.	Drugs - Large Volume Parenterals/ Sera and Vaccines/Recombinant DNA derived drugs specified in Schedules C and C1 excluding those in Schedule X	Form 27-D	Form 28-D	Rs 6000 + Rs 1500
9.	Operation of Blood Bank and processing of whole blood or preparation of Blood Components	Form 27-C	Form 28-C	Rs 6000 + Rs 1500
10.	Blood Products	Form 27-E	Form 28-E	Rs 6000 + Rs 1500
11.	Mfg. of drugs for purpose of examination, test/analysis	Form 30	Form 29	Rs 250 for every application
12.	Cosmetics	Form 31	Form 32	Rs 2500 + Rs 1000
13.	Loan licence for manufacturing of Cosmetics	Form 31A	Form 32-A	Rs 2500 + Rs 1000

Drugs and Cosmetics Prohibited to be Manufactured and Sold under the Drugs and Cosmetics Act, 1940

No person shall himself or by any other person on his behalf:

(a) Manufacture for sale or for distribution, or sell, stock or exhibit or offer for sale, or distribute:
  (i) Any drug which is not of standard quality or is misbranded, adulterated or spurious.
  (ii) Any cosmetic which is not of a standard quality, or is misbranded, adulterated or spurious.
  (iii) Any patent or proprietary medicine whose complete formula is not disclosed on the label or container.
  (iv) Any drug which purports, or claims to prevent, cure or mitigate any disease specified in Schedule J.
  (v) Any cosmetic containing any ingredient which may render it unsafe or harmful for use under the directions indicated or recommended.
  (vi) Any drug or cosmetic in contravention of the Act or Rules thereunder.
(b) Sell or stock or exhibit or offer for sale or distribute any drug or cosmetic, which has been imported or manufactured in contravention of the provisions of this Act or Rules thereunder.
(c) Manufacture for sale or for distribution, or sell, stock or exhibit or offer for sale, or distribute any drug or cosmetic, except under and in accordance with the conditions of a licence issued for such purpose.

However, nothing in this section shall apply to the manufacture, subject to prescribed conditions, of small quantities of any drug for the purpose of examination, test or analysis. The Central Government may however permit the manufacture for sale or for distribution, sale, stocking or distribution of any drug or class of drugs, not being of standard quality.

I. Manufacture of drugs other than those specified in Schedules C, C1 and X

Application for the grant or renewal of a licence for the manufacture of drugs other than those specified in Schedules C, C1 and X should be made to the Licensing Authority in Form 24 and for the manufacture of drugs not specified in Schedules C and C1 but specified in Schedule X in Form 24F. The respective licences are issued in Forms 25 and 25F.

Conditions for Grant of Licence

Before a licence in Forms 25 or 25F is granted or renewed the following conditions must be satisfied by the applicant:

(i) The manufacture shall be conducted under the active direction and personal supervision of competent technical staff consisting of at least one person who is a whole-time employee and who is:
   (a) A graduate in Pharmacy or Pharmaceutical Chemistry of a recognized university and has had at least 18 months practical experience, after graduation, in the manufacture of drugs. The period of experience may be reduced by six months if the person has undergone training in manufacture of drugs for a period of six months during his graduation; or
   (b) A graduate in Science of a recognized university with Chemistry as a principal subject and who has had at least 3 years' practical experience in the manufacture of drugs, after his graduation; or
   (c) A graduate in Chemical Engineering or Chemical Technology or Medicine of a recognized university with general training and practical experience of not less than three years in the manufacture of drugs, after his graduation; or
   (d) Holding any foreign qualification, comparable to any of the above in quality and content of training, and is permitted to work as competent technical staff under this Rule by the Central Government.
   For drugs other than those specified in Schedules C, C1 and X and meant for veterinary use, the whole-time employee under whose supervision the manufacture is conducted, may be a graduate in Veterinary Science or Pharmacy or General Science or Medicine of a recognized university and who had at least three years practical experience in the manufacture of drugs excluding graduate in Pharmacy, who shall have 18 months practical experience in manufacture of drugs.
   Provided that any person, not having the above qualifications but having adequate experience of manufacturing, may also be permitted by the Licensing Authority to actively direct and personally supervise the manufacture of disinfectant fluids, insecticides, liquid paraffin, medicinal gases, non-chemical contraceptives, Plaster of Paris and surgical dressings, for the manufacture of which the knowledge of pharmacy or pharmaceutical chemistry is not essential.
(ii) The factory premises shall comply with the conditions prescribed in Schedule M.
(iii) The applicant shall provide adequate space, plant and equipment for the manufacturing operations as given in Schedule M.
(iv) The applicant shall provide and maintain adequate staff, premises and laboratory equipment for carrying out tests of the strength and purity of the substances at a testing unit, which shall be separate

from the manufacturing unit and the head of the testing unit shall be independent of the head of the manufacturing unit. Tests, requiring sophisticated instrumentation techniques or biological or microbiological methods other than sterility, may be permitted by the Licensing Authority to be conducted at institutions approved for this purpose. The head of the testing unit shall possess a degree in Medicine or Science or Pharmacy or Pharmaceutical Chemistry of a recognised university and adequate experience in the testing of drugs.

(v) The applicant shall make adequate arrangements for the storage of drugs manufactured by him.

(vi) While applying for a licence to manufacture patent or proprietary medicines the applicant shall furnish to the Licensing Authority evidence and data justifying that the patent or proprietary medicines:

   (a) Contain the constituent ingredients in therapeutic/prophylactic quantities, as determined in relation to the claims or conditions for which the medicines are recommended for use or claimed to be useful.

   (b) Are safe in the context of the vehicles, excipients, additives or pharmaceutical aids used in the formulation and under conditions in which the formulations are recommended for administration and use.

   (c) Are stable under the conditions of storage recommended.

   (d) Contain such ingredients and in such quantities for which there is therapeutic justification.

(vii) The licensee shall comply with the requirements of "Good Manufacturing Practices" as laid down in Schedule M.

A licence in Forms 25 or 25F remains valid for a period of five years from date of issue, unless suspended or cancelled earlier. If the application for renewal of licence is made before its expiry, or if the application is made within six months of its expiry, after payment of the additional fee, the licence shall continue to be valid until orders are passed on the application. The licence shall be deemed to have expired if the application for its renewal is not made within six months of its expiry.

Conditions of licence

A licence in Forms 25 and 25-F shall be subject to the following conditions:

(i) The licensee shall provide and maintain an adequate staff and premises and plant for the proper manufacture and storage of substances.

(ii) The licensee shall comply with the provisions of the Act and Rules and with such further requirements as may be specified.

(iii) The licensee shall, either in his own laboratory, or in any other approved laboratory test each batch or lot of the raw materials used by him for the manufacture of his product and also each batch of the final product and shall maintain records and registers, showing the particulars in respect of such tests as specified in Schedule U. The records or registers shall be retained for a period of 5 years from the date of manufacture.

(iv) The licensee shall allow an Inspector authorised by the Act to enter, with or without prior notice, any premises where the manufacture is carried on and to inspect the premises, and the process of manufacture and the means employed in standardizing and testing the drugs.

(v) The licensee shall allow an Inspector to inspect all records and registers maintained under the Rules and to take samples of the manufactured product and shall supply any other relevant information.

(vi) The licensee shall from time to time inform the Licensing Authority any change in the expert staff and any material changes in the premises or plant since the date of the last inspection made on behalf of the Licensing Authority.

(vii) On request by the Licensing Authority, the licensee shall furnish from every batch a sample of adequate quantity for any examination and, if required, full protocol of the tests which have been applied.

(viii) If directed by the Licensing Authority, the licensee shall not sell any batch in respect of which a sample is furnished for examination, until a certificate authorising the sale of the batch has been issued to him.

(ix) If any part of the batch of any substance is found by the Licensing Authority not to conform with the standards of strength, quality and purity specified and on being directed to do so, the licensee shall withdraw the remainder of the batch from sale and recall all issues already made from that batch.

(x) The licensee shall maintain an inspection book to enable an Inspector to record his impression and defects noticed.

(xi) The licensee shall maintain reference samples from each batch of drugs manufactured by him in a quantity twice than that sufficient for conducting all the tests. In case of drugs bearing an expiry date the reference samples shall be maintained for a period of three months beyond the date of expiry and in case of other drugs, for a period of three years from the date of manufacture.

(xii) In case of Schedule X drugs other than those specified in Schedules C and C1, the licensee shall forward to the Licensing Authority of the state, a statement of the sales effected to the manufacturers, wholesalers, retailers, hospitals, dispensaries, nursing homes and RMPs every three months. He shall also maintain accounts of all transactions giving details as indicated below in a bound and serially numbered register and retain the same for a period of five years or one year after the date of expiry, whichever is later.

(xiii) The licensee shall comply with the requirements of Good Laboratory Practices (Schedule L-I) and of Good Manufacturing Practices (Schedule M)

II. Manufacture of Drugs those are Specified in Schedules C and C1 Excluding Part X-B and Schedule X Drugs

Application for the grant or renewal of licence to manufacture drugs specified in Schedules C and C1, excluding those specified in Schedule X, shall be made to the Licensing Authority in Form 27 and for drugs specified in Schedules C, C1 and X, in Form 27B. Application for manufacturing large volume parenterals, recombinant DNA derived drugs and sera and vaccines should be made in Form 27D. Respective licences are issued in Forms 28 and 28B and 28D.

Conditions for grant of Licence

The following conditions should be complied with, by the applicant, before a licence is granted or renewed:

(i) The manufacturing shall be conducted under personal supervision and active direction of competent technical staff consisting at least of one person who is a whole-time employee and who is:

(a) A graduate in pharmacy or pharmaceutical chemistry of a recognised university with at least 18 months' practical experience after the graduation in the manufacture of drugs to which this licence applies. This period of experience may however be reduced by six months if the person has undergone training in manufacture of drugs to which this licence applies for a period of six months during his university course; or

(b) A graduate in science of a recognised university, who for the purpose of his degree has studied Chemistry or Microbiology as a principal subject and has had at least three years' practical experience in the manufacture of drugs to which this licence applies after his graduation; or

(c) A graduate in medicine from a recognised university with at least three years' experience in the manufacture and pharmacological testing of biological products after his graduation; or

(d) A graduate in Chemical Engineering of a recognised university with at least three years' practical experience in the manufacture of drugs to which this licence applies after his graduation; or

(e) Holding any foreign qualification comparable in quality, content and training with above qualifications and is permitted to work as competent technical staff by the Central Government. For drugs specified in Schedules C and C1 meant for veterinary use, the whole-time employee under whose supervision the manufacture is conducted, may be a graduate in Veterinary Science or General Science or Medicine or Pharmacy of a recognised university and who had at least three years' experience in the manufacture of biological products.

For medical devices specified in Schedule C, the whole-time employee, under whose supervision the manufacture is conducted, may be a graduate in Science with Physics or Chemistry or Microbiology as one of the subjects; or graduate in Pharmacy; or degree/diploma holder in Mechanical or Chemical or Plastic Engineering of a recognised university.

(ii) The factory premises shall comply with the conditions prescribed in Schedule M (and Schedule M-III in respect of medical devices).

(iii) The applicant shall provide adequate space, plant and equipment for any or all the manufacturing operations as prescribed in Schedule M and Schedule M-III.

(iv) The applicant shall provide and maintain adequate staff, premises and laboratory equipment for carrying out such tests for the strength, quality and purity of the substances as required under the Rules including proper housing for animals, used for the purposes of such tests, the testing unit being separate from the manufacturing unit and the head of the testing unit being independent of the head of the manufacturing unit.

Provided that for tests requiring sophisticated instrumentation techniques or biological or microbiological methods other than sterility, the Licensing Authority may permit such tests to be conducted by approved institutions.

The head of the testing unit should possess a degree in Medicine or Science or Pharmacy or Pharmaceutical Chemistry of a recognized university and shall have adequate experience in the testing of drugs.

(v) The applicant shall make adequate arrangements for the storage of drugs manufactured by him.

(vi) The applicant shall furnish to the Licensing Authority, if required, data on the stability of drugs which are likely to deteriorate for fixing the date of expiry, which shall be printed on the labels of such drugs on the basis of data so furnished.

(vii) While applying for the licence to manufacture patent or proprietary medicines, the applicant should furnish to the Licensing Authority evidence and data justifying that the patent or proprietary medicines:

    (a) Contain the constituent ingredients in therapeutic/prophylactic quantities as determined in relation to the claims or conditions for which the medicines are recommended for use or claimed to be useful.

    (b) Are safe for use in the context of the vehicles, excipients, additives and pharmaceutical aids used in the formulations, and under the conditions in which the formulations for administration and use are recommended.

    (c) Are stable under the conditions of storage recommended.

    (d) Contain such ingredients and in such quantities for which there is therapeutic justification.

(viii) The licensee shall comply with the requirements of "Good Manufacturing Practices" as laid down in Schedule M.

A licence in Forms 28, 28B or 28D remains valid for a period of five years from date of issue. Provided that, if the application for renewal of licence is made before its expiry, or if the application is made within six months of its expiry. after payment of additional fee, the licence shall continue to be in force until orders are passed on the application. If the application for its renewal is not made within six months of its expiry, the licence shall be deemed to have expired.

Conditions to be complied for manufacturing

Schedules C and C1 and X and LVP sera and vaccines and R-DNA derived drugs after grant of Licence

After the grant of licence, the licensee has to comply with such special conditions as set out in Schedules F or F1, as the case may be, and to the following general conditions:

(i) (a) The licensee shall provide and maintain an adequate staff and adequate premises and plant for the proper manufacture and storage of substances.

    (b) Every holder of a licence, who for any purpose engaged in the culture or manipulation of pathogenic spore-bearing micro-organisms, shall provide to the satisfaction of the Licensing Authority, separate laboratories and utensils and apparatus required for the culture and manipulation of such micro-organisms, the laboratories, utensils, and apparatus so provided not being used for any other purpose.

(ii) The licensee shall provide and maintain staff, premises and equipment as specified.
(iii) (a) The licensee shall maintain records of manufacture as per particulars given in Schedule U.
(b) The licensee shall, either in his own laboratory or in any other approved laboratory, test each batch or lot of the raw material used by him for manufacture of his product and also each batch of the final product, and shall maintain records and registers showing the particulars in respect of each test as specified in Schedule U. The records shall be retained in the case of a substance for which a potency date is fixed for a period of two years from the expiry of such date, and in the case of other substances for a period of five years from the date of manufacture.
(iv) The licensee shall allow an Inspector appointed under the Act to enter any premises, where the manufacture is carried on, and to inspect the premises and in the case of substance specified in Schedules C and C1, to inspect the plant and the process of manufacture and the means employed for standardizing and testing the substance.
(v) The licensee shall allow an Inspector to inspect all registers and records, maintained under these Rules, and to take samples of the manufactured product and shall supply any other relevant information as may be required.
(vi) The licensee shall from time to time inform the Licensing Authority any changes in the expert staff and material changes in the premises or plant since the date of last inspection made on behalf of the Licensing Authority, before the issue of the licence.
(vii) The licensee shall, on request, furnish to the Licensing Authority, a sample of adequate quantity from every batch of drugs manufactured, for any examination along with full protocols of the test which have been applied.
(viii) If directed by the Licensing Authority, the licensee shall not sell, or offer for sale any batch in respect of which a sample is furnished for examination, until a certificate authorising the sale of the batch has been issued to him.
(ix) If any part of the batch of any substance is found by the Licensing Authority not to conform with the standards of strength, quality, or purity specified, on being directed so to do, the licensee shall withdraw the remainder of the batch from sale and recall all issues already made from that batch.
(x) No drug manufactured under the licence shall be sold unless the precautions, necessary for preserving its properties, have been observed throughout the period after manufacture.

(xi) The licensee shall comply with the requirements of the Act and the Rules and any additional requirement which may be specified.
(xii) The licensee shall maintain an inspection book to enable an inspector to record his impression and defects noticed.
(xiii) The licensee shall maintain reference samples from each batch of drugs manufactured by him in a quantity twice than that sufficient for conducting all the tests. In case of drugs bearing an expiry date, the reference samples shall be maintained for a period of three months beyond the date of expiry and in case of other drugs, for a period of three years from the date of manufacture.
(xiv) In case of manufacture of drugs those specified in Schedules C and C1 and X, the licensee shall forward to the Licensing Authority of the State a statement of the sales effected to the manufacturers, wholesalers, retailers, hospitals, dispensaries, nursing homes and RMPs every three months. He shall also maintain accounts of all transactions giving details as indicated below in a bound and serially numbered register and retain the same for a period of five years or one year after the date of expiry of potency, whichever is later.
(xv) The licensee shall store drugs specified in Schedule X in bulk form and when any such drug is required, for manufacture, it shall be kept in a separate place under direct custody of a responsible person.
(xvi) The licensee shall comply with the requirements of "Good Laboratory Practices" as laid down in schedule L-I and "Good Manufacturing Practices" as laid down in Schedule M.

III. Manufacture of drugs specified in Schedule X

(i) All conditions stated for Schedules C and C1 drugs are applicable for Schedule X drugs, except that the application is made in Form 27-B.
(ii) The licensee shall furnish to the Licensing Authority every three months a statement of sales effected to the manufacturers, wholesalers, retailers, hospitals, dispensaries, nursing homes and Registered Medical Practitioners along with copies of invoices.
(iii) Maintain an accounts register as given thereunder.
(iv) The licensee shall not manufacture drugs specified in Schedule X for use as "Physicians Sample".

A. Accounts of drugs specified in Schedule X used for the manufacture

(a) Date of issue.
(b) Name of drug.
(c) Opening balance of stock on the production day.

(d) Quantity received, if any, and sources of supply.
(e) Quantity used in manufacture.
(f) Balance quantity in hand at the end of production day.
(g) Signature of the person in-charge.

B. Accounts of production

(a) Date of manufacture.
(b) Name of drug.
(c) Batch number.
(d) Quantity of raw material used in manufacture.
(e) Anticipated yield.
(f) Actual yield.
(g) Wastage.
(h) Quantity of manufactured goods transferred to stock.

C. Accounts of manufactured drugs

(a) Date of manufacture.
(b) Name of drug.
(c) Batch number.
(d) Opening balance.
(e) Quantity manufactured.
(f) Quantity sold.
(g) Name of purchaser and his address.
(h) Balance quantity at the end of the day.

IV. Manufacture of drugs for examination, test or analysis

A licence is necessary to manufacture any drug in small quantity for the purpose of examination, test or analysis. If a person proposing to manufacture does not hold a licence to manufacture drugs specified in Schedules C and C1 or to manufacture drugs other than those specified in Schedules C, C1 and X, he shall obtain a licence in Form 29 before commencing such manufacture.

In case of drugs not specified as safe for use, a licence in Form 29 can be granted only on producing a no objection certificate from the Licensing Authority appointed by the Central Government. Application should be made by or countersigned by the head of the institution or director of the firm or the company which proposes to undertake manufacture. The licence remains valid for a period of one year unless sooner cancelled and may thereafter be renewed for periods of one year at a time. Any drug manufactured for the purpose of examination, test or analysis shall be kept in containers bearing labels indicating the purpose for which it has been manufactured. When such drugs are supplied to any other manufacturer, the containers shall bear label stating the name and the address of the manufacturer, scientific name of the substance or reference enabling the substance to be identified, and the purpose for which it has been manufactured.

Conditions of Licence

A licence in Form 29 should fulfill the following conditions:
  (i) The licensee shall use the drugs, manufactured under the licence, exclusively for purpose of examination, test or analysis and shall carry on the manufacture and examination, test or analysis at the place specified in the licence.
  (ii) The licensee shall allow an Inspector to inspect the premises and to satisfy himself that only examination, test or analysis is being conducted.
  (iii) The licensee shall keep a record of the quantity of drugs manufactured and of any person or persons to whom the drugs have been supplied.
  (iv) The licensee shall maintain an inspection book to enable an Inspector to record his impression and defects noticed.
  (v) The licensee shall comply with such further requirements as may be specified and of which the Licensing Authority has given him not less than one month's notice.

V. Manufacture on Loan Licences

If an applicant does not have his own arrangements for manufacture, but who intends to avail himself the manufacturing facilities owned by another licensee, a loan licence may be issued by Licensing Authority. A loan licence means a licence issued by a Licensing Authority to a person who does not have his own manufacturing facilities (premises, plant and machinery), but who intends to avail himself of the manufacturing facility of another person, having the licence in Form 25 or Form 28.

Type of Loan Licence

Two types of loan licence are issued – one for all drugs other than those specified in Schedules C, C1 and X, and the other for the drugs specified in Schedules C and C1. There is no provision for manufacture of Schedule X drugs under loan licence.
1. Application for grant of loan licence shall be made in Forms 24A or 27A, as the case may be.
2. Before the grant of a loan licence the Licensing Authority shall get the premises inspected by one or more inspectors with or without an expert in the concerned field. The inspector shall examine all portions of the premises, plant and appliances, process of manufacture, means for standardizing and testing the drugs.

3. The Licensing Authority, before grant of loan licence, shall satisfy by himself that the principal manufacturing unit has adequate staff, capacity for manufacture and facilities for testing, to undertake the manufacture on behalf of the applicant for a loan licence.
4. For manufacturing of additional items on a loan licence, an application shall be made to the Licensing Authority. The licensee is required to test each batch of the raw material and the finished product and to maintain the relevant records as specified in Schedule U. Such records shall be maintained for a period of five years from the date of manufacture.
5. In case the Loan licence is cancelled or suspended of the lending person, whose manufacturing facilities are to be utilized by the loan licensee, then the loan licence is deemed to be cancelled or suspended automatically.
6. The loan licensee shall maintain an inspection book.

V. Repacking Licences

Repacking licences are granted for the purpose of breaking up any drug other than those specified in Schedules C and C1, on application to the Licensing Authority in Form 24B and the licence is issued in Form 25B subject to satisfying the following conditions:

(i) The repacking operation shall be carried out under hygienic conditions and under the supervision of a competent person, namely:
   (a) A person who holds Diploma in Pharmacy approved by Pharmacy Council of India or is a Registered Pharmacist; or
   (b) A person who has passed the intermediate examination, with chemistry as one of the principal subjects or an equivalent recognised examination; or
   (c) A person who has passed the matriculation or equivalent recognised examination and has at least four years' practical experience in the manufacture, dispensing or repacking of drugs.
(ii) The factory premises shall comply with the conditions prescribed in Schedule M.
(iii) The licensee shall make adequate arrangements for the storage of drugs.
(iv) The licensee shall comply with the provisions of the Act and Rules and with such further requirements as may be specified.
(v) The licensee shall either in his own laboratory or in any other approved laboratory test each batch or lot of the raw materials used by him for repacking and also each batch of the product thus packed and shall maintain records and registers showing the particulars in

respect of such tests as specified in Schedule U. The records or registers shall be retained for a period of 5 years from the date of repacking.

(vi) The licensee shall allow any inspector authorised by the Act to enter, with or without prior notice, any premises where the packing of drugs is carried on and to inspect the premises and to take samples of repacked drugs.

(vii) The licensee shall maintain an inspection book to enable an inspector to record his impression and defects noticed.

(viii) The licensee shall maintain reference samples from each batch of drugs repacked by him in a quantity twice than that sufficient for conducting all the tests. In case of drugs bearing an expiry date the reference samples shall be maintained for a period of three months beyond the date of expiry and in case of other drugs, for a period of three years from the date of manufacture. The licence remains valid for a period of five years from date of issue. For repacking any additional items, advance applications have to be made to the Licensing Authority. Apart from the other particulars, the label on the repacked drugs shall mention the name and address of the licensee, and his licence number preceding by the word "Rpg. Lic. No.".

VI. Manufacture of New Drugs

A 'new drug' is defined as:

(a) A new substance of chemical, biological or biotechnological origin; in bulk or prepared dosage form; used for prevention, diagnosis, or treatment of disease in man or animal, which, except during local clinical trials, has not been used in the country to any significant extent; and which, except during local clinical trials, has not been recognised in the country as effective and safe for the proposed claims.

(b) A drug already approved by the Licensing Authority for certain claims, which is now proposed to be marketed with modified or new claims, namely, indications, dosage, dosage form (including sustained release dosage form) and route of administration.

(c) A fixed dose combination of two or more drugs, individually approved earlier for certain claims, which are now proposed to be combined, for the first time, in a fixed ratio, or if the ratio of ingredients in an already marketed combination is proposed to be changed, with certain claims, viz., indications, dosage, dosage form (including sustained release dosage form) and route of administration.

For the purpose of this Rule, all vaccines and recombinant DNA (r-DNA) derived drugs shall be new drugs unless certified otherwise by the

Licensing Authority and a new drug shall continue to be considered as new drug for a period of four years from the date of its first approval.

Following provisions are applicable for the manufacture of a new drug whether classifiable under Schedules C and C1 or otherwise:

(a) No 'new drug' can be manufactured unless prior approval of the Licensing Authority is taken.
(b) A manufacturer of a new drug, when applying for approval, shall submit data as given in Appendix I to Schedule Y including the results of clinical trials carried out in the country as per format given in Appendix II to Schedule Y.
(c) While applying for a licence to manufacture a 'new drug' or its preparations, an applicant shall produce along with his application, evidence of safety data of drug that the drug has already been approved. The requirement of submitting the results of local clinical trials may not be necessary, if the drug is of such a nature that the Licensing Authority may, in public interest, decide to grant permission on the basis of data available from other countries. The requirement of submission of data relating to animal toxicology, reproduction studies, teratogenic studies, perinatal studies, mutagenicity and carcinogenicity may be modified or relaxed in case of new drug, approved and marketed for several years in other countries, if he is satisfied that there is adequate published evidence regarding the safety of the drug.

VII. Special provisions related to Biological and other Special Products

No substance specified in Schedule C can be sold unless it has been sealed in a previously sterilized container made of glass or other suitable material approved by the Licensing Authority. This condition is however not required, if the substance is to be terminally sterilized. In case of multidose containers for liquids, the liquid shall contain a sufficient proportion of some antiseptic to prevent the growth of any organism which may be accidentally introduced in the process of removing a portion of the contents of the container. This condition is however not applicable to Penicillin suspension in oil and wax. The containers shall comply with the requirements of Schedules F or F1, as the case may be. The tests, if any, required for determining the strength and quantity of each substances specified in Schedules C and C1 are those specified in Schedules F or F1 as specified.

If a substance is required in an emergency by a RMP but the licensee has no filled containers in stock, the licensee may issue the substance from a batch, which has already passed the test for sterility and freedom from abnormal toxicity, without completing the sterility test on the filled container, provided that he shall complete the sterility test on the filled containers and report any visible growth immediately to the Licensing Authority. The licensee shall also maintain records of emergency issues and of the sterility tests run by him. The records relating to sterility test shall contain following particulars:

  (i) Serial number.
  (ii) Name of the product, its batch number and batch size.
  (iii) Whether in bulk or final containers.
  (iv) Number of samples used for the test.
  (v) Name of the antiseptic, if any, and its concentration.
  (vi) Volume of inoculums and culture media.
  (vii) Date of inoculation.

Test for Freedom from Abnormal Toxicity

Each batch of serum should be tested for freedom from abnormal toxicity by giving a dose of 0.5 c.c. subcutaneously into a normal mouse or a dose of not less than 5 c.c. subcutaneously or intraperitoneally into a normal guinea pig. If no death or serious symptoms are produced in the animal within seven days, the serum is treated to have passed the test.

Test for Pyrogens

Solutions for parenteral administration, in doses of 10 ml or more at a time, should be tested for freedom from pyrogens. Water or other solvent supplied along with the substances for preparing solutions should also be free from pyrogens.

QUESTIONS FOR REVISION

1. Define the term 'manufacture' as per Drugs and Cosmetics Act and mention the different types of licences available for the manufacture of drugs.
2. What are the general conditions to be fulfilled for the grant of licence for the manufacture of drugs?
3. What are the conditions for issuing licence to manufacture drugs other than those specified in Schedules C, C1 and X?
4. Write briefly the conditions to be observed for issue of licence to manufacture Schedules C and C1 drugs? How their quality is controlled before marketing?
5. Give an account of the conditions and regulations prescribed for the manufacture of Schedule X drugs.

6. Explain the procedure to be adopted to obtain a licence for the manufacture of biological and other special products. What conditions must be fulfilled before such a licence is granted?
7. Write the conditions and regulations for manufacture of drugs for examination, test and analysis.
8. What are the conditions for issuing licence to manufacture blood products?
9. What are loan licences and repacking licences? Discuss the conditions specified relating to their issue.
10. Write short notes on:
    (a) Loan licence
    (b) Repacking of drugs
    (c) Central Licence Approving Authority.
11. Give the procedure for getting loan licence.
12. What is the procedure to be followed to obtain necessary licence for repacking of drugs for distribution?
13. Write a brief note on qualified person. What qualifications have been prescribed for technical personnel to supervise the manufacture of drugs?

SALE OF DRUGS

Sale may be defined as a contract whereby the seller transfers or agrees to transfer the property in goods to the buyer for a price. Sale of drugs can be by way of:

(i) Wholesale from the stockists to the shopkeepers.
(ii) Retail sale from the shopkeeper to the patients.

With the enforcement of the Drugs and Cosmetics Act, 1940, the sale of drugs has become a restricted practice and only those persons who have been granted licences by the Licensing Authorities of the States, can engage themselves in the wholesale, retail, compounding or dispensing of drugs. The premises for the retail sale of drugs are required to be specified as a Drug Store or Chemist and Druggist or Pharmacy.

Definitions

Drug Store

These retail shops do not require the services of a "Qualified Person" and can sell only such drugs which do not require any technical supervision. Some OTC products, certain products exempted in Schedule K and external preparations like pain balm can be sold here.

Chemists and Druggists

These retail shops have to employ the services of a "Registered Pharmacist" and can sell all types of drugs except those drugs which have to be compounded against prescriptions.

Pharmacy or Dispensing Chemist

These retail shops employ "Qualified Person" and engage in the compounding of drugs. These are required to maintain equipments and space as laid down in Schedule N. The name "Pharmacy" or "Pharmaceutical Chemist" or "Dispensing Chemist" shall be prominently displayed on the premises.

Registered Pharmacist (Earlier as Qualified person)

One who has acquired the minimum qualification and got his name entered in the Register of Pharmacists of State Pharmacy Council in which he is residing and practising profession of Pharmacy.

Registered Medical Practitioner (RMP)

A person who is:

(a) holding a qualification granted by an authority specified in the Schedules of the Indian Medical Council Act 1956; or
(b) registered or eligible for registration in a medical register of state; or
(c) registered or eligible for registration in the register of Dentist of a state under the Dentists Act; or
(d) engaged in the practice of veterinary medicine and possesses qualifications approved by State Government.

Itinerant Vendor

One who has no specified place of business and who will be licensed to conduct business in a particular area within the jurisdiction of Licensing Authority.

For the purpose of granting sale licences, the drugs have been divided into the following categories:

  (i) Drugs specified in Schedules C and C1 but excluding those specified in Schedule X.
  (ii) Drugs specified in Schedule X.
  (iii) Drugs other than those specified in Schedules C, C1 and X.

The retail and wholesale licences are granted with respect to all the above three categories. The wholesale and distribution of drugs specified in Schedules C and C1 and other than those specified in Schedules C, C1 and X are also permitted from motor vehicles provided a licence is taken for the same. No licence is, however, required for the free distribution of samples of medicines to the medical practitioners, hospitals, dispensaries, etc. by agents of licensed manufacturers or licensed importers of drugs.

A licence for the sale of drugs remains valid for a period of five years from date of issue. Application for the renewal of the licence may be made within six months of the date of its expiry. In the event of any change in constitution of a licensed firm, the licensee shall inform the Licensing Authority. Licences of such firms are deemed to be valid for a period of three months from the date of change unless in the meantime a fresh licence has been obtained from the Licensing Authority.

FORMS OF LICENCES

The following forms are required for the issuing of licences in the different categories (Table 4.5).

Table 4.5. Sale Application Form, Licence Form and Fees for Renewal

S. No.	Category	Type of Sale	Application Form	Licence issued in Form	Fees for grant or renewal
1.	Drugs other than those specified in Schedules C, C1 and X	Wholesale	19	20B	1500
		Retail	19	20	1500
		Restricted (Gen Store)	19A	20A	500
2.	Drugs specified in Schedules C and C1 but excluding those specified in Schedule X	Wholesale	19	21B	1500
		Retail	19	21	1500
		Restricted (Gen Store)	19A	21A	500
3.	Drugs specified in Schedule X	Wholesale	19C	20G	500
		Retail	19C	20F	500
4.	Sale of Drugs from motor vehicles 1. Drugs other than those specified in Schedules C and C 1 2. Drugs specified in Schedules C and C1	Wholesale	19AA	21BB	500
		Retail	19AA	21BB	500
5.	Homoeopathic Medicines	Wholesale	19B	21D	250
		Retail	19B	21C	250

RETAIL SALE OF DRUGS

It means a sale to a purchaser for the purpose of consumption or use and for not for resale. Two types of licences are granted for the retail sale of drugs:

(a) General Licences.
(b) Restricted Licences.

(a) General Licences

General Licences are granted to persons who have premises for the business and who engage the services of a "Qualified Person" to supervise the sale of drugs and do the compounding and dispensing. For the purpose of granting general licences for retail sale, the drugs have been divided into the following categories:

  (i) Licence for drugs other than those in Schedules C, C1 and X (issued in Form 20).
  (ii) Licence for drugs in Schedule X (issued in Form 20-F).
  (iii) Licence for drugs in Schedules C and C1 but excluding those specified in Schedule X (issued in Form 21).

(b) Restricted Licence

It is granted to persons who deal in retail sale of drugs which do not require the services of a qualified person. For the purpose of granting restricted licences for retail sale, the drugs have been divided into the following categories:

  (i) Licence for drugs other than those in Schedules C, C1 and X (issued in Form 20A)
  (ii) Licence for drugs in Schedules C and C1 but excluding those specified in Schedule X (issued in Form 21A).
  (iii) No licence is granted for drugs specified in Schedule X.

Conditions for the grant of general licences for retail sale

Separate licence is required to be taken for the retail sale of Schedules C and C1 drugs, Schedule X drugs and drugs other than those listed in Schedules C, C1 and X. The following conditions shall be fulfilled for the grant of the licences:

  (i) Premises shall be adequate (not less than 10 square metres) and equipped with facilities for proper storage of drugs.
  (ii) A competent qualified person shall be incharge of sale and distribution.

(iii) Licence shall be displayed in a prominent part of the premises open to the general public.
(iv) No drug shall be sold unless such drug is purchased under cash or credit memo from a duly licensed dealer.
(v) No Physician's Sample (not for sale) or expired drugs will be stocked on the sale premises.
(vi) Drugs will be sold in accordance with the provisions of the Drugs and Cosmetics Act, 1940 and Rules made thereunder.
(vii) The licence will get renewed as and when required.
(viii) Any change in "Qualified Person" shall be notified to the Licensing Authority within thirty days.
(ix) Drugs would be sold on a cash or credit memo in which following details be recorded:
  (1) Serial number.
  (2) Date of supply.
  (3) Name and address of Patient.
  (4) Name and address of Doctor.
  (5) Quantity and name of the drug, batch number, expiry date and price.
  (6) Signature of the "Qualified Person".
(x) No drug meant for free distribution under schemes ESI, CGHS, Armed Forces Medical Store or a Government Hospital shall be stocked in the licensed premises.
(xi) In case of a Pharmacy, the compounding of the prescription would be done under the personal supervision of a Qualified Person.
(xii) All registers and records required to be maintained under the Act would be preserved for a period of at least 2 years from the date of the last entry therein.

Conditions for the grant of Restricted Licence for retail sale

The following conditions are required to be fulfilled for the grant of Restricted Licence:

(i) The licensee would deal only in such drugs as can be sold without the supervision of a Registered Pharmacist.
(ii) The licensee shall have adequate premises equipped with storage facilities for proper storage of drugs.
(iii) The licence would be displayed in a prominent part of the premises.
(iv) The licensee shall purchase drugs only from a duly licensed dealer or manufacturer.
(v) The licensee would comply with the provisions of the Drugs and Cosmetics Act and Rules thereunder, in force from time to time.

(vi) Drugs would be sold in their original containers. Before granting a restricted licence, the Licensing Authority may take into account the number of licences granted in a locality during the last one year and the occupation, trade or business of the applicant.

WHOLESALE OF DRUGS

It means the selling of goods in relatively large quantities and at generally lower prices than retail. This also includes sale of drugs to hospitals, dispensaries, medical, educational and research institutions and to persons who purchase it for resale.

Categories of licence for wholesale of drugs

Licences under the following three categories are granted for the wholesale of drugs:

(a) Licence for the wholesale of drugs other than those specified in Schedules C, C1 and X (issued in Form 20-B).
(b) Licence for the wholesale of Schedule C and Schedule C1 drugs but excluding those specified in Schedule X (issued in Form 21-B).
(c) Licence for the wholesale of Schedule X drugs (issued in Form 20-G).
(d) Drugs other than those in Schedules C and C1 from a motor vehicle (issued in Form 20-BB).
(e) Drugs specified in Schedules C and C1 from a motor vehicle (issued in Form 21-BB).

Conditions for grant of licence for wholesale of drugs

(i) A licence to sell, stock, exhibit or offer for sale or distribute drugs shall be granted or renewed if the premises are well equipped with proper storage conditions.
(ii) The Licensing Authority shall have regard to the occupation, trade or business carried out by the applicant.
(iii) In respect of an application for grant of licence in Form 20-B or Form 21-B or both, the Licensing Authority shall satisfy in terms of premises and competent persons.

Conditions of licence for the wholesale of drugs other than those specified in Schedules C, C1 and X

(a) The licence shall be displayed in a prominent part of the premises.
(b) Drugs would be purchased only from a duly licensed dealer or manufacturer.
(c) The licensee would comply with the provisions of the Drugs and Cosmetics Act and Rules, as applicable from time to time.

(d) The drugs would only be sold to persons licensed to retail them. However, this condition shall not apply to:
   (i) Hospitals, medical, educational or research institutions or an RMP for the purpose of supply to his patients.
   (ii) Manufacturers of hydrogenated vegetable oils, beverages, confectionery or other non-medicinal products where such drugs are needed for processing their products.
   (iii) An officer or authority purchasing on behalf of the Government.

Conditions for the grant of Licence for the wholesale of Schedules C and C1 drugs (excluding Schedule X drugs)

(a) The licensee shall have adequate premises (not less than 10 square metres) equipped with facilities for the proper storage of drugs.
(b) The licence shall be displayed in a prominent part of the premises open to the public.
(c) No drug would be sold unless due precautions have been taken in order to ensure its preservation.
(d) The drugs would only be sold to persons licensed to retail them. However, this condition shall not apply for sale to:
   (i) Hospitals, medical, educational or research institutions or an RMP for the purpose of supply to his patients.
   (ii) Manufacturers of hydrogenated vegetable oils, beverages, confectionery or other non-medicinal products where such drugs are needed for processing their products.
   (iii) An officer or authority purchasing on behalf of the Government.
(e) The licensee shall obtain prior permission of the Licensing Authority for the purpose of selling any additional category of drugs not specified in his licence.
(f) The licensee shall maintain records of all purchases and sales of drugs by way of wholesale under the following headings:
   (i) The date of purchases and sale.
   (ii) Names and addresses of the firms from whom purchased and the firms to whom sold.
   (iii) Names and quantities of the drugs and their batch numbers.
   (iv) Names of the manufacturers of the drugs.
(g) Such records would be preserved for a period of at least three years from the date of sale.

Conditions of Licence for the wholesale of Schedule X drugs

(a) The licence shall be displayed in a prominent part of the premises open to the public.

(b) Drugs would be purchased only from a duly licensed dealer or manufacturer.
(c) The licensee would comply with the provisions of the Drugs and Cosmetics Act and Rules, as applicable.
(d) The drugs would only be sold to persons licensed to sell or distribute drugs specified in Schedule X. However, this condition shall not apply to:
　(i) Hospitals, medical, educational or research institutions or an RMP for the purpose of supply to his patients.
　(ii) An officer or authority purchasing on behalf of the Government.
(e) The licensee would forward to the Licensing Authorities copies of the invoices of sale made to the retail dealers.

Wholesale of Drugs from Motor vehicles

Licences can also be obtained for the distribution of drugs from motor vehicles. Separate licences are necessary for:

　(i) Drugs other than those specified in Schedules C and C1 [Form 20-BB].
　(ii) Drugs specified in Schedules C and C1 [Form 21-BB].

　The conditions applicable to these licences are similar to the conditions applicable for the wholesale of drugs.

(a) Drugs would be purchased only from a licensed manufacturer or wholesaler and can be distributed to only such persons who have valid licence for retail sale of drugs.
(b) The licence would be displayed in a prominent place in the vehicle.
(c) No drug would be sold unless due precautions have been taken in order to ensure its preservation.
(d) The licensee would obtain prior permission of the Licensing Authority for the purpose of selling any additional category of drugs not specified in his licence.
(e) Wholesale or resale can be made to an officer or person purchasing on behalf of a government or a hospital, medical, educational or research institutions or an RMP for the purpose of supply to his patients.
(f) The drugs may also be distributed to manufacturers of hydrogenated vegetable oils, beverages, confectionery or other non-medicinal products where such drugs are needed for processing their products.
(g) The licensee would inform the Licensing Authority, in writing, in case of any change in the ownership of the vehicle specified in the licence within 7 days of such change.

SUPPLY OF SCHEDULE C AND C1 DRUGS

Retail supply of such Schedule C and C1 drugs except by way of wholesale or on the prescription of an RMP should be recorded at the time of supply either in a register or in a cash or credit memo book specially maintained for this purpose in which the following particulars should be entered:

(i) Serial number of the entry,
(ii) Date of supply,
(iii) Name and address of the purchaser,
(iv) Name and quantity of the drug supplied,
(v) Name of the manufacturer,
(vi) Batch number and date of expiry,
(vii) Signature of the qualified person under whose supervision the drug was sold.

Carbon copies of the cash or credit memo retained by the licensee should be maintained in a legible manner.

SUPPLY OF SCHEDULE H AND X DRUGS

Substances specified in Schedules H and X should not be sold by retail except on the prescription of an RMP and in case of substances specified in Schedule X, prescriptions should be in duplicate, one copy of which shall be retained by the licensee for a period of 2 years.

A prescription for Schedule H and X drugs should be:
(i) In writing and signed by the prescriber and dated by him.
(ii) Specify the name and address of the owner of the animal if the drug is meant for veterinary use.
(iii) Indicate the total amount of medicine to be supplied and the dose to be given.

The supply of drugs specified in Schedules H or X to RMP, hospitals, dispensing and nursing homes shall be made only against the signed and written order which should be preserved by the licensee for a period of 2 years.

The prescriptions for Schedule H and X drugs must not be dispensed more than once unless the prescriber has stated thereon that it may be dispensed more than once; however, it may be dispensed at stated number of times or at stated intervals of time in accordance with the directions of the prescriber. At the time of dispensing, it must be noted on the prescription above the signature of the prescriber, the name and address of the seller and the date of dispensing.

No person dispensing a prescription containing substances specified in Schedule H and X may supply any other preparation whether containing the same substances or not in lieu thereof.

Supply of Schedule X drugs should be recorded at the time of supply in a bound and serially numbered register maintained for this purpose and separate pages should be allotted for each drug. The following particulars should be entered in the said register:

(i) Date of purchase,
(ii) Quantity received, if any, the name and address of supplier and the licence number of the supplier,
(iii) Name and quantity of the drug supplied,
(iv) Manufacturer's name, batch or lot number,
(v) Name and address of the patient/purchaser,
(vi) Reference number of the prescription against which supplies were made,
(vii) Bill number and date of receipt of purchase and supply made by him,
(viii) Signature of the person under whose supervision the drugs have been supplied.

RECORDS OF PURCHASES OF DRUGS

Records of all drugs purchased, whether intended to be sold by retail or wholesale, should be maintained under the following headings:

(i) Date of purchase
(ii) Name and address of the licensee from whom purchased and No. of relevant licence held by him,
(iii) Name and quantity of the drug and its batch number,
(iv) Name of the manufacturer of the drugs.

Purchase bills, including cash/credit memos should be kept as records.

STORAGE OF SCHEDULE X DRUGS AND DRUGS WITH EXPIRY DATES

Drugs specified in Schedule X should be stored under lock and key in either a drawer or a cupboard reserved for the storage in a part of the establishment which is separate for the remainder of the premises and to which the customers have no access.

STORAGE OF VETERINARY MEDICINES

Drugs meant for veterinary use should be stored in a separate drawer or cupboard solely reserved for their storage in a part of the premises to which the customers have no access.

OFFENCES AND PENALTIES WITH RESPECT TO SALE OF DRUGS

Table 4.6 shows the offences and penalties with respect to sale of drugs.

Table 4.6. Offences and penalties with respect to sale of drugs

Offence	Penalty
1. Sale, stocking, exhibition or offer for sale of drugs likely to cause death or grievous hurt as per Sec. 320 of IPC.	Imprisonment from 5 years to life and not less than Rs. 10,000 fine.
2. Sale, stocking, exhibition or offer for sale of spurious drugs.	Imprisonment from 1 to 3 years and at least Rs. 5000 fine on first conviction and 2 to 6 years and fine of Rs. 10,000 on subsequent convictions.
3. Sale, stocking, exhibition or offer for sale of spurious drugs.	Imprisonment from 3 to 5 years (less for adequate reasons) and subsequent offences 2 to 6 years and Rs. 10,000 fine.
4. Sale, stocking, exhibition or offer for sale in contravention of any other provision.	Imprisonment from 1 to 2 years and fine (less on adequate reasons) for subsequent offence 2 to 4 years and/or Rs. 5000 fine.
5. Failure to keep records or disclose required information.	Imprisonment up to 1 year and/or fine up to Rs. 1000.
6. Use of reports of government analysts or Central Drug Laboratory for advertising.	Fine up to Rs. 500 on first conviction and imprisonment up to 10 years or fine or both on subsequent convictions.

Note: Pharmacies, chemists and druggists approved by Government can stock, sell drugs labelled as 'Central Government Medical Stores', department and other government departments under health schemes.

SUSPENSION AND CANCELLATION OF LICENCES

The licences, issued for the sale or distribution of drugs, may be cancelled or suspended by the Licensing Authority at any time if the licensee fails to observe any of the conditions of the licence after giving an opportunity to the licensee to show cause. The cancellation or suspension may relate to all drugs or only to some of them.

If, however, the contravention is due to an act or omission on the part of an agent or employee of the licensee, the licence may not be cancelled or suspended, if the Licensing Authority is satisfied:

(i) That the act or omission was not instigated by the licensee, and if the licensee be a firm or a company by a partner of the firm or a director of the company;

(ii) That the licensee or an employee or an agent of his has not been guilty of a similar act within 12 months of the date on which contravention in question took place or where the employee has been guilty

the licensee did not or could not reasonably have had knowledge of any previous contravention;
(iii) That the act or omission was not a continuing act or omission or if it was so, the licensee could not reasonably have had knowledge of the previous act or omission;
(iv) That the licensee had used due diligence to ensure that the conditions of the licence and the provisions of the Act and the Rules were being observed.

A licensee, whose licence has been suspended or cancelled by the Licensing Authority, has the right to appeal against the decision of the Licensing Authority to the State Government within 3 months of the order.

The Licensing Authority may also refuse to grant licence to an applicant or refuse to renew the licence of a licensee, if it is satisfied that the person has been convicted of an offence under the Act or the Rules or that his licence has been previously suspended or cancelled and such person was not a fit person for the grant of a licence for the sale of drugs. Any person, who is not satisfied with such an order of the Licensing Authority, may appeal to the State Government within a month of the communication of such an order to him. The decision of the State Government shall be final.

QUESTIONS FOR REVISION

1. Define the following:
    (a) Registered Medical Practitioner
    (b) Qualified person for retail sale of drugs
2. Explain the following terms:
    (a) Drug store
    (b) Chemists & Druggists
    (c) Pharmacy.
3. Describe briefly the types of licences issued for the sale of drugs. Describe procedure and conditions for obtaining a general licence for the sale of drugs.
4. Write a note on:
    (i) Sale of Schedule H and X drugs
    (ii) Role of Retail Pharmacist while selling drugs
    (iii) Offences and penalties
    (iv) Suspension and Cancellation of Licences
5. What is the procedure to be followed to obtain necessary licences for:
    (a) Distribution of drugs in motor vehicle.
    (b) Distribution of drugs without the supervision of a qualified pharmacist.

6. Discuss the conditions for the grant of licence for wholesale of Schedule C and C1 drugs.
7. What classes of drugs are prohibited to be sold, distributed, stocked or offered for sale?
8. What are the requirements of a Retail shop to sell drugs as per the Drugs and Cosmetics Act and Rules made thereunder?
9. Mention the classes of drugs prohibited to be sold, distributed or exhibited for sale.
10. Enumerate the classes of drugs prohibited to be sold. What records are required to be maintained for sale of various categories and schedules of drugs?

LABELLING AND PACKING OF DRUGS

Labelling

It refers to all labels and other written, printed or graphic matter up or in any package or wrapper in which it is enclosed. The label contains the name of preparation, percentage content of a drug of a liquid preparation, amount of active ingredient of a dry preparation, the route of administration, storage condition, expiry date, name of manufacturer or distributor and an identifying lot number.

Packing

It refers to the science, art and technology of enclosing or protecting products for distribution, storage, sale and use. It also includes the process of design, evaluation and production of packages.

LABELLING OF DRUGS

A. General Requirements of Labelling

The following particulars shall be printed or written in indelible ink and shall appear in a prominent place on the label of the innermost container of drug and on every other covering like carton.
1. Proper name of the drug along with trade name, if any.
2. The abbreviated name of pharmacopoeia like I.P., B.P., U.S.P., etc. and for other drugs the approved scientific name.
3. Net contents in terms of weight or volume in metric units or the number of units. Any information relating to potency standards.
4. The content of active ingredients in terms of 5 ml for liquid orals, per tablet or capsule and per ml in case of injections or percentage of volume for single dose container.
5. Distinctive Batch No. or Lot No.

6. Manufacturing licence number.
7. Date of manufacture and expiry date as per Schedule P.
8. Manner of use of drug and directions for storage.
9. Precautions related to handling, use, distribution, etc.
10. Name and address of manufacturer.
11. Sample packs meant for free distribution to medical professionals shall be overprinted in indelible ink as "Physician's Sample – Not to be sold" across the pack.
12. Retail price of the pack.
13. Presence of non-vegetarian ingredients, if any, to be mentioned.

Table 4.7 gives the significant labelling requirements of drugs.

Table 4.7. Significant labelling requirements of drugs

Category	Legal Requirements to be mentioned

Schedule G	(i) **Any drug**
	    (a) Name of the drug
	    (b) Potency in units
	    (c) Date of expiry
	    (d) Manufacturing or import licence number
	    (e) Batch number
	(ii) **Medicines made up for internal use in human ailments**
	    (a) The words "Caution: It is dangerous to take this preparation except under medical supervision", written conspicuously on the label and surrounded by a line
	    (b) A red vertical line, not less than 1 mm thick, on the left side of the label.

Schedule H	(i) **Medicines made up for internal use in human ailments**
	    (a) "Schedule H Drug - Warning: To be sold on the prescription of a Registered Medical Practitioner only.", written conspicuously on the label and surrounded by a line.
	    (b) Symbol R displayed conspicuously on the left top corner of the label.
	    (c) A red vertical line, not less than 1 mm thick, on the left side of the label.
	(ii) **Medicines falling under the Narcotic Drugs and Psychotropic Substances Act**
	    (a) Schedule H Drug - Warning: To be sold on the prescription of a RMP only.", written conspicuously and surrounded by a line
	    (b) Symbol NRx conspicuously displayed on the left top corner
	    (c) A red vertical line, not less than 1 mm thick, on the left side of the label.

(Contd.)

Category	Legal Requirements to be mentioned

Schedule X	(i) **Medicines made up for internal use in human ailments**
	  (a) "Schedule X Drug - Warning: To be sold on the prescription of a RMP only", written conspicuously and surrounded by a line
	  (b) Symbol XRx conspicuously displayed on the left top corner
	  (c) A red vertical line, not less than 1 mm thick, on the left side
	(ii) **In bulk form**
	  Symbol XRx conspicuously displayed in red.

Schedule C	(a) Name of the substance in addition to any patent or proprietary name (b) Statement of potency in units wherever required by the Rules (c) Name and address of the manufacturer of the final product (d) Date of manufacture (e) Date of expiry wherever prescribed (f) Where a test for maximum toxicity is prescribed, a statement that the drug has passed the test (g) Nature and percentage of antiseptic added, if any (h) Precautions necessary for preserving the properties of the drug (i) Licence No. under which manufactured or imported (j) Batch No. or Lot. No.
Large volume parenterals	(a) Strength of active ingredients expressed in % w/v. (b) Concentration of electrolyte expressed in millimoles per litre. (c) Solutions containing visible particles must not be visible. (d) Unused portion of solution to be discarded.
Ophthalmic ointments	(a) Warning: If irritation persists or increases discontinue use and consult physician (b) Special instructions about storage where applicable.

Ophthalmic solutions and suspensions	(a) **Warning**
	  (i) Use within one month of opening. Not for injection.
	  (ii) Name and concentration of preservative.
	  (iii) NOT FOR INJECTION
	  (iv) Special storage instructions if any.
	(b) **Instructions**
	  (i) If irritation persists or increases discontinue use and consult physician. Keep the container tightly closed.
	  (ii) Do not touch the dropper tip/other dispensing tip to any surface as this may contaminate. "Before fixing the dropper, scrub hands with soap and rinse with water.

Veterinary drugs	(a) **Warning:** "Not for human use. For animal treatment only." (b) Shall bear symbol depicting head of any domestic animal only.

B. Labelling requirement of other drugs

(i) **Patent and proprietary drugs:**
   (a) Name and quantities of the active ingredients.
   (b) Name and address of the manufacturer.
   (c) In case of vitamins, following may be written, "For therapeutic use only", "For prophylactic use", "For paediatric use" and age of child/infant.

(ii) **Alcoholic preparations containing not less than 3% v/v alcohol:** Statement of quantity of alcohol as average % of absolute alcohol by volume.

(iii) **Medicines containing industrial methylated spirit:** The words "Contains industrial methylated spirit" and "FOR EXTERNAL USE ONLY".

(iv) **Non-sterile surgical ligature and suture:** Words to be printed in red ink as "Non-sterile surgical ligature (suture). Not to be used for operations upon the human body unless efficiently sterilized".

(v) **Mechanical contraceptives:**
   (a) Particulars specified in Schedule R.
   (b) Date of manufacture and date upto which it is expected to retain its potency.
   (c) Storage conditions necessary for the preservation of its properties.

(vi) **Disinfectants:**
   (a) Name and nature of the product
   (b) Grade and phenol coefficient
   (c) Its method of use.

(vii) **Pharmacopoeial drugs:**
   (a) Name or synonym as specified in the Pharmacopoeia followed by the letters: IP, BP, BPC, USP, NF, etc., as the case may be, or description of the substance (proper name being not less conspicuous than trade name, if any).
   (b) Net amount of the drug in terms of weight or measure in metric system or units of activity or, in case of tablets, capsules, etc., the quantity in each.
   (c) Amounts of active ingredients (content per single dose in oral preparations and in terms of volume in case of parenteral preparations). For preparations of antibiotics, hormones and other drugs for parenteral use, whose dosage is expressed in units or by weight, total units or quantity in each container or number of units or weight per gm or ml (not necessary in case of pharmacopoeia preparations).
   (d) Name and address of manufacturer.
   (e) Manufacturing Licence No. and Batch No.

Labels for products extemporaneously prepared and dispensed in pharmacy shops

The requirement for this differs from that of the drugs industrially manufactured. They shall be labelled with the following:
   (i) Name of the patient
   (ii) Quantity of the medicine supplied
   (iii) Serial number as entered in the dispensing register
   (iv) Dose, if for internal use
   (v) The words, "For External Use Only", if for external application
   (vi) Name and address of the supplier (Pharmacy)
   (vii) Any other directions given in the prescription by the Medical Practitioner.

Prohibited in the Labelling

   (i) No drug may purport or claim to prevent or cure or may convey to the user that it may prevent or cure, one or more of the diseases or ailments specified in the Schedule J.
   (ii) No drug may purport or claim to procure or assist to procure, or may convey to the user thereof any idea that it may procure or assist to procure, miscarriage in women.

Few specimen labels have been shown on pages 107 and 108.

PACKING OF DRUGS

Packing of drugs is a coordinated system of preparing goods for transport, warehousing, logistics, sale and end use.

The pack sizes of drugs meant for retail sale shall be as prescribed in Schedule P1 to the Rules.

For drugs not covered by Schedule P1, the pack sizes shall be as given below:

   (i) For Tablets/Capsules less than 10, the packing shall be by the integral number. For numbers above 10, the pack sizes shall contain multiples of 5.
   (ii) The pack sizes for Liquid Oral Preparations shall be 30 ml (paediatric only), 60 ml, 100 ml, 200 ml, 450 ml.
   (iii) The pack sizes for Paediatric Oral Drops shall be 5 ml, 10 ml, 15 ml.
   (iv) The pack sizes for Eye, Ear, Nasal Drops shall be 3 ml, 5 ml, 10 ml.
   (v) The pack sizes for Eye Ointment shall be 3 gm, 5 gm, 10 gm.

However, the provisions of the pack sizes covered under this Rule shall not apply to the following:

   (i) The imported formulations in finished form.
   (ii) Preparations intended for veterinary use.

SPECIMEN LABELS

℞   10 Tablets

Cetirizine hydrochloride
Tablets I.P. 10 mg

Each film-coated tablet contains:
Cetirizine hydrochloride I.P. 10 mg
Colour: Titanium dioxide I.P.
Dosage: As directed by physician
Store below 20°C. Protect from moisture

> **Schedule H Drug**
> **Warning:**
> To be sold by retail on the prescription of a
> Registered medical Practitioner only

Rs 10 for 10 Tabs (Incl. of All Taxes)
Mfg. Lic. No. 3/8506
Batch No. 240
Mfg. Date: Dec. 10   Exp. Date: Nov. 16
Manufactured by: Dheer Pharmaceuticals Ltd.
RICO Indl. Area, Jaipur

℞   10 Tablets

Erythromycin stearate
Tablets I.P. 250 mg

Each uncoated tablet contains:
Erythromycin stearate I.P. equivalent to Erythromycin 250 mg
Colour: Titanium dioxide I.P.
Dosage: As directed by physician
Store at cool place protected from light

> **Schedule H Drug**
> **Warning:**
> To be sold by retail on the prescription of a
> Registered medical Practitioner only

Rs 40 for 10 Tabs (Incl. of all Taxes)
Mfg. Lic. No. 4/282
Batch No. 120
Mfg. Date: Jan. 2012   Exp. Date: Dec. 2016
Manufactured by: Dheer Pharmaceuticals Ltd.
RICO Indl. Area, Jaipur

SPECIMEN LABELS

XR$_x$ 1 ml

Pentobarbitone sodium
Injection U.S.P.

Each ml contains:
Pentobarbitone sodium U.S.P. 50 mg
For intramuscular injection only
Dosage: As directed by physician

> **Schedule X Drug**
> **Warning:**
> To be sold by retail on the prescription of a
> Registered medical Practitioner only

The injection should be discarded if any precipitate is observed
Mfg. Lic. No. 140/Raj
Batch No. 120
Mfg. Date: Jan. 2012   Exp. Date: Dec. 2016
Manufactured by: Dheer Pharmaceuticals
12 E, 22 Godam, Jaipur

---

10 gm

Povidone-Iodine
Ointment U.S.P.

Composition:
Povidone-Iodine U.S.P. 5% w/w
(Available iodine 0.5% w/w)
Water-soluble ointment base q.s.
Store below 25°C. Do not freeze. Protect from light.
For external use only
Mfg. Lic. No. 120/Raj
Batch No. 140
Mfg. Date: Jan. 2012   Exp. Date: Dec. 2016
Manufactured by: Dheer Pharmaceuticals
12 Godam, Jaipur - 4

(iii) Preparations intended for export.
(iv) Vitamins, tonics, cough preparations, antacids, laxatives in liquid oral forms.
(v) Pack sizes of dosage forms meant for retail sale to hospitals, RMPs, nursing homes.

(vi) Physician's Samples.
(vii) Pack sizes of large volume intravenous fluids.
(viii) Pack sizes or dosage forms not covered by the above provisions of this Rule.

Packing of drugs specified in Schedule X

The drugs specified in Schedule X shall be marketed in packings not exceeding:

(i) 100 unit doses in the case of tablets/capsules.
(ii) 300 ml in the case of oral liquid preparations.
(iii) 5 ml in case of injections.

However, this Rule shall not apply to packing meant for use of a hospital or a dispensary provided such supplies are made by the manufacturers or distributors directly to the hospital or dispensaries.

QUESTIONS FOR REVISION

1. Describe the labelling conditions specified in the Drugs and Cosmetics Act.
2. Write short notes on:
    (a) Labelling of Schedule C, C1, Schedule H and Schedule G drugs.
    (b) Labelling and packing of Schedule X drugs.
    (c) Labelling of ophthalmic preparations.
    (d) Labelling of veterinary preparations.
    (e) Packing of ophthalmic preparations
3. Describe the method of fixing the date of manufacturing of different products.
4. Write short note on labelling of medicines extemporaneously prepared and dispensed in a pharmacy.
5. Write short note on the provisions for packing of drugs for sale.
6. Write a note on labelling of veterinary products for sale coming under Schedule O.

PROVISIONS APPLICABLE TO AYURVEDIC, SIDDHA AND UNANI DRUGS

Ayurveda and Siddha systems of medicine are as old as the Indian civilization. Ayurveda is a sub-section of the 'Atharvaveda', one of the four Vedas which are the repositories of the ancient wisdom and learning of this country. This system still retains its popularity and large section of the population seeks cure of ailments in Ayurveda. Siddha system is in southern regions of the country. The Government of India has given extensive and outstanding place to the Indian system of medicine. To achieve this, extensive provisions have been introduced in the Drug and Cosmetics Act regarding the manufacture, standardization of drugs of these classes. An expert committee in respect of Ayurveda, Siddha and Unani has been given a prominent place in the execution of the Act's purpose and policy.

The Unani System which originated in the Western Asia, chiefly in Arabia, had travelled to India along with the conquerors from that part of the world who later became rulers of the country. It gained lot of popularity from 12th century A.D. up to the end of Moghul rule. It still retains its popularity in few ancient centres of Muslim rule like Delhi, Hyderabad, Lucknow, etc.

There has been a recent amendment in the Drugs and Cosmetics Act. It has made some of its provisions applicable to the Ayurvedic, Siddha and Unani drugs, which are defined to include medicines for internal or external use in human beings for diagnosis, prevention, mitigation or treatment of diseases and which are mentioned in and are manufactured exclusively in accordance with the formulae described in literature listed in Schedule I to the Act. Years back, the manufacture of the Ayurvedic and Unani drugs was confined to the Vaidyas and Hakims only who compounded the drugs for the use of their own patients. But now, commercial organizations have been entering into the field of manufacture of these drugs and are marketing them throughout the country.

The Government appointed a committee (Udupa Committee) to enquire into the manufacture of Ayurvedic and Unani drugs and the committee disclosed that substances like gold, musk, saffron, etc. which were important components of such drugs were largely faked. So the need was felt to bring Ayurvedic and Unani drugs within the scope of the Drugs and Cosmetics Act.

In the Drugs and Cosmetics Amendment Act, 1982 definitions of misbranded, adulterated and spurious Ayurvedic, Siddha and Unani drugs have been included which are exactly parallel to the definitions of corresponding allopathic drugs.

ADMINISTRATIVE AGENCIES

1. Advisory Bodies

(a) Ayurvedic, Siddha and Unani Drugs Technical Advisory Board

The Central Government shall constitute an Ayurvedic, Siddha and Unani Drugs Technical Advisory Board to advise the Central and the State

Governments on technical matters relating to such classes of drugs and perform such other functions as assigned to it by the Central Government. The Board is required to be constituted of the following members:

Ex-officio
(i) Director General of Health Services
(ii) Drugs Controller of India
(iii) Director, Central Drugs Laboratory Ex-officio
(iv) Principal Officer dealing with the indigenous systems of medicine in the Ministry of Health

Nominated by the Central Government
(v) A government analyst for Ayurvedic and Unani drugs
(vi) A pharmacognosist
(vii) A phytochemist
(viii) Four persons, two from amongst the members of the Ayurvedic Pharmacopoeia Committee, and one each from the members of the Siddha/Unani Pharmacopoeia Committees
(ix) One person who is a teacher in Dravyaguna and Bhaishjya Kalpana
(x) One teacher in Ilm-ul-advia and Taklis-wa-dawa salt
(xi) Three persons, one from each to represent Ayurvedic and Unani systems of medicine. The Central Government is required to appoint one of the members as the Chairman and to provide the Board with Secretary and other necessary clerical staff.
(xii) One teacher in gunapadam.
(xiii) Three persons, one each to represent the Ayurvedic, Siddha and Unani drug industry.

(b) Ayurvedic, Siddha and Unani Drugs Consultative Committee

An Ayurvedic, Siddha and Unani drugs consultative committee shall be constituted consisting of two nominees of the Central Government and one nominee of each of the State Governments. Like the committee for allopathic drugs, this committee has to secure uniformity in the administration of the Act throughout India with reference to the Ayurvedic, Siddha and Unani drugs.

2. Analytical

Drug control laboratories specified for allopathic drugs have to also analyse and report on drugs of these categories.

Government analysts

A person to be appointed as Government Analyst shall possess the qualifications as prescribed for appointment of Government Analyst for allopathic drugs or holding a degree in Ayurvedic, Siddha or Unani systems of medicine with not less than 3 years' experience in the analysis of drugs acquired under:

(i) Government analyst, or
(ii) Chemical examiner to the Government, or
(iii) Head of an institution specially approved for the purpose.

Persons having any financial interest in the manufacture or sale of drugs cannot be appointed.

3. Executive

The Licensing Authorities for all categories of drugs and cosmetics are common.

Licensing Authority

The Central or State Government appoints a person, as it thinks fit, and has the prescribed qualification as Licensing Authority. Any application for grant or renewal of a licence for import, manufacturing or sale, etc., of Ayurvedic, Siddha and Unani drugs is to be made to the Licensing Authority.

A person appointed as Licensing Authority shall possess:

(a) The Ayurvedic, Siddha and Unani qualifications as per Schedule II of CCIM Act, 1970 (the Indian Medicine Central Council Act, 1970)/ B.Pharma (Ayurveda of a recognised university).
(b) At least 5 years experience in the Ayurvedic, Siddha and Unani drug manufacturing or testing of these drugs or enforcement of provisions relating to Ayurvedic, Siddha and Unani drugs of Drugs and Cosmetics Act, 1940 and Rules made thereunder or teaching/research on clinical practice of Ayurveda, Siddha and Unani system.

Drug inspectors

The Central or State Government appoints a person, as it thinks fit, and has the prescribed qualifications as Inspector. Persons having any financial interest in the manufacture or sale of drugs cannot be appointed. Every Inspector shall be deemed to be a public servant.

A person appointed as an Inspector shall possess:

(i) Qualifications for appointment as inspectors for allopathic drugs and have undergone practical training in manufacture of Ayurvedic, Siddha or Unani drugs or have a degree or diploma in Ayurvedic, Siddha or Unani system of medicine, or
(ii) Degree or Diploma in Ayurvedic, Siddha or Unani systems or degree awarded in Ayurved Pharmacy, as the case may be.

Duties of Inspector

Duties of Inspectors are similar to Inspectors appointed for allopathic system of medicine.

IMPORT

There are no provisions for import of Ayurvedic, Siddha and Unani drugs. The drugs being indigenous to the country are not manufactured outside India and as such no provisions for their import have been made.

MANUFACTURE OF AYURVEDIC, SIDDHA AND UNANI DRUGS

At the moment the Ayurvedic, Unani and Siddha drugs are required to be manufactured according to the formulae prescribed in the First Schedule (list of authoritative books of Ayurvedic, Siddha and Unani Tibb systems of medicine) to the Act. Those medicines (excepting parenteral products) which are not made in accordance with the formulae in the books listed in Schedule I but contain ingredients specified therein are to be deemed to be patent and proprietary medicines. A licence is required for the manufacture of these drugs and a separate licence is required for the manufacture of these drugs at different premises. Application for grant of licence shall be made in Form No. 24-D (24-E for loan licence) and licence issued in Form No. 25-D (25-E for loan licence). Applications shall be accompanied with the prescribed fees. Licences granted remain valid upto 31st December of the year following in which the licence was granted. Loan licences can also be issued for manufacture of Ayurvedic, Siddha and Unani drugs.

The manufacture of drugs should be carried out under the direction and supervision of competent technical staff at least one of whom should be wholetime employee possessing either of the following qualifications:

1. A degree or diploma in Ayurveda or Ayurvedic pharmacy or Siddha or Unani system of medicine recognised by the Central or the State Governments.
2. A degree in pharmacy or pharmaceutical chemistry with at least one year's experience or a degree in chemistry or botany with at least 2 years' experience in the manufacture of Ayurvedic, Siddha or Unani drugs.
3. Vaid or Hakim with at least 4 years' experience in the manufacture of Ayurvedic, Siddha or Unani drugs.
4. Qualified pharmacist in Ayurvedic, Siddha or Unani system of medicine with at least 8 years' experience in the manufacture of drugs.

The following further conditions must be satisfied by persons licensed to manufacture these drugs:

1. The manufacturing premises should conform to the requirements of factory premises and hygienic conditions specified in Schedule T.
2. Proper records of the details of manufacture and tests run on raw materials and finished goods should be maintained.
3. The licensee should allow the Inspectors, duly authorised, to inspect the premises and records and to take samples of raw materials and finished drugs.

The raw materials used for the manufacture of drugs shall be identified and tested for their genuineness wherever tests are available and records of such tests and methods used for testing should be maintained. Those Vaidyas and Hakims who manufacture drugs for the use of their patients are, however, exempt from the provisions relating to the manufacture of these drugs. A small quantity of drug manufactured for the purpose of examination, test or analysis, is also exempted from the provisions of manufacture.

LABELLING AND PACKAGING

Following particulars shall be displayed on the containers of Ayurvedic (including Siddha) and Unani drugs:

1. List and quantities of all ingredients used in the manufacture and a reference to the method of preparation as detailed in the Standard Text and Adikarana. The list of ingredients should be in the normal course displayed on the label but in case it is too large to be accommodated there the same may be printed and enclosed with the packing and a reference to this effect made on the label.
2. If medicine is for internal use containing any substance specified in Schedule E(I) it should be labelled with the words: Caution: "To be taken under medical supervision" both in English and Hindi.

Following particulars shall be written or printed in indelible ink, and appear in a conspicuous manner on the label of innermost container and coverings:

1. Name of the drug as mentioned in literature in the First Schedule.
2. Net contents in terms of weight or volume in metric system.
3. Number of licence under which the drug is manufactured preceded by the words Manufacturing Licence Number (Mfg. Lic. No. or MI:).
4. "Batch" or "Lot Number" or any other distinguishing prefix.
5. Name and address of the manufacturer and address of the premises where manufactured.
6. Date of manufacture.
7. Words "Ayurvedic medicine", "Siddha medicine" or "Unani medicine", as the case may be.

8. The words "FOR EXTERNAL USE ONLY" if the medicine is meant for external application.
9. The words "Physician's Sample. Not to be sold", if the drug is intended for free distribution to the members of the medical profession.

STANDARDS

Standards to be complied with in the manufacture or sale or distribution of Ayurvedic, Siddha and Unani drugs are given in Table 4.8.

Table 4.8. Standards to be complied with in the manufacture or sale or distribution of Ayurvedic, Siddha and Unani drugs

Class of Drugs	Standards to be complied with
1. Drugs included in Ayurvedic Pharmacopoeia	The standards for identity, purity and strength as given in the editions of Ayurvedic Pharmacopoeia of India for the time being in force.
2. Asavas and Arishtas	The upper limit of alcohol as self-generated alcohol should not exceed 12% v/v, except those that are otherwise notified by the Central Government from time to time.

LOAN LICENCE

Similar to allopathic drugs manufacture, a facility is available to manufacture Ayurveda, Siddha and Unani medicines under loan licence.

EXCISE DUTY

Excise duty is payable on products containing alcohol (both self-generated as well in added alcohol preparations) as stipulated in Medicinal and Toilet Preparations Act and Rules.

DEPARTMENT OF AYUSH

The name of the department of Indian Systems of Medicines and Homoeopathy, which comes under the Ministry of Health and Family Welfare, is changed as the Department of Ayush. Under the 'Golden Triangle' project of the Government, Deptt. of Ayush will carry out scientific validation of ISM and Homoeopathic medicines and prepare protocols of tests. With the help of CSIR, it will undertake pharmacological studies in scientific way similar to modern medicines.

SALE OF AYURVEDIC, SIDDHA AND UNANI DRUGS

No licence is required for effecting sale of Ayurvedic, Siddha or Unani drugs but dealers in such drugs can sell only products manufactured by a person licensed to manufacture drugs under the Act.

OFFENCE AND PENALTIES

(i) Any person who manufactures any spurious drug shall be liable to imprisonment from 1 to 3 years and a fine of not less than Rs. 5,000 on first conviction and to imprisonment between 2 and 6 years and a minimum fine of Rs. 10,000 on any subsequent convictions. The trying courts may, however, for any special reasons impose sentences of less than 1 or 2 years or fines less than those prescribed.

(ii) Manufacture of adulterated drugs or manufacture without valid licence, imprisonment up to 1 year and a fine of at least Rs. 2,000 on first conviction and imprisonment up to 2 years and a fine of at least Rs. 2,000 for any subsequent conviction are prescribed. The courts, however, have discretion to impose less severe penalties for any special reasons.

(iii) For manufacture of drugs in contravention of any other provision a minimum imprisonment of 3 months and a fine of at least Rs. 500 may be awarded on first conviction and imprisonment up to 6 months and a fine of a least Rs. 1,000 on any subsequent conviction. The drugs in respect of which an offence has been committed are liable to confiscation. The Licensing Authority may cancel or suspend a licence for valid reasons. A licensee who is aggrieved by this decision of the Licensing Authority may, however, appeal to the State Government within 3 months of the date of suspension or cancellation.

QUESTIONS FOR REVISION

1. What are the conditions imposed in the manufacture of Ayurvedic, Siddha and Unani medicines by the Licensing Authority?
2. Discuss labelling of Ayurvedic, Siddha and Unani drugs in the light of Drugs and Cosmetics Rules, 1945.
3. Write short notes on:
   (a) Standards of Ayurvedic, Siddha and Unani drugs.
   (b) Packaging and labelling requirements of Ayurvedic medicines.
4. Write the constitution and composition of Ayurvedic, Siddha and Unani Drugs Technical Advisory Board. What are its functions?
5. Write short notes on AYUSH department of the Government.

PROVISIONS APPLICABLE TO HOMEOPATHIC MEDICINES

Dr. Hahnemann is considered as the father of Homeopathy and it originated in Germany. It is based on the principle of 'like cures like' and as of now has global clientele. If one views this system of medicine from modern view point it may be difficult to explain action of homeopathic drugs on the basis of pharmacological rationale. But it is popular in many parts of world. Homeopathic medicines have been defined to include drugs recorded in homeopathic provings or drugs whose therapeutic efficacy has been established through long clinical experience (as recorded in Indian or foreign homeopathic literature) and which are prepared according to techniques of homeopathic pharmacy. However, drugs administered by parenteral routes are excluded from the lists of homeopathic medicines.

IMPORT

No licence is required to import the homeopathic drugs in India. For the purpose of import they are classed with such allopathic drugs for the import of which no licence is necessary. However, new homeopathic medicines (meaning medicines not specified in the homeopathic pharmacopoeias of U.S.A. or U.K., or not recognized as efficacious in authoritative homeopathic literature under recommended conditions of use) cannot be imported without the permission of the Licensing Authority. For obtaining such a permission the importer has to furnish to the Licensing Authority evidence, including the minimum provings carried out with it, as may be required for assessing efficacy of the medicine. All imported homeopathic medicines should be labelled and packed in accordance with the Rules.

MANUFACTURE

A licence is required for the manufacture of homeopathic medicines and can be obtained from the Licensing Authority on payment of the requisite licence and inspection fees as necessary for undertaking manufacture of homeopathic mother tinctures and potentised preparations. The fees for manufacture of Mother Tinctures is more than the fees for the manufacture of potentised preparations. Licences for the manufacture of potentised preparations can also be granted to homeopathic pharmacies holding licence for the retail of homeopathic medicines provided they ensure that manufactured products conform to claims on their labels.

Licence for manufacture is granted in Form 25C. A separate licence is required for the manufacture of these drugs at different premises. Licence granted remains valid upto 31st December of the year following in which the licence was granted.

New homeopathic medicines can be manufactured only with prior approval of the Licensing Authority. The manufacture of homeopathic medicines should be carried out:
(i) In hygienic conditions under the direction and personal supervision of competent technical staff at least one of whom should be a whole-

time employee and is a graduate in science with chemistry as one of the subjects and 3 years experience in manufacture of homeopathic medicines or graduate in pharmacy with 18 months experience or holds qualifications as per subclause (g) of clause 1 of Sec. 2 of Homeopathic Central Council Act 1973 and 18 months experience.

However, persons already employed in manufacture of homeopathic medicines and have 5 years experience and were recognized for manufacture will be deemed to the competent technical staff.

(ii) The manufacturing premises should be distinct and separate from residential premises.
(iii) The premises used for the manufacture should be in accordance the directions given in schedule M-1 unless relaxed or suitably altered in a particular case for reasons to be recorded in writing by the Licensing Authority.
(iv) There should be proper facilities for storage of the drugs and inspectors should be allowed to inspect the premises and take samples of manufactured drugs.
(v) An inspection book should also be maintained wherein the inspectors may record their impression and defects noticed.
(vi) Manufacturers of mother tinctures should maintain adequate facilities for identifying the crude drugs and for ascertaining the total solid and alcohol contents of the mother tinctures or should make suitable arrangements for such tests and records maintained for a period of five years, with the institutions approved by the Licensing Authority.
(vii) Mother tinctures should be preferably filled in containers of neutral glass and should be free from any sort of impurities.
(viii) Records of sale of homeopathic medicines containing alcohol should be maintained showing the quantities sold and the name and address of the parties to whom sold.
(ix) No colour shall be added in homeopathic medicines, except caramel may be added in combinations of homeopathic preparations with syrup base.

Rules applicable to the cancellation and suspension of licences of allopathic drugs hold good for homeopathic medicines as well.

SALE

A licence is required for the wholesale or retail sale of homeopathic medicines which can be obtained from the Licensing Authority on prepayment of requisite fees. Application for issue of licence can be made in Form 19E along with the prescribed fees and it is issued in Form 20C for retail and Form 20D for wholesale. A separate licence is required for the sale of these drugs at different premises.

A person licensed to sell homeopathic medicines should maintain the premises in clean condition and sale must be supervised by a person competent to deal in homeopathic medicines. The licensee should allow Inspectors to inspect the licensed premises and records relating to purchase and sale of medicines containing alcohol should be maintained. However, no such records need be maintained in respect of potentised preparations packed in containers of 30 ml or less and mother tinctures packed in containers up to 60 ml capacity.

Homeopathic medicines containing more than 12% v/v alcohol packed in containers of more than 30 ml capacity can be sold. However, such medicines packed in bottles to 100 ml can be sold to hospitals/dispensaries.

Other conditions relating to duration, cancellation, suspension etc. of the licence are similar to those for allopathic drugs.

LABELLING

The following particulars are required to appear on the labels of homeopathic medicines and on all subsequent coverings:

(i) Name of the medicine as specified in the homeopathic pharmacopoeias of U.S.A. or U.K. for drugs specified therein or a name descriptive of the true nature of a drug and those with 2 or more ingredients their names, potency and proportion.
(ii) Potency in decimal, centesimal or millesimal systems.
(iii) Name and address of the manufacturer or in case a medicine is not sold in its original container the name and address of the seller.
(iv) Percentage of alcohol, if the medicine contains it, but the alcoholic content of medicines contained in containers of up to 30 ml capacity need not be stated.
(v) The words, "Homeopathic medicine".
(vi) Manufacturing licence No. preceded by the words Mfg. No. or M.N. and batch number preceded by the words Batch or Lot No. or Lot.
(vii) Proprietary name, if any (no medicines containing a single ingredient can be labelled with such a name).
(viii) Labels shall be printed or written in indelible ink.
(ix) Net content and MRP shall be mentioned.

QUESTIONS FOR REVISION

1. What are homeopathic medicines? Give an account of the manufacture, sale and provisions applicable to the homeopathic medicines.
2. Write short notes on:
   (i) Schedule M1
   (ii) Labelling requirements of homeopathic medicines.

PROVISIONS APPLICABLE TO COSMETICS

COSMETICS

The word cosmetic originates from a Greek root "Kosmetikos" meaning 'to adorn'. The use of cosmetics, which at one time was confined to royal and rich ladies, has now percolated to all in a big way. Even the males are using them to a great extent at par with the females.

Cosmetics, as defined in the Act, mean articles meant to be rubbed, poured, sprinkled or sprayed or introduced into or otherwise applied to the human body or any part thereof for cleansing, beautifying, promoting attractiveness or altering the appearance. In the last few years the consumption of cosmetics has touched new heights and the curve is shooting upwards and hence the controls sought to be exercised on the drugs have been extended to a certain extent to the cosmetics.

IMPORT

No licence is require for purposes of import of the cosmetics but the importer shall follow all rules applicable to import of such classes of drugs which are imported without licence. However, the import of the following classes of cosmetics is prohibited:

(i) Misbranded cosmetics meaning cosmetics which contain colours other than those prescribed or are not labelled in the prescribed manner or make any false or misleading claims.
(ii) Spurious cosmetics meaning cosmetics which are imitations or substitutes for other cosmetics or resemble other cosmetics in a manner likely to cause deception or are imported under names of other cosmetics or bear names of manufacturers which are fictitious or who are truly not the manufacturers.
(iii) Cosmetics not of standard quality.
(iv) Cosmetics containing any harmful or unsafe ingredients.
(v) Cosmetics containing prescribed colours which contain more than 2 p.p.m. of arsenic or 20 p.p.m. of lead or 100 p.p.m. of heavy metals other than lead.
(vi) Cosmetics intended for use on the eyebrows or eyelashes or around the eyes containing coal tar dyes or intermediates.
(vii) Cosmetics coloured with arsenic or lead compounds.
(viii) Cosmetics containing hexachlorophene or mercury compounds.
(ix) Cosmetics whose use is likely to involve any risk to the users.
(x) Tooth paste/tooth powder containing tobacco.

However, small quantities of cosmetics whose import is otherwise prohibited may be imported if they are meant for personal use and form part of a passenger's baggage and are declared to the customs authorities on being directed to do so.

Cosmetics can be imported
(a) by sea at Chennai, Kolkata, Mumbai, Cochin, Nhova Sheva and Kandla;
(b) by air at Chennai, Kolkata, Mumbai, Delhi, Ahmedabad and Hyderabad.

Procedure for Import of Cosmetics

All imported consignments shall be accompanied by a statement or invoice showing the name and quantities of cosmetic preparations along with name and address of manufacturer.

The importer shall give a declaration that no cosmetics prohibited under the Drugs and Cosmetics Act, 1940 are being imported.

Samples may be drawn, if the Customs Officer suspects about the quality.

MANUFACTURE

For manufacturing cosmetics, a licence obtainable from the Licensing Authority is now essential. If the cosmetics are manufactured in more than one premise, a separate licence for each is required. The licensee may be applied in Form 31 (31A for loan licence) and licence is issued in Form 32 (32 A for loan licence). The licence is valid upto 31st December of year following the year in which it was granted.

The licences are granted on payment of requisite fees and fulfillment of other prescribed conditions and, in general, rules applicable to the licences granted for the manufacture of allopathic drugs are applicable to these licences as well. Manufacture of cosmetics containing hexachlorophene or mercury compounds or misbranded or spurious cosmetics or cosmetics which are not of standard quality is prohibited. A person licensed to manufacture cosmetics should fulfill following conditions:

(i) Clean conditions should be maintained in the factory premises. It should be situated in hygienic surroundings, and should be distinct and separate from premises used for residential purposes.
(ii) Adequate space and staff should be provided. The manufacture of cosmetic should be conducted under the direction and personal supervision of competent technical staff at least one of whom should be a wholetime employee and should either hold diploma in pharmacy approved by the Pharmacy Council of India or be a registered pharmacist under the Pharmacy Act or should have passed intermediate examination with chemistry as one of the subjects. However,

for small scale manufacturers, employing not more than 5 persons, a person with general training and experience, extending over not less than 4 years in the manufacture of cosmetics, may be deemed to be competent technical staff by Licensing Authority.
(iii) Adequate facilities should be provided on the premises for the testing of raw materials and manufactured products or suitable arrangements should be made with approved institutions for the purpose. Records relating to such tests should be maintained for at least 3 years from the date of manufacture.
(iv) Cosmetics containing colours other than those specified by Bureau of Standards or colours which contain more than 2 p.p.m. of arsenic or more than 20 p.p.m. of lead or more than 100 p.p.m. of heavy metals other than lead and for eyebrows or eyelashes, etc. containing any coal tar colour should not be manufactured. The use of arsenic or lead compounds for coloring cosmetics is also prohibited.
(v) The licensee should allow inspectors to inspect premises, records etc., and to take samples of manufactured products. An inspection book should also be maintained wherein the inspectors can enter their remarks.
(vi) The licensee should maintain records or registers of raw materials used in manufacture, tests carried out of final product, etc. and should be kept as per Schedule U(1) for at least 3 years.

As in the case of drugs, licences for the manufacture of cosmetics remain valid up to 31st December in the year following the year of issue and may be suspended or cancelled if the licensee fails to observe any of the conditions discussed above. In case a licensee is aggrieved by this decision he can appeal to the State Government within 3 months of suspension or cancellation. Cosmetics can also be manufactured under loan licences as is the case with drugs.

Anyone manufacturing any spurious cosmetic shall be punishable with imprisonment up to 3 years and fine. Persons convicted of manufacture of cosmetics in contravention of any other provision are liable to imprisonment for a term up to 1 year and/or fine up to Rs. 1,000.

SALE

Licence is not necessary for the sale of cosmetics but the dealers in cosmetics can sell only such products which do not contravene any provisions of the Drugs and Cosmetics Act and the Rules. If a dealer is required to disclose the name and other particulars of the person from whom he obtained cosmetics, he shall legally comply with such directions. Anyone who fails to disclose the name of manufacturer or sells any cosmetic in contravention of the Act and the Rules may be imprisoned for 1 year or fined Rs. 500 on first conviction or imprisoned for 2 years and fined up to Rs. 1,000 on any subsequent conviction.

The manufacture and sale of the following classes of cosmetics is prohibited:
   (i) Misbranded or spurious cosmetics and cosmetics which are not of a standard quality.
  (ii) Cosmetics containing any ingredient which makes them unsafe or harmful for use under the directions indicated or recommended.
 (iii) Cosmetics imported or manufactured in contravention of any provision of the Act and the Rules.

The inspectors may require a person not to dispose any stock of cosmetics.

LABELLING AND PACKING

Cosmetics sold or distributed in India, whether they are of Indian origin or imported from outside, should be labelled and packed in accordance with the following provisions (Tables 4.9 and 4.10):

In addition, the following instructions in English and local language should appear on each package of hair dyes.

"This preparation may cause serious inflammation of the skin in some cases and hence a preliminary test should always be carried out to determine whether or not special sensitivity exists. To make the test, clean a small area behind the ear or upon the inner surface of the forearm using either soap or water or alcohol. Apply a small quantity of the hair dye as prepared for use to the area gently with soap and water. If no irritation or inflammation is apparent it may be assumed that no hypersensitivity exists. The test should however be carried out before each and every application. The preparation should on no account be used for dyeing eyebrows or eyelashes since severe inflammation of the eye or even blindness may result".

Standards

The standards of cosmetics shall be as prescribed in Schedule S or as laid down by the Bureau of Indian Standards (BIS).

QUESTIONS FOR REVISION

1. Define cosmetics, misbranded cosmetics and spurious cosmetics.
2. What are the restrictions imposed in the import of cosmetics.
3. Discuss cosmetics with respect to manufacture, labelling, packing and standards.
4. Write short notes on labelling of cosmetics.

Table 4.9. Labelling and packing of cosmetics

Class of cosmetics	Labelling particulars (on both inner and outer labels)
Cosmetics in general	1. Name of the cosmetic and name and address of the manufacturer. 2. Manufacturing Licence No. preceded by the letter M and Batch number preceded by the letter B if the cosmetic is packed in containers having more than 10 gm. **On the Outer Labels** Net contents of the package expressed as weight for solids and semi-solids, as volume for liquids or as numerical counts, if the cosmetic is subdivided provided that this statement need not appear if the contained cosmetic is not more than 60 ml/30 gm. **On Inner Label Only** In addition should indicate: Adequate directions for safe use; warning caution or special directions; names and quantities of ingredients that are hazardous.
Hair dyes containing paraphenylene di-amine or other coal tar dyes, colours and pigments	With the words: Caution. This product contains ingredients which may cause skin irritation in certain cases and so a preliminary test according to the accompanying directions should be made. This product should not be used for dyeing the eyelashes or eyebrows as such use may cause blindness. (Equivalent labelling in local languages is also mandatory).

Note: If the cosmetic has only one label, all the information required to be disclosed on the inner or outer labels shall be displayed on this label.

Table 4.10

Alcoholic fragrance solutions such as eau-de-cologne containing diethyl phthalate	(i) The words: HARMFUL IF TAKEN INTERNALLY (ii) Content of diethyl phthalate in each ml.
Cosmetics for export	(i) Specific requirements, if any (ii) Name and address of manufacturer and name of cosmetic or a code No. approved by the licensing authority.
Soaps containing hexachlorophene	Contains hexachlorophene; not to be used on babies
Tooth pastes containing fluorides	(i) Content of fluoride in p.p.m. (max. 1000 ppm) (ii) Date of expiry.

Note: No soap is permitted to contain more than 1% hexachlorophene.

5. What are the requirements that should be met for the manufacture of cosmetic?
6. What are the restrictions imposed in the manufacture of cosmetics in Drugs and Cosmetics Act?
7. What type of cosmetics are prohibited from manufacture?

GENERAL PROVISIONS ABOUT OFFENCES

(i) In case a person is convicted of an offence under the Act, the convicting court may order that the offender's name, place of residence and the offence committed shall be published at the expense of the convicted person in such newspapers as the court may direct.

(ii) Where an offence is committed under the Act by a company, every person, who was at the time in charge of company and responsible for its business, shall be deemed guilty of the offence and shall be liable to punishment, unless the officer can prove that he was ignorant of the offence and that he had used due diligence to prevent the commission of the offence. 'Company' for the purpose of the Act means a body corporate and includes a firm or other association of individuals.

(iii) No suit, prosecution or other legal proceedings shall lie against any person for anything done in good faith.

(iv) Offences by Govt. Departments: Where offences are committed by Government Departments relating to sale, manufacture, etc. of the drugs, the head of that department shall be deemed to be guilty of that offence unless he proves that he had exercised due diligence to prevent the commission of the offence.

(v) Confiscations: When a person is convicted of an offence, the Court may order confiscation of the stocks of drugs as well as of vessels, vehicles, etc. used for the commitment of the offence. The confiscated drugs may be referred to a drug inspector and if he reports them to be sub-standard the same may be ordered to be destroyed. However, if the drugs are standard and safe for use the same may be ordered to be given to hospitals, dispensaries supported by Govt. or to charitable institutions.

DIRECTIONS OF CENTRAL GOVERNMENTS TO STATE GOVERNMENTS

The Central Government can issue directions to any of the State Governments for executing any of the provision of the Act or of any Rules made under it. The Central Government may also appoint Analysts and Inspectors of its own in addition to those appointed by the various State

Governments. Though the Central Government can have the licensed establishments inspected and the sample of drugs analysed, yet it cannot take action such as suspension or cancellation of licences, since the licensing powers are vested in the State Governments. So, to overcome these short-comings and anomalies that the Central Government has been empowered to issue directions to the State Governments.

SUMMARY TRIALS OF OFFENCES

A recent amendment of the Act provides that all offences under the Act punishable with imprisonment not exceeding 3 years (excepting offences related to manufacture of spurious Ayurvedic, Siddha and Unani drugs) may be tried in a summary way under Sections 262 to 265 of the Code of Criminal Procedure 1973. But, whatsoever in such trials magistrates can impose imprisonment not exceeding one year. Whenever the magistrates feel that sentences of more than 1 year have to be awarded the cases shall be tried in the normal manner.

MISCELLANEOUS

STANDARDS

The Indian Pharmacopeia, the United States Pharmacopeia, the National Formulary of the United States of America, the British Pharmacopeia and the British Pharmaceutical Codex, the International Pharmacopeia, the Russian Pharmacopeia, the National Formulary of India, the Swiss and French Pharmacopoeias are deemed to be books of standards for purposes of the Act. The drugs for which no standards of identity, quality and strength are prescribed in the latest editions of B.P., but are specified in the B.P.C., the standards shall be deemed to be those prescribed in the latter. Those drugs for which no standards have been prescribed either in the latest edition of the B.P. or the B.P.C. but are specified in the earlier editions the standards shall be deemed to be those which are specified in the earlier edition of the B.P. or the B.P.C. All other drugs must comply with the following standards (Table 4.11):

The Central Government may, in consultation with the D.T.A.B. and after giving at least 3 months' notice to this effect, amend the Schedule of Standards.

LIST OF COLOURS PERMITTED TO BE USED IN DRUGS

The following colours may be added to medicines, provided the common name and the percentage of the colour are stated on the label of the container. The medicines to which these colours are added shall not be deemed to be misbranded only because of the fact of addition of colours therein:

Table 4.11. Standards used in different classes of drugs

S. No.	Class of drugs	Standards
1.	Patent or proprietary medicines	The formula or the list of the active ingredients should be displayed on the label of the container, in the prescribed manner and they should comply with such other standards as may be prescribed.
2.	Vaccines, sera, toxins toxoids, antitoxins, antigens and other biological products of such nature	The standards maintained at the laboratory for Biological Standards Serum Institute, Copenhagen and such further standards of strength, quality and purity as may be prescribed.
3.	Vitamins, hormones and analogous products	The standards maintained at the National Institute for Medical Research, London and such further standards as may be prescribed.
4.	Patent and proprietary medicines containing vitamins for prophylactic, therapeutic or paediatric use excepting those having single vitamin or meant for parenteral use	Standards as laid down in Schedule V.
5.	Substances, other then food, intended to affect the structure on and function of the human body, commonly known as chemical contraceptives	As may be prescribed or the formula approved as safe by the Central Government and displayed in the prescribed manner.
6.	Substances for destroying insects or vermin which cause diseases in human beings or animals	Standards as laid down in the prescribed pharmacopoeia or a list of ingredients displayed in the prescribed manner on the label of the container.
7.	Disinfectants	Standards as laid down in Schedule O.
8.	Ophthalmic preparations	Standards as per Schedule FF.
9.	Mechanical contraceptives including condoms, diaphragms and intrauterine devices	Standards as per Schedule R.

1. Natural colours: Annatto, carotene, cochineal, curcumin, chlorophyll, red oxide of iron, yellow and black oxide of iron, titanium dioxide.
2. Artificial colours: Caramel.
3. Coal tar colours (Table 4.12).

Table 4.12

Common Name of Colour	Colour Index Number	Chemical Name
GREEN		
Quinazarine Green SS	61565	1,4-bis (p-Toluino) anthraquinone
Alizarin Cyanine Green F	61570	Disodium salt of 1,4-bis (o-sulfo-p-tulouino)
Fast Green FCF	42053	Anthraquinone
Green S	44090	
YELLOW		
Tartrazine	19140	Trisodium salt of 3-carboxy-5-hydroxy-1-p-sulfopheny1-4-p-sulfophenyl-azopyraozle
Sunset Yellow FCF	15985	Disodium salt of 1-p-sulfophenyl-azo-2-naptho-1-6 sulfonic acid
Quinoline	47005	Disodium salt of Yellow WS disulfonic acid of 2(2-Quinoly1)-1,3-indardoine
RED		
Amaranth	16185	trisodium salt of 1(4-sulfo-Inaphthylazo) 2-naptho-1-3,6-disulfonic acid
Erythrosine	45430	Disodium salt of 9-0-carbo-xyphenyl-6-hydroxy-2,4,5,7-tetrabromo-3-isoxanthone.
Eosin YS or Eosine G	45380	Disodium salt of 2,4,5,7 or Eosine G-tetrabromo-9-p-carboxy-phenyl-6-hydroxy-3-isoxanthone
Toney Red or Sudan III	26100	1-p-phenylazophenylazo- -2-naphtho
Ponceau 4 R	18255	Trisodium salt of 1-(4-sulpho-1-naphthyl-azo)-2-naphto-1-6,8 disulphonic acid
Carmoisine	147720	Disodium salt of 2-(4-sulpho-1-4 sulphonic acid
Fast Red E	16005	Disodium salt of 2-(4-sulpho-1-naphthyl-azo)-2-naphthol-6-sulphonic acid
BLUE		
Indigo Carmine	73015	Disodium salt of indigotin
Brilliant Blue FCF	42090	-5:5-Disulphonic acid
VIOLET		
Alizurol Purple	60725	Disodium salt of 1-phenylazo-2-naptho-6,8-disulphonic acid

(Contd.)

Common Name of Colour	Colour Index Number	Chemical Name
BROWN		
Resorcin Brown	20170	Monosodium salt of 4 p-sulfophenylazo 2(2,4-xylylazo)1,3-resorcinol
BLACK		
Naphthol Blue	20470	Disodium salt of 8 amino 7-5-nitro-phenylazo-2-phenylazo-2-phenylazo-1-naphthol-3,6-disulfonic acid

LIST OF COLOURS, DYES AND PIGMENTS USED IN SOAPS

As specified by Bureau of Standards.

Chapter 5

Medicinal and Toilet Preparations (Excise Duties) Act, 1955 and Rules, 1956

Alcohol is being used since time immemorial as an euphoric drink. Drinking alcohol, for pleasure sake, can be an abuse but for preparing medicines is a necessity. It has an excellent property of a good solvent, a preservative and widely used in manufacturing of pharmaceuticals. It is also employed in the manufacture of toilet preparations, which may be classed as a luxury. Alcohol used for toilet preparations such as perfumes, deodorants, etc. and drinking purpose are subject to higher excise duty as compared to that which is used for manufacturing of medicinal preparations. Hence, in order to have control on the alcohol which is obtained at a low rate of excise duty and prevent its misuse, it was made essential to control the availability and transport of alcohol on government level. Prior to the enactment of this Act, the control of spirituous medicinal preparations was a State subject and each State had a different set of Rules. Therefore, each preparation was subject to different rates of excise duty in different states and this led to a large scale inter-State smuggling of such preparations.

In order to curtail this evil and repeal all laws in force in any State, before the enforcement of this Act, "The Medicinal and Toilet Preparations Act" was passed in 1955, and the Rules passed in 1956 to bring uniformity in duty leviable on all such preparations throughout the country. The Act extends to whole of India and came into force on 1st April, 1957.

OBJECTIVES

The Medicinal and Toilet Preparations (Excise Duties) Act, 1955 was passed with the following objectives:

- To provide for the collection of levy and duties of excise on medicinal and toilet preparations containing alcohol, opium, Indian hemp or other narcotic drugs or narcotics.
- To provide for uniformity in the Rules and rates of excise duties leviable on such preparations throughout the country.

DEFINITIONS

a. **"Dutiable Goods"** means the medicinal and toilet preparations specified in the Schedule, as being subject to the duties of excise levied under this Act.

   Dutiable goods said to be manufactured in bond within the meaning of this Section, if they are allowed to be manufactured without payment of any duty of excise leviable under any law, for the time being in force in respect of alcohol, opium, Indian hemp or other narcotic drug or narcotic, which is to be used as an ingredient in the manufacture of such goods.

b. **"Excise Officer"** means an officer of the Excise Department of any State and includes any person empowered by the Collecting Government to exercise all or any of the powers of an excise officer under this Act.

c. **"Medicinal Preparation"** includes all drugs which are a remedy or "prescription" prepared for internal or external use of human beings or animals and all substances intended to be used for or in the treatment, mitigation or prevention of disease in human beings or animals.

d. **"Narcotic Drug"** or **"Narcotic"** means a substance which is coca leaf, or coca derivative, or opium or derivative of opium, or Indian hemp and shall include any other substance, capable of causing or producing in human beings dependence tolerance and withdrawal syndromes, and which the Central Government may, by notification in the official gazette, declare to be a narcotic drug or narcotic.

e. **"Toilet Preparation"** means any preparation which is intended for the use in toilet of the human body or in perfuming apparel of any description, or any substance intended to cleanse, improve or alter the complexion, skin, hair or teeth, and includes deodorants and perfumes.

f. **"Bonded Manufactory"** means the premises or any part of the premises approved and licensed for the manufacture and storage of medicinal and toilet preparations containing alcohol, opium, Indian hemp and other narcotic drugs or narcotics on which duty has not been paid.

g. **"Non-bonded Manufactory"** means the premises or any part of the premises approved and licensed for the manufacture and storage of medicinal and toilet preparations, containing alcohol, opium, Indian hemp and other narcotic drugs or narcotics on which duty has been paid.

h. **"Denatured Spirit"** or **"Denoted Alcohol"** means alcohol of any strength which has been rendered unfit for human consumption by the addition of substances approved by the Central Government or by the State Government with the approval of the Central Government.

i. **"Gauge"** means to determine the quantity of alcohol or dutiable goods contained in, or taken from, any cask or receptacle or to determine the capacity of any cask or receptacle.

j. **"Restricted Preparation"** means every medicinal preparation specified in the schedule and includes every preparation declared by the Central Government as restricted preparation under the Rules.

k. **"Unrestricted Preparation"** means any medicinal preparation containing alcohol but other than a restricted preparation or a spurious preparation.

l. **"Spirit Store"** means that portion of the bonded or non-bonded manufactory which is set apart for the storage of alcohol, opium, Indian hemp and other narcotic drugs or narcotic purchased free of duty or at prescribed rates of duty specified in the Schedule to the Act.

m. **"Standard Preparation"** means a preparation other than a 'sub-standard preparation'.

n. A **"Sub-standard Preparation"** is:
   i. A pharmacopoeial preparation in which the amount of any of the various ingredients is below the minimum that the pharmacopoeial composition would require.
   ii. A proprietary medicine which does not conform to the formula or the list of ingredients disclosed on the label on the container or on the container.

MANUFACTURING

The manufacture of spirituous and other narcotic preparations can be done only after obtaining a licence from the authority for this purpose. Licence for the manufacture of alcoholic medicinal preparations can be granted by the authority, only to the applicant who already holds the requisite licence for the manufacture of drugs under the Drugs and Cosmetics Act. The procedures which should be followed for the manufacture of Homeopathic and Ayurvedic preparations, removal of goods from bonded laboratories and inter-state movements of excisable preparations, etc. are laid down in the Act. The manufacture of alcoholic preparations can be done 'in bond' or 'outside bond'.

Requirements for getting licence to manufacture alcoholic and narcotic preparations in or outside bond

(i) Application for the licence to manufacture dutiable goods in or outside bond or for its renewal is to be made to Licensing Authority, along with the required documents and information. The Licensing Authority is the Excise Commissioner in the case of a bonded manufactory or warehouse and in other cases, an authorized officer by the State Government.

(ii) A separate application is to be made if more than one kind of licence is desired. Where the applicant has more than one place of business, he should obtain a separate licence in respect of each such place of business.

The applicant shall furnish a list of all preparations which he proposes to manufacture and/or those manufactured during the preceding year, showing the percentage or proportion of alcohol in alcohol preparations or opium, Indian hemp or other narcotic drug in terms of weight in proportions containing those substances, quoting the pharmacopoeia, under which such preparations are/were proposed to be manufactured.

On receipt of the application, the Licensing Authority shall ensure qualifications and previous experience of technical personnel, the equipments present and applicant's financial position and may issue the licence.

The licence cannot be sold or transferred and should be exhibited in a conspicuous part of the licensed premises. The licensee shall inform the Licensing Authority, within stipulated time any change in constitution of firm address, etc. A licence can be revoked, or suspended, by the Licensing Authority if the licensee or any other person in his employment is found to have committed a breach of the prescribed conditions or any of the provisions of the Act or Rules, or has been convicted of an offence; after giving him a reasonable opportunity of showing cause against the action proposed to be taken.

I. MANUFACTURE OF ALCOHOLIC PREPARATIONS IN BOND (BONDED LABORATORY)

Preparations are deemed to be manufactured in bond, when they are manufactured in a premise, licensed or approved for this purpose, using alcohol, on which duty has not been paid under excise supervision and on which excise duty is paid while removing the finished products from the licensed premises.

Manufacturer uses the alcohol without paying the duty and enters into a bond by applying in the prescribed form to the Excise Commissioner

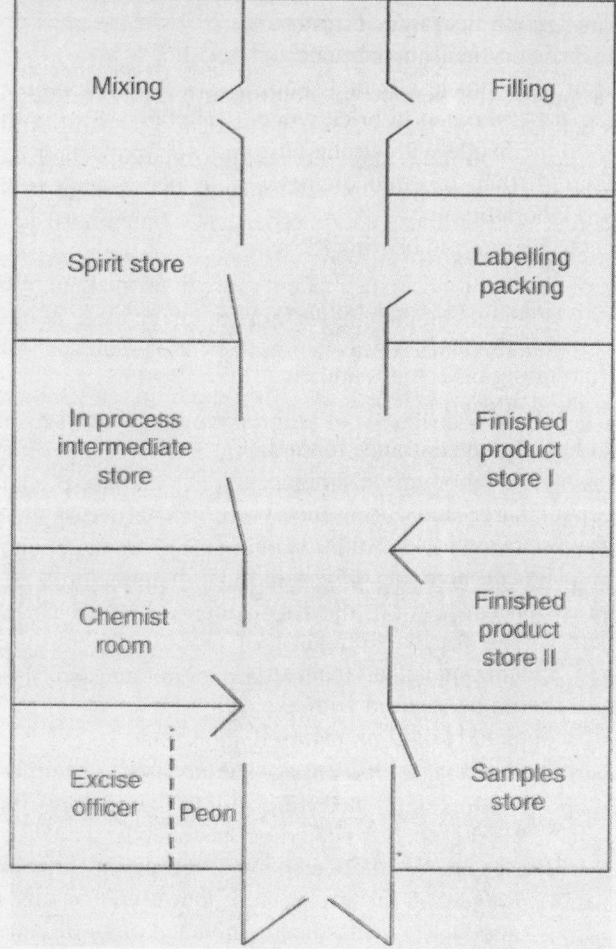

Fig. 5.1. Plan 1 of a typical bonded laboratory.

with sufficient security, towards due payment of the duty before removing the finished products from the premises and observance of the rules.

A bonded laboratory should have the following provisions:

a. A spirit store, in case the laboratory is not attached to a distillery or a spirit warehouse.
b. A large room for the manufacture of medicinal preparations with separate arrangement for manufacture of toilet preparations.
c. One or more separate rooms for the storage of finished medicinal or toilet preparations.

d. Accommodation with necessary furniture for the officer-in-charge of the bonded laboratory near its entrance.
e. Malleable iron rods, not less than 1.9 cm in thickness, set not more than 10 cm apart, embodied in brick work to a depth of at least 5 cm and covered on the inside with strong wire netting or expanded metal of a mesh not more than 2.5 cm in diameter or length, in every window of the bonded laboratory.
f. A board outside every room bearing the name and serial number of the room.
g. All pipes from sinks inside the laboratory, connected with the general drainage system of the premises.
h. Provisions for cutting off the gas and electric supply to the laboratory at the end of the day's work.

There should be only one entrance to the laboratory and door for each of its compartments. The laboratory can be opened only in the presence of the excise officer-in-charge and during his absence, all the doors should be secured with excise ticket locks. Addition or alteration to the permanent fixture in the premises can be made only with the previous permission of the Excise Commissioner.

The permanent vessels for the storage of alcohol, narcotic drugs and narcotics received, under bond and all the finished products on which duty has not been paid, should be secured with excise ticket locks. All vessels intended to hold alcohol and liquid preparations, should bear a distinctive serial number and their full capacity distinctly and indelibly marked on them.

Steps to be followed for manufacture of alcoholic preparations in bond

1. Procurement of spirit from a distillery or spirit warehouse

Rectified spirit required for the manufacture of medicinal and toilet preparations can be obtained on an indent countersigned by the officer-in-charge of the laboratory, from any approved distillery or spirit warehouse either situated in the same State or in another State. The officer of the distillery or spirit warehouse, on receipt of the duplicate copy of the indent, shall issue the spirit in duly sealed containers and send an advice of the consignment to the excise officer-in-charge of the bonded laboratory.

2. Verification and storage of spirit received

Consignments of spirit received at the laboratory is verified in volume and strength by the excise officer and then stored in the spirit store, from where it can be issued from time to time to the manufacturer on his requisition.

3. Issue of spirit from the spirit store for manufacture

Calculated quantities of spirit can be obtained by the manufacturer on a requisition to the officer-in-charge, who shall then issue the same from the spirit store. The spirit so issued has to be immediately mixed with other ingredients of the preparation in the presence of the officer-in-charge. The percolators or other vessels charged with the spirit should be labeled with the following particulars:

(i) Name and batch number of the preparation.
(ii) Description and quantity of alcohol put in it.
(iii) Date of removal of preparation and the quantity of such preparation removed.

As soon as the manufacture of a preparation has been completed, it should be removed to the finished goods store, measured and stored in the vessels provided for the purpose. Details of the preparation should also be entered in a register and it should be given a batch number. The excise officer-in-charge may permit the manufacturer to take a sample of not more than 250 ml for analysis purpose, free of duty. A separate account must be maintained by the manufacturer regarding the amount of samples used by him for analysis and any amount left over after analysis should be mixed with the main bulk of the batch.

4. Storage of finished product

All finished preparations should be stored in bulk in jars or bottles, each containing not less than 2.25 litres of the preparation. Every container should be labelled with the name of the preparation, its batch number, strength, date of storage and actual content in bulk litres. The containers should be so arranged in suitable racks so as to allow ready identification of each batch. A record of all deficiencies in bulk content of finished preparations, should be kept by the officer-in-charge and reported to the excise commissioner quarterly. If the excise commissioner is satisfied that the deficiency reported was due to some unavoidable reasons, he may remit the duty payable. Otherwise, such loss is subject to levy of duty at penal rate which shall not be more than double the prescribed rates.

5. Issue of alcoholic preparations from bonded laboratories

Alcoholic preparations from a bonded laboratory can be taken out by the manufacturer by making an application to the officer-in-charge and after payment of the excise duty. Duty is payable even on Physician's free samples. However, preparations issued to bonded warehouse or for export to a place outside India or to institutions authorized to receive duty free preparations may be issued without payment of duty. *Supply of preparations exempted from excise duty payment are:*

(a) To hospitals and dispensaries working under Central or State Government.
(b) To hospitals and dispensaries subsidized by Central or State Government.
(c) To charitable hospitals and dispensaries under the control and management of a local body.
(d) To Medical Stores Depot of Central or State Governments.
(e) To Institutions which supply medicines freely to the poor and certified to that effect by the Principal Medical Officer of the District.

6. Wastage of spirit during manufacture

The permissible percentage of wastage of alcohol during the manufacture of a particular medicinal or toilet preparation is fixed by the State Government from time to time. Any wastage exceeding the permissible limit and not properly accounted for, shall be charged with the duty together with such penalty not exceeding the duty leviable thereon as the excise commissioner may deem fit.

7. Remission of duty in case of loss due to accident

In case of any accidental loss of alcohol in bonded manufactory (except on account of theft), the excise commissioner may remit the duty on the alcohol so lost, if he is advised by the excise officer-in-charge of the laboratory that the loss was beyond the control of the manufacturer.

Disposal of Sub-standard Preparations

A finished medicinal or toilet preparation that is or is suspected to have deteriorated in quality, may be destroyed by the manufacturer, with the permission of the excise commissioner. The excise commissioner may also allow the manufacturer to reprocess a sub-standard preparation. The excise commissioner shall waive the duty on the alcoholic content of the preparation so destroyed if he is satisfied that the deterioration of the preparation, or its improper manufacture, was due to reasons beyond the control of the manufacturer.

Disposal of Recovered Alcohol

Alcohol recovered in the course of production of a medicinal or toilet preparation may be used for subsequent production of the same preparation provided such alcohol is collected and accounted for separately. Where the alcohol, recovered from a preparation liable to duty at the lower rate is sought to be used in the manufacture of a preparation subject to higher rate of duty, the duty on the preparation so manufactured shall be collected after determining the spirit strength of the preparation. An account of recovered alcohol shall be maintained by the officer-in-charge in the prescribed form. Recovered alcohol, unfit for the consumption, shall be destroyed by the manufacturer in the presence of office-in-charge. No rebate of duty shall, however, be allowed on recovered alcohol so destroyed.

II. MANUFACTURE OF ALCOHOLIC PREPARATIONS OUTSIDE BOND (NON BONDED LABORATORY)

In case when spirit is obtained from the distillery after paying the duty (duty paid spirit), execution of bond does not arise. Preparations that are deemed to be manufactured in a licensed or approved premises, where duty paid spirit is used for the preparation is called as "manufactured without bond" or "outside bond" and the laboratory is called the "Non-Bonded Laboratory".

Licence is issued by the Excise Commissioner for the manufacture of preparations. Application is made in the prescribed form along with the required fees and other detailed – building plan, list of equipments, constitution of firm, etc.

General description of a non-bonded laboratory

The laboratory should have the following:

1. It should be separate and independent from other activities.
2. It shall have only one main entrance to the laboratory and one door each to the compartments like spirit store, mixing, finished store, etc.
3. Each window should be provided with 19 mm thick malleable iron rods, set 102 mm apart and shall be covered outside with strong iron netting of mesh not exceeding 25 mm.
4. The pipes from sink or wash basins inside the laboratory should discharge directly into the general drainage.
5. The electric and gas connections should be cut off at the end of the day's work.
6. Separate store rooms should be there for spirit purchased at the rate of Rs 10, Rs 20 and Rs 80 per litre.
7. Separate finished products store room should be there for medicinal and toilet preparations.
8. Alterations, if any, should be made only with the previous sanction of the Excise Commissioner.

Steps to be followed for manufacture of alcoholic preparations outside bond

1. Procurement of spirit

Rectified spirit, for manufacture, can be obtained from a distillery or a spirit warehouse on an indent prepared in triplicate. The original copy should be sent to the distiller or spirit warehouse-keeper while the triplicate copy should be retained by the manufacturer. The duty should be paid to the Government Treasury and a challan in token of such payment should be enclosed with the duplicate copy of the indent and sent to the officer-in-charge of the distillery or spirit warehouse. The treasury officer shall also send an advice to the officer-in-charge of the distillery or spirit warehouse, who shall issue the spirit together with a permit covering the issue. The spirit brought into the manufactory has to be immediately transferred to the spirit store and the necessary details entered into the prescribed register.

2. Manufacture and storage

The manufacture of the preparations from duty paid spirit should be carried out only at the licensed premises. Each preparation, soon after its manufacture, should be registered and given a distinct batch number. All finished preparations should be transferred to the finished goods store and should be so arranged that the checking of stock of every batch of preparation from the register is facilitated. Preparations stored in bulk should be measured in the storage vessel nearest to the fluid ounce and sealed. The quantities, taken out from time to time, should be entered in the stock card, maintained for the purpose.

3. Sampling

The Excise officer may, without any prior notice to the manufacturer, take samples of not less than 10% and not more than 15% of the total number of batches manufactured, once every month. These samples are forwarded to the chemical examiner for the verification of alcoholic contents thereof. If the report of the chemical examiner differs by more than 3° proof strength on either side from the strength declared by the manufacturer, the manufacturer is liable to pay a penalty at the rate of 10 times the difference in duty on the quantity so manufactured but not exceeding Rs. 2000. Frequent occurrence of such offences shall be a ground for the cancellation of the licence held by the manufacturer.

All samples are to be taken by the excise officer personally and in the presence of the manufacturer or his authorised agent. Every sample should be taken in duplicate and the cork of each bottle should be fixed with the officer's personal seal. Label of the bottle should be signed by the officer taking the sample. The manufacturer can also affix his seal and sign the labels. Duplicate samples are to be preserved carefully under lock and key and returned promptly to the manufacturer, when needed no more. The manufacturer is not entitled to any compensation for the samples taken for analysis.

4. Returns

The manufacturer should maintain up-to-date and proper accounts of the transactions of business in his manufactory and deliver them to proper officer by the 5th of each month. The manufacturer is also required to furnish a list of all his employees who are required to enter non-bonded manufactory, to the excise commissioner and only such persons should be allowed to enter the laboratory.

5. Inspection

The non-bonded laboratory can be inspected by the excise commissioner and other officers having jurisdiction over the area in which the manufactory is situated. It shall be inspected at least once every month by the proper excise officer. The State Government may authorise inspection of the non-bonded establishment by any officer of prohibition, land revenue or medical and public health departments.

MANUFACTURE OF AYURVEDIC, HOMOEOPATHIC PREPARATIONS AND PATENT AND PROPRIETARY PREPARATIONS

(i) Ayurvedic Preparations

Ayurvedic preparations containing alcohol are generally of two types:

(i) Those containing self-generated alcohol, such as 'Asavas' and 'Aristas'; and

(ii) Those which are either prepared by distillation or to which alcohol is added at any stage of the manufacture.

Ayurvedic preparations containing self-generated alcohol, in which the alcohol content does not exceed 2% proof spirit, are deemed to be non-alcoholic for the purposes of this Act and are, therefore, exempt from the payment of excise duty.

Preparations containing more than 2% alcohol, but which are not capable of being consumed as ordinary alcoholic beverage, are also exempt from excise duty.

The preparations which can be consumed as alcoholic drinks are liable to duty of Rs. 2.50 per L.P. litre.

(iii) However, Ayurvedic practitioners, registered under any law for the time being in force, are allowed to manufacture and dispense such preparations free of duty, provided they take a licence from the excise authorities and use such preparations only for their patients. The practitioner is however required to allow excise officers to take samples of the preparations manufactured by them and also maintain accounts of the quantities manufactured and dispensed to the patients, together with the name and addresses of the patients. Ayurvedic preparations, which are either made by distillation or to which alcohol is added at any stage of their manufacture, are treated as preparations capable of being used as ordinary alcoholic beverages and hence are liable to a duty of Rs. 80 per L.P. litre. *They may be manufactured in bond or without bond.*

(ii) All homoeopathic preparations

All homoeopathic preparations containing alcohol are classified as being capable of being consumed as ordinary alcoholic beverages and attract duties prescribed for such class of preparations falling under the category of restricted preparations.

(iii) Patent and Proprietary preparations

All allopathic preparations, containing alcohol, can be categorized into the following two categories:

(a) Official preparations made according to the formulae given in the current editions of B.F., B.P.C., I.P., U.S.P., the National Formulary of the United States or Veterinary Codex, etc. approved by the Government or any other pharmacopoeia recognized under the Drugs and Cosmetics Act, 1940.

(b) Non-Official allopathic preparations also known as proprietary preparations.

All official and non-official preparations, which are capable of being consumed as ordinary alcoholic beverages, are known as 'Restricted preparations' and are listed in the Schedule to the Act. All other standard preparations and proprietary preparations which are not capable of being consumed as alcoholic beverages are referred to as 'Unrestricted preparations'. Any of the unrestricted preparations, if widely misused, may be declared to be restricted preparations by the Central Government, either on the request of the State Government or on its own or on the advice of the Standing Committee.

Any new proprietary preparation containing alcohol is deemed to be a restricted preparation, until it has been declared to be otherwise by the

Central Government on the advice of the Standing Committee. Any manufacturer, if wants to manufacture a proprietary preparation, should submit two samples of the same together with its formula to the State Government. The State Government, after seeking the advice of the Standing Committee, will declare whether the sample is to be classified as a restricted or as an unrestricted preparation.

The Standing committee consists of:

(i) The Drugs Controller of India.
(ii) The Chief Chemist, Central Revenues Laboratory.
(iii) One pharmacologist nominated by the Central Government.
(iv) The advisor in Indigenous System of Medicine, Ministry of Health.

The Committee advises the Central Government on all matters connected with the technical aspects of administration of the Act and the Rules and particularly whether a preparation is to be treated as a genuine medicinal or toilet preparation for the purpose of the Act, and if so, whether it should be treated or continue to be treated as a restricted or unrestricted preparation.

WAREHOUSING OF ALCOHOLIC PREPARATIONS

The manufacturers or dealers in alcoholic preparations can establish bonded warehouse, anywhere in India for depositing goods on which duty has not been paid. Licence for establishing a private warehouse for this purpose is issued by the excise commissioner. The excise commissioner, before granting the licence, may require the licensee to furnish a bond with security, binding him to pay duty on the goods deposited in the warehouse and for the due observance of the terms, conditions and requirements of the Act and the Rules. The excise commissioner may also direct in what manner, and on what terms, dutiable goods should be stored and how and in what manner such warehouse should be secured by locks or fastening.

Movements of goods from one warehouse to another and receipt and dealing with warehoused goods

All goods received at the warehouse should be produced to the excise officer-in-charge together with the transport permit and should be weighed, gauged in his presence and assessed to duty prior to entry in the warehouse. The description and quantity of goods, marks and numbers of the packages, the number and date of the permit and the amount of duty leviable thereon should be noted in the warehouse register. At the warehouse, these goods should be kept separate from other goods until the receipt account has been taken by the officer-in-charge. The warehouse owner may separate, pack or repack the goods and make necessary alterations therein for the preservation, sale or disposal of such goods with the sanction of the proper officer. *No goods, other than the dutiable ones, can be deposited in a licensed warehouse.*

No goods can be removed from any warehouse without the payment of duty, unless they are removed for the purpose of export from India or for transfer to another bonded warehouse. Any goods warehoused may be left in the warehouse for a period of three years or such extended period as allowed by the excise commissioner. If any goods are lost or destroyed in the warehouse due to some unavoidable reason, the excise commissioner may remit the duty thereon, provided a notice is given to the officer-in-charge of the warehouse immediately on discovery of such loss or destruction. The licensee of the warehouse shall be responsible for the safety of the goods lodged at the warehouse.

Clearance on payment of duty

For removal of goods on payment of duty the licensee should make an application in triplicate to the officer-in-charge at least twelve hours before he intends to remove the goods. The officer then assesses the amount of duty leviable on the goods and on production of evidence that the sum has been paid, allows the goods to be cleared.

Returns

The licensee must submit details of the transactions made in the warehoused goods and such other details as prescribed by the State government in this behalf, within seven days after the close of every month.

Transport of alcoholic goods

When warehoused goods are desired to be moved from one warehouse to another, the consigner or the consignee of the goods, has to enter into a bond with the excise commissioner and furnish a security to the extent of at least twice the amount of duty payable on such goods. The bond shall remain valid, until the officer-in-charge of the warehouse, from which goods were removed, has received a certificate from the officer-in-charge of the destination warehouse saying that the goods have been re-warehoused. The excise commissioner may however permit a person to remove warehoused goods from one warehouse to another by entering into a general bond with security, similar to above, so that goods can be removed from time to time.

EXPORT OF ALCOHOLIC PREPARATIONS

(i) Under bond
(ii) Under claim for rebate of duty.

No duty is required to be paid on alcoholic preparations, which are exported from India. Such preparations can be exported in either of the following two ways:

(i) Under bond (directly from a bonded laboratory without payment of duty), or

(ii) Under claim for rebate of duty.

(i) Export under Bond

Only those persons who either have a bonded laboratory or a bonded warehouse can export alcoholic preparations under bond. The exporter should present an application in triplicate to the officer-in-charge of the laboratory or warehouse, stating whether the goods are to be exported by land, sea, air or by post parcel. A separate application is required in respect of each consignment. The officer-in-charge sends the original copy of the application to the customs officer or the border examiner or the post master, as the case may be, at the place of export. The duplicate is delivered to the consigner and the triplicate is retained as the office copy. Goods for export should be packed in cases or packages and should be legibly marked in ink or oil colour with the following particulars:

(i) Serial number commencing with I for each year.
(ii) Owner's name and special mark, if any.
(iii) Total quantity of dutiable goods with their alcohol content in L.P. litres.

After verifying the particulars entered in the application, the officer-in-charge may get the following particulars noted on the body of each package:

(i) Name and address of the consignee.
(ii) Description of the goods.
(iii) Total quantity of goods packed.
(iv) Gross weight of the package.

The said officer shall then seal each package with his official seal in such a manner that the package cannot be tempered with, without breaking the seal. The officer shall also endorse all the copies of the application and specify the period within which the goods should be actually exported and return the duplicate copy to the consigner. After despatching the goods, the consigner should enter the number and date of railway receipt or bill of lading on the duplicate copy and communicate these particulars to the proper officer for entry in the other copies.

If the goods are being sent by post, the exporter should present the duplicate copy of his application, duly endorsed by the excise officer, to the post master at the office of booking together with relevant packets or packages. Postmaster of the destination post office should certify on the duplicate application that the goods have been duly exported out of India and return the same through the post master at the post office of booking, to the exporter who shall present it to the officer-in-charge of his laboratory or warehouse.

(ii) Export of duty Paid Goods

Goods on which duty has already been paid can be exported under claim for rebate of duty. The owner of a non-bonded manufactory or a warehouse dealer, who wants to export duty-paid goods, should give at least 48 hours notice to the concerned excise officer for supervising the packing of goods to be exported. The consigner should present the entire consignment before the proper officer who shall take samples of the goods and send to the chemical examiner for analysis. On receipt of reports from the chemical examiner, he shall enter the alcoholic content of the goods in the duplicate copy of the application. This copy of the application should be presented by the exporter to the excise commissioner for claiming rebate of excise duty. After verifying the particulars entered in the application, the officer-in-charge may get the following particulars entered on the body of each package:

(i) Name and address of the consignee.
(ii) Description of the goods.
(iii) Total quantity of goods packed and their alcoholic content in L.P. litres.
(iv) Gross weight of the package.

The officer-in-charge should then seal each package with his official seal, so as to make them temper-proof. The packages can then be exported in the same manner as in case of the bonded goods.

Claim for rebate of duty has to be made within one month of the issue of export certificate, by presenting the duplicate certified application to the excise commissioner. The rebate is sanctioned by the excise commissioner if he is satisfied that the claim is in order. The excise commissioner may extend the period within which such claim for rebate shall be made.

PROCEDURES

Regulatory powers of excise officer

Inspection

Any officer, authorised in this behalf by the Excise Commissioner, can at all reasonable times, enter any premises licensed for manufacture or storage of dutiable goods with or without notice. He may inspect the building, plant, machinery, etc. and check the records and registers, with a view to ascertain the accuracy of returns submitted under these Rules. Any person who wilfully obstructs the officer in the performance of his duties, or giving any false or misleading information, shall be liable to be punished under the Rules.

Entry, Search and Seizure

Excise officers, not below the rank of sub-inspectors, are authorised to stop and search any vessel, vehicle, car, etc., and also to enter and search, whether by day or by night, any land, building, enclosed space, vessels, conveyance, etc., if they have reason to believe that durable goods are being stored, manufactured or carried, in contravention of the Act and the Rules thereunder. In case of any resistance, the officer can break open the door and remove other obstacles. The officers can also seize any goods, in respect of which they believe that the duty has not been paid or which appears to them to be in contravention of the Act. Any receptacles, packages or coverings in which contraband goods are contained, together with any implements or machinery used in their manufacture or any animals, vehicles or other conveyance used for carrying them, may also be seized by the excise officer. The articles seized by an officer must be handed over to the officer-in-charge of the police station, who shall keep the same in custody, pending orders of a magistrate. The articles may be sealed by the seizing officer.

Detention of Persons

All excise officers, duly empowered in this behalf by the State Governments, may stop and detain any person found carrying goods, for the transport of which a permit is required. They may require the production of permits from persons in possession of dutiable goods and may examine the goods with a view to ascertain whether they are in conformity with the permit or not. Excise officers, not below the rank of sub-inspectors, can arrest any person whom they believe to be liable to punishment under the Act or any person who refuses to give his name and address or gives a name and address which appears to be false.

Disposal of Seized Articles

The officers-in-charge of all police stations should take charge of and keep in safe custody, all articles seized under the Act or Rules, which may be declared to them. The articles seized by the officers should be disposed of speedily according to provisions of the law. In the case of seizure of an animal, the owner of the animal should provide for its day to day keep, failing which the animal may be sold by public auction and the expenses incurred, in keeping the animal, realized from the proceeds of the sale. Articles, which were seized but subsequently released, should be collected by their owners within one month of the order of release and any penalties or charges due thereof should be paid. If the owner fails to do so, the articles may be disposed of by public auction and any penalties or other changes, defrayed from the proceeds of the sale.

Disposal of Arrested Persons

Every person arrested should be forwarded without delay to the nearest excise officer empowered to produce persons before a magistrate or where there is no excise officer within reasonable distance, to the officer-in-charge of the police station.

Offences and Penalties

(i) Failure to observe conditions of a licence or to pay duty: Any person who:
   a. Either manufactures dutiable goods without a licence or fails to observe any condition of the licence granted to him;
   b. Evades any payment of duty due from him;
   c. Fails to supply information asked for or supplies false information;
   d. Attempts or commits or abets the commission of any offence
   shall be liable to imprisonment upto six months or a fine upto Rs. 2000 or both.
(ii) Sale of dutiable goods (except in prescribed containers bearing the labels): If any dealer of dutiable goods is found in possession of goods which are not wrapped or labelled as prescribed or whose label or wrapper is torn, or whose containers bear marks of having been opened or tampered with, shall be liable to a fine upto Rs. 1000.
(iii) Obstructing officers and giving false information: Any person who wilfully obstructs or offers any resistance or gives any false or misleading information to any excise officer, shall be liable to a fine of up to Rs. 5000.
(iv) Disclosure of information by excise officers: Any officer disclosing information acquired by him in his official capacity in respect of any goods (except in the discharge of his duty, in good faith), shall be liable to a fine of up to Rs. 1000.

Prosecutions

(i) Prosecutions: No prosecutions under the Act can be instituted, except by an Excise Officer, not below the rank of a sub-inspector.

(ii) **Confiscations:** When an article is confiscated under the Act or Rules, the article shall vest in the collecting Government and may be disposed of according to its direction.
(iii) **Attachment of properties:** The excise commissioner can detain any machinery, plants, goods, etc. in lieu of duty that may be due to the Government and such direction shall have effect notwithstanding any change in the ownership of the trade or business.
(iv) **Appeals:** An appeal against a decision of an excise officer can be made to the excise commissioner. An appeal against the decision of the latter should be made to the State Government. Appeals should be filed within three months of the date of the decision appealed against. The decision of the authorities, to whom appeals are directed, shall be full and final. Each appeal should be accompanied by a copy of the decision or the order by which the appellant is aggrieved.

The Central Government can reserve or revise any decision of the State Government or of the excise commissioner on appeal made to it.

QUESTIONS FOR REVISION

1. What are the objectives of Medicinal and Toilet Preparations Act?
2. Define Bonded and Non-bonded Laboratory and Toilet preparations.
3. Explain the terms – manufacture in bond and manufacture outside bond. Describe the procedure to obtain a licence for the establishment of a bonded laboratory and outline the layout and working schedule of the bonded laboratory while manufacturing alcoholic preparations.
4. Give a brief account of manufacture in bonded laboratory and briefly describe the procedure to be followed for obtaining spirit from a distillery and issue of finished products from a bonded laboratory.
5. Write short note on non-bonded laboratory.
6. Write a note on the warehousing of alcoholic preparations. How the goods are moved from one warehouse to another?
7. What are the procedures to be followed by excise personnel for inspection of premises? Explain the duties and powers of an Excise Commissioner.

Chapter 6

The Narcotic Drugs and Psychotropic Substances Act, 1985

The use of opium in the country could be traced back as far as 1000 AD where it finds mention in ancient texts such as Dhanvantari Nighantu as a remedy for variety of ailments. Coca, opium and hemp, though excellent drugs are habit forming substances and their unrestricted use is a serious problem for the society. The menace of drug trafficking and drug abuse is not only a serious issue plaguing our nation but is destroying mankind globally. On one hand the lure of vast sums of money has enticed people to take desperate risks. More and more sophisticated methods of modus operandi, along with organized international syndicates, having no geographical boundaries or shackled by race, religion or creed have made the task of law enforcement agencies more complicated and difficult. On the other hand, the evolving modern-day societies, along with development, both mental and physical, also have an intrinsic negative superficial aspect where, unfortunately, drug abuse has become fashionable and at times, a mark of high society as well. For others, though ephemeral, a 'high' is still worth it.

To effectively tackle this extremely serious issue, both within the country and beyond the cultivation of poppy was brought under control in India in 1857, when the Opium Act was enacted to regulate the production of opium. This was followed by the Opium Act, 1878, in which restrictions were imposed on the possession, sale, supply, etc. of opium. The Narcotic Drugs and Psychotropic Substances Act, 1985 was enacted consolidating and amending the provisions for the control and regulation of operation relating to narcotic drugs and psychotropic substances under the Opium Act, 1878 and the Dangerous Drugs Act, 1930. This Act was amended once in 1989 and subsequently in 2001. Prior to 1950, the administration of the Narcotics Laws, namely, the Opium Act of 1857 & 1878 and the Dangerous Drugs Act, 1930 vested with the Provincial Government. The amalgamation of these Agencies laid the foundation of the Opium Department in November, 1950, which is presently known as Central Bureau of Narcotics (CBN). The CBN Headquarters was shifted from Shimla to Gwalior in 1960.

The amending Act of 2001 rationalised the sentence structure so as to ensure that while drug traffickers, who traffic in significant quantities of drugs are punished with deterrent sentences, the addicts and those who commit less serious offences are sentenced to less severe punishment. Provisions for tracing and seizing of illegally acquired properties, pursuant to drug trafficking activity, were introduced in the principal Act by way of amendment in 1989 and were further strengthened in the amending Act of 2001. To address the anomalies arising out of the amendments made in 2001, the Narcotic Drugs and Psychotropic Substances (Amendment) Bill, 2014 ("NDPS") was passed by Parliament and The Narcotic Drugs and Psychotropic Substances (Ammendment) Act, 2014 received the assent of the President on 7th March, 2014, and was published in the Gazette of India, Extraordinary, Part II Section 1, No. 17 dated 10th March, 2014. INDIAN PARLIAMENT ACT No. 16 OF 2014.

The amendments make important and path-breaking changes for medical access to narcotic drugs by removing barriers that date back to 1985, when the Act was first introduced. The amendments also include provisions to improve treatment and care for people dependent on drugs, moving away from abstinence oriented services to treating drug dependence as a chronic, yet manageable condition.

India is a signatory to The UN Single Convention on Narcotics Drugs 1961, The Convention on Psychotropic Substances, 1971 and The Convention on Illicit Traffic in Narcotic Drugs and Psychotropic Substances, 1988 which prescribe various forms of control aimed to achieve the dual objective of limiting the use of narcotics drugs and psychotropic substances for medical and scientific purposes as well as preventing the abuse of the same.

The Narcotic Drugs and Psychotropic Substances Bill, 1985 was passed by both the Houses of Parliament and it was assented by the President on 16th September, 1985. It came into force on 14th November, 1985 as ***The Narcotic Drugs and Psychotropic Substances Act, 1985 (61 of 1985)***.

Amending Act

1. The Narcotic Drugs and Psychotropic Substances (Amendment) Act, 1988 (2 of 1989).

2. The Narcotic Drugs and Psychotropic Substances (Amendment) Act, 2001 (9 of 2001).
3. The Narcotic Drugs And Psychotropic Substances (Ammendment) Act, 2014

The Narcotic Drugs and Psychotropic Substances Act, 1985

It extends to the whole of India and it applies also-

(a) to all citizens of India outside India;
(b) to all persons on ships and aircrafts registered in India, wherever they may be.

Objectives

Main objectives of the Narcotic Drugs and Psychotropic Substances Act, 1985 are:

(i) to consolidate and amend the law relating to narcotic drugs, and to make stringent provisions for the control and regulation of operations relating to narcotic drugs and psychotropic substances,
(ii) to provide for the forfeiture of property derived from, or used in, illicit traffic in narcotic drugs and psychotropic substances,
(iii) to implement the provisions of the International Convention on Narcotic Drugs and Psychotropic Substances and for matters connected therewith.

Definitions

(i) "**Cannabis (hemp)**" means
  (a) charas, that is, the separated resin, in whatever form, whether crude or purified, obtained from the cannabis plant and also includes concentrated preparation and resin known as hashish oil or liquid hashish;
  (b) ganja, that is, the flowering or fruiting tops of the cannabis plant (excluding the seeds and leaves when not accompanied by the tops), by whatever name they may be known or designated; and
  (c) any mixture, with or without any neutral material, of any of the above forms of cannabis or any drink prepared therefrom.
(ii) "**Cannabis plant**" means any plant of the genus cannabis.
(iii) "**Coca derivative**" means
  (a) crude cocaine, that is, any extract of coca leaf which can be used, directly or indirectly, for the manufacture of cocaine;
  (b) ecgonine and all the derivatives of ecgonine from which it can be recovered;

(c) cocaine, that is, methyl ester of benzoyl-ecgonine and its salts; and

(d) all preparations containing more than 0.1 percent of cocaine.

(iv) "**Coca leaf**" means
   (a) the leaf of the coca plant except of a leaf from which all ecgonine, cocaine and any other ecgonine alkaloids have been removed;
   (b) any mixture thereof with or without any neutral material, but does not include any preparation containing not more than 0.1 per cent of cocaine.

(v) "**Coca plant**" means the plant of any species of the genus Erythroxylon.

(vi) "**Commercial quantity**", in relation to narcotic drugs and psychotropic substances, means any quantity greater than the quantity specified by the Central Government by notification in the Official Gazette.

(vii) "**Manufacture**", in relation to narcotic drugs or psychotropic substances, includes
   (1) all processes other than production by which such drugs or substances may be obtained;
   (2) refining of such drugs or substances;
   (3) transformation of such drugs or substances; and
   (4) making of preparation (otherwise than in a pharmacy on prescription) with or containing such drugs or substances.

(viii) "**Manufactured drug**" means
   (a) all coca derivatives, medicinal cannabis, opium derivatives and poppy straw concentrate;
   (b) any other narcotic substance or preparation which the Central Government, by notification in the Official Gazette, has declared it to be a manufactured drug.

The Central Govt. under Notification dated November 14, 1985 declared certain drugs to be "Manufactured Drugs".

These include "Methyl Morphine" commonly known as 'Codeine' and Ethyl morphine and their salts (including Dionine), all dilutions and preparation. Except those which are compounded with one or more other ingredients and containing not more than 100 milligrams of drugs per dosage unit and with a concentration of not more than 2.5% in the dose 1 of 3 undivided preparation and which have been established in therapeutic practice.

Therefore any preparation containing not more than 100 mg (per dosage unit of codeine) and with a concentration of not more than 2.5% in therapeutic practice is not a narcotic drug.

(ix) "**Medicinal cannabis**", that is, medicinal hemp, means any extract or tincture of cannabis (hemp).

(x) "**Narcotic Commissioner**" means the Narcotics Commissioner appointed under section 5.

(xi) "**Narcotic drug**" means coca leaf, cannabis (hemp), opium, poppy straw and includes all manufactured goods.

(xii) "**Opium**" means
   (a) the coagulated juice of the opium poppy; and
   (b) any mixture, with or without any neutral material, of the coagulated juice of the opium poppy, but does not include any preparation containing not more than 0.2 per cent of morphine.

(xiii) "**Opium derivative**" means
   (a) medicinal opium, that is, opium which has undergone the processes necessary to adapt it for medicinal use in accordance with the requirements of the Indian Pharmacopoeia or any other pharmacopoeia notified in this behalf by the Central Government, whether in powder form or granulated or otherwise or mixed with neutral materials;
   (b) prepared opium, that is, any product of opium by any series of operations designed to transform opium into an extract suitable for smoking and the dross or other residue remaining after opium is smoked;
   (c) phenanthrene alkaloids, namely, morphine, codeine, thebaine and their salts;
   (d) diacetylmorphine, that is, the alkaloid also known as diamorphine or heroin and its salts; and
   (e) all preparations containing more than 0.2 per cent of morphine or containing any diacetylmorphine.

(xiv) "**Opium poppy**" means
   (a) the plant of the species *Papaver somniferum* L.; and
   (b) the plant of any other species of *Papaver* from which opium or any phenanthrene alkaloid can be extracted and which the Central Government may, by notification in the Official Gazette, declare to be opium poppy for the purposes of this Act.

(xv) "**Poppy straw**" means all parts (except the seeds) of the opium poppy after harvesting whether in their original form or cut, crushed or powdered and whether or not juice has been extracted therefrom.

(xvi) "**Poppy straw concentrate**" means the material arising when poppy straw has entered into a process for the concentration of its alkaloids.

(xvii) "**Preparation**", in relation to a narcotic drug or psychotropic substance, means any one or more such drugs or substances in dosage form or any solution or mixture, in whatever physical state, containing one or more such drugs or substances.

(xiii) **"Psychotropic substance"** means any substance, natural or synthetic, or any natural material or any salt or preparation of such substance or material included in the list of psychotropic substances specified in the Schedule.

The Central Government has the power to add to or omit from the list of psychotropic substances, if satisfied that it is necessary or expedient so to do on the basis of information and evidence of its being abused or having the scope for abuse or the modifications or provisions (if any) which have been made to, in International Convention. The list of Psychotropic substances is given in **Appendix C**.

Prohibition of certain operations under the Act

No person shall-

(a) cultivate any coca plant or gather any portion of coca plant; or
(b) cultivate the opium poppy or any cannabis plant; or
(c) produce, manufacture, possess, sell, purchase, transport, warehouse, use, consume, import inter-State export, inter-State import into India, export from India or transship any narcotic drug or psychotropic substance, except for medical or scientific purposes and in the manner and to the extent provided by the provisions of this Act or the Rules or Orders made thereunder and in a case where any such provision imposes any requirement by way of licence, permit or authorization also in accordance with the terms and conditions of such licence, permit or authorization.

Officers and Administrative Agencies

The NDPS Act divides the powers and responsibility of regulation of licit activities. The Act has listed various activities which the Central Government can, by Rules, regulate while there are various activities which the State Governments can, by Rules, regulate. Thus, we have NDPS Rules of the Central Government and the State NDPS Rules framed by each State Government under the same Act. These are enforced by the Central or concerned State Government.

The Central Government appoints a Narcotics Commissioner and subordinate officers for the purpose of preventing and combating abuse and illicit traffic of the narcotic and psychotropic substances. The Narcotics Commissioner, either by himself or through his officers, shall control the cultivation of the opium poppy and production of opium and shall also exercise and perform other functions, which may be entrusted to him by the Central Government.

The State Government may also appoint officers with such designations as it thinks fit for the purpose, who shall be subject to the general control and direction of the State Government.

The Narcotic Drugs and Psychotropic Substances Consultative Committee

"The Narcotic Drugs and Psychotropic Substances Consultative Committee", constituted by Central Government, an advisory committee, having a chairman and a maximum of 20 members, advises the Central Government on such matters relating to the administration of this Act.

Deaddiction Centers and National Fund for Control of Drug Abuse

The Central and State Governments have to establish necessary centers for identification, treatment, etc. of persons addicted to narcotic and psychotropic materials and to control supply of drugs to such persons.

The National Fund for Control of Drug Abuse shall meet the expenditure incurred in measures, taken in combating illicit traffic and control of abuse.

Power of Central Government to permit, control and regulate

The Central Government may, by Rules

(a) permit and regulate-
   (i) the cultivation, or gathering of any portion (such cultivation or gathering being only on account of the Central Government) of coca plant, or the production, possession, sale, purchase, transport, import inter-State, export inter-State, use or consumption of coca leaves;
   (ii) the cultivation (such cultivation being only on account of Central Government) of the opium poppy;
   (iii) the production and manufacture of opium and production of poppy straw;
   (iv) the sale of opium and opium derivatives from the Central Government factories for export from India or sale to State Government or to manufacturing chemists;
   (v) the manufacture of manufactured drugs (other than prepared opium) but not including manufacture of medicinal opium or any preparation, containing any manufactured drug from materials, which the maker is lawfully entitled to possess;
   (vi) the manufacture, possession, transport, import inter-State, export inter-State, sale, purchase, consumption or use of psychotropic substances;

(vii) the import into India and export from India and transhipment of narcotic drugs and psychotropic substances;
(b) prescribe any other matter requisite to render effective the control of the Central Government over any of the matters specified in clause (a).

Power of State Government to permit, control and regulate

The State Government may, by Rules

(a) permit and regulate-
   (i) the possession, transport, import inter-State, export inter-State, warehousing, sale, purchase, consumption and use of poppy straw;
   (ii) the possession, transport, import inter-State, export inter-State, sale, purchase, consumption and use of opium;
   (iii) the cultivation of any cannabis plant, production, manufacture, possession, transport, import inter-State, export inter-State, sale, purchase, consumption or use of cannabis (excluding charas);
   (iv) the manufacture of medicinal opium or any preparation containing any manufactured drug from materials which the maker is lawfully entitled to possess;
   (v) the possession, transport, purchase, sale, import inter-State, export inter-State, use or consumption of manufactured drugs other than prepared opium and of coca leaf and any preparation containing any manufactured drug;
   (vi) the manufacture and possession of prepared opium from opium lawfully possessed by an addict registered with the State Government on medical advice for his personal consumption;
(b) prescribe any other matter requisite to render effective the control of the State Government over any of the matters.

Cultivation, Production, Sale, etc. of Opium

In India, opium poppy cultivation is prohibited, under Section 8 of the Narcotics Drugs and Psychotropic Substances (NDPS) Act, 1985, except under a licence issued by the Central Bureau of Narcotics (CBN). At present, the licit opium cultivation is permitted by the Government of India in selected tracts in three traditionally opium growing States namely Madhya Pradesh, Uttar Pradesh and Rajasthan. As a signatory to the United Nations Single Convention on Narcotics Drugs, 1961 and as a licit producer of opium, India is required to adhere to the regulations under the said convention. The NDPS Act, 1985 was amended twice in 1989 and 2001. The NDPS (Amendment) Act, 2011, passed on 21 February 2014, aimed at ensuring availability of essential opioid medicines for medical use and private sector involvement.

The control mechanism is exercised by the Central Government over opium poppy cultivation which is carried out in terms of the provisions under the Act and Rules, 1985 made thereunder. The actual control mechanism adopted by CBN is aimed at strict control over the activities of the cultivation right from the stage of issue of licence till final collection of opium.

The following timeline is followed for opium crop cycle (Table 6.1):

Table 6.1

1. Finalization of opium policy	August to September
2. Issue of licences to cultivate opium poppy	October
3. Sowing period	October to November
4. Measurement of fields by range officer	Mid December to Mid January
5. Test measurement of poppy fields by senior officers	Mid January to 2nd week of February
6. Lancing and collection of opium and checking of Preliminary Weighment Register	Mid February to 3rd week of March
7. Uprooting of unlanced damaged crop	On receipt of applications
8. Weighment Operation (collection of opium and 90% payment to cultivators based on provisional analysis)	April 1st week to April end
9. Analysis of opium in Government factories and updating of records for calculation of Average Yield and balance payment due to cultivators	May to end of 3rd week of July

The opium can be cultivated only on behalf of the Central Government under a licence, granted by district opium officer, who may also designate one of the licensed cultivators as Lambardar, who may discharge duties specified by Narcotic Commissioner. The licences granted, may be withheld or cancelled, by higher officers, after giving one chance and if any opium is cultivated under a licence which is subsequently cancelled, the crop shall be destroyed.

Production of Opium

Cultivators during harvesting should take each day's collection to Lambardar for weighment and entry in records which should be jointly attested, every day by Lambardar and cultivator. These records shall be checked by the officers and if any discrepancy is found in quantity produced and quantity entered an enquiry shall be carried out to determine the liability on the cultivator as punishment.

All opium produced has to be given to the district opium officer to weigh, examine and classify the same in the manner specified. If a cultivator is dissatisfied with the classification, he may have the opium forwarded to government opium factory. All opium forwarded to the government opium factory has to classified by its General Manager.

If the district opium officer suspects that adulterated opium is delivered to him, he may send it to the government opium factory after sealing it in the presence of the cultivator and Lambardar. The adulterated opium is liable to confiscation after giving a hearing to the cultivator.

Cultivators aggrieved by the orders of cancellation or withdrawal of licences, may appeal to the Narcotic Commissioner and those aggrieved by the decisions of opium factory may appeal to the Chief Controller of Factories.

Manufacture of Opium

The opium collected from the farmers by the CBN is sent to Government Opium and Alkaloid works (GOAW) Neemuch and Ghazipur which are under the control of the Chief Controller of Factories (CCF) under the Narcotic Control Division (NCD).

Sale of Opium

Sale of opium to the State Government or manufacturing chemist can be made only from the Government Opium factory, Ghazipur. The sale to the manufacturing chemist is possible only under the permit from concerned State Government, three copies of which are sent to the opium factory. The sale price shall be fixed from time to time.

MANUFACTURE OF MANUFACTURED DRUGS AND PSYCHOTROPIC SUBSTANCES

1. Manufacture of Cocaine, Morphine, etc.

Manufacture of crude cocaine, ecgonine and its salt and diacetylmorphine is strictly prohibited. Cocaine hydrochloride can be manufactured by chemical staff of the Central Board of Excise and Customs from confiscated cocaine, while morphine, codeine, thebaine and some other alkaloids of opium can be manufactured only by the Government Opium Factory.

2. Manufacture of Medicinal Hemp

Medicinal hemp can be manufactured only in accordance with the condition of a licence granted by the chief excise authority of State Government on payment of fees and in accordance with conditions laid down in this behalf.

3. Manufacture of Other Narcotic Drugs

Such materials can be manufactured only in accordance with a licence granted by the Narcotic Commissioner or any other officer authorized by the Central Government. Licence shall be issued only to persons holding licence under the Drugs and Cosmetics Act, 1940 for manufacture of drugs, and on furnishing a security deposit as stated. For manufacture only lawfully possessed materials can be used. The quantities manufactured cannot exceed limits as permitted by the Licensing Authority or the estimated requirements for one year of the country. The licensee has to provide for adequate security and has to give notice of 15 days before commencement of manufacture and one months notice before cessation.

True accounts of all transactions have to be maintained and returns submitted to the Narcotic Commissioner as specified. Sale and distributions shall be done only in accordance with the Rules made by the State Governments.

4. Manufacture of Psychotropic Substances

Psychotropic substances have several medicinal uses but they are also liable to be abused. Hence, manufacture of psychotropic substances is regulated. All psychotropic substances have been listed in the Schedule to the NDPS Act, 1985. These may be categorized into:

Psychotropic substances whose manufacture is completely prohibited

These substances are listed in Schedule I of the NDPS Rules, 1985.

Psychotropic substances whose manufacture is permitted but only for export

These are the substances listed in Schedule III. These are not medically used in India but they are so used in some other countries. Hence, any company interested in manufacturing these can do so but only for export purposes.

Psychotropic substances which can be manufactured for sale in India or for export

Any psychotropic substance not listed in Schedule I and Schedule III of the NDPS Rules, 1985 can be manufactured (for sale in India or for export) after obtaining a licence from the State Drugs Controller under the Drugs and Cosmetics Act and Rules.

Possession of Psychotropic Substances

No person can possess any psychotropic substance unless he is lawfully authorized to possess such substance. However, this rule shall not apply to any research institute or hospital or dispensary maintained or supported by the Government or local body or charity or local subscription or to any person requiring a reasonable quantity for genuine scientific or medical requirement. The research institution, hospital or dispensary shall maintain proper accounts and records in relation to purchase and consumption of the psychotropic substance in their possession.

Conditions for Issue of Licence for the Manufacture of Synthetic Manufactured Drugs

1. The licensee should have Drug Manufacturing Licence granted to him by the Authority under the Drugs and Cosmetics Act, 1940.
2. The licensee should make a deposit of Rs. 5,000 as security in the manner specified by the issuing authority.
3. The licence is granted keeping in view the total quantity of the drug manufactured during any one year, and which does not exceed the estimated requirements of the country for the relevant year, as furnished to the International Narcotics Control Board.
4. Necessary security arrangements in the manufacturing premises shall be made as specified by the date of commencement of manufacture of the drug and at least one month's notice before he ceases to manufacture the same.
5. The licensee shall give an advance notice of 15 days, in writing, to licence issuing authority, from the date of commencement of manufacture of the drug and at least one month's notice before he ceases to manufacture the same.
6. The licensee is required to maintain necessary accounts giving full details regarding:
   (a) Materials used for manufacture of drug,
   (b) Quantity manufactured,
   (c) Quantity sold or disposed of and also furnish returns in a manner prescribed by the Narcotics Commissioner.
7. The licensee shall permit the inspector/officer concerned to inspect the premises at all reasonable times with or without prior notice and to check and verify all the records.

Import, Export, Transshipment of Narcotic Drugs and Psychotropic Substances

Narcotic drugs and psychotropic substances can be imported and exported subject to the following restrictions:

1. Import and export of narcotic drugs and psychotropic substances listed in Schedule I to the NDPS Rules is prohibited.

2. Import of opium, concentrate of poppy straw, and morphine, codeine, thebaine and their salts, is prohibited except by the Government Opium Factory. However, certain manufacturers who require these substances only for export, and importers of samples of these substances up to 1 kg in a year, can import the substances after following the due procedure, provided they are notified by the Government to do so.
3. To import any narcotic drug or psychotropic substance, one should apply for and obtain an import certificate from the Narcotics Commissioner for each consignment.
4. Export of some psychotropic substances is not permitted to specific countries. These substances and the countries to which each substance cannot be exported are listed in Schedule II of the NDPS Rules, 1985.
5. Narcotic drug or psychotropic substances specified in Schedule II can be exported only under authorizations issued by proper authority. These applications have to be accompanied by required excise permit from State Government and "Import Certificate" from countries of export.
6. Psychotropic substances which are listed in Schedule III can be exported by declaration in a prescribed form after the same has been duly endorsed by the country of export and returned.
7. To export any narcotic drug or psychotropic substance, one should apply for and obtain an export authorization, from the Narcotics Commissioner for each consignment.
8. Opium can be exported only on behalf of the Central Government.
9. Export through post offices/bank cannot be done.

Transshipment

No consignment containing any Schedule II drug can be transshipped at any port without custom collector permission and until he is satisfied that the consignment is covered by valid authorization of the exporting country. Normally no consignment can be transshipped to country other than its original destination. It can be diverted only if the export authorization specially permit it to be diverted.

SCHEDULES

The Schedule in the Act gives the list of psychotropic substances. As on today one hundred and ten (110) substances are covered, with their salts and preparations also. The Rule has got four Schedules and seven Forms.

Schedule I

Gives the list of narcotic drugs and psychotropic substances that are prohibited from import into and export from India. The psychotropic substances listed, are prohibited from manufacture, possession, transport, sale, purchase, consumption or use. Drugs listed in this Schedule are like (ND) Coca leaf, Cannabis, Heroin, Etorphine. (PS) Lysergide, Methaqualone, Bromazepam, Camazepam, Haloxazolam, Tetrazepam, etc.

Schedule II

The psychotropic substances listed under this Schedule can be imported into India and exported from India, after obtaining certificate from authorities in Forms 4 or 5 respectively.

Schedule III

The schedule gives the list of drugs which require special compliance for export, after obtaining permission in Form 5. Declaration is to be made in quadruplicate. The original and duplicate copies are to be submitted immediately by the exporter to the Narcotics Commissioner of India at Gwalior, the third copy is to be sent along with the consignment and the fourth copy is to be retained by him for own records. The Narcotic Commissioner will send the duplicate copy to the concerned authority of the importing country, requesting him to certify the actual quantity of psychotropic substances imported and return the said copy. This has been provided to safeguard that no pilferage or misuse takes place during the transshipment of the drug.

PROCEDURES

Power to issue warrant for search, arrest, seizure, etc. and authorization

1. A Metropolitan Magistrate or a Magistrate of the First Class or any Magistrate of the Second Class, specially empowered by the State Government in this behalf, may issue a warrant for the arrest of any person or for search.
2. Gazetted officers of the departments of central excise, narcotics, customs, revenue intelligence or any other department of the Central Government or of the Border Security Force are empowered to arrest a person, if they have reasons to believe from personal knowledge or information received or they may search a building, conveyance or place whether by day or by night.

Females cannot be searched by anyone except females. Provisions of Code of Criminal Procedures, 1973 are applicable to warrants, arrests, searches seizures, etc.

Reports of arrests, seizures, etc. have to be made within 24 hrs. to immediate superior official. All officers of the various departments are required to assist each other in carrying out the provisions of this Act.

Power of entry, search, seizure and arrest without warrant or authorization

The authorized officer, if he has reason to believe from personal knowledge or information given by any person and taken down in writing, that any narcotic drug, or psychotropic substance, in respect of which an offence punishable has been committed, may, between sunrise and sunset-

(a) enter into and search any such building, conveyance or place;
(b) in case of resistance, break open any door and remove any obstacle to such entry;
(c) seize such drug or substance and all materials used in the manufacture thereof and any other article, any document and any animal or conveyance which he has reason to believe, to be liable to confiscation under this Act; and
(d) detain and search, and, if he thinks proper, arrest, any person whom he has reason to believe to have committed any offence punishable relating to such drug or substance.

The authorized officer has the power of seizure and arrest in public places which may include any public conveyance, hotel, shop, or other place intended for use by, or accessible to, the public.

Procedure where seizure of goods liable to confiscation not practicable

Where it is not practicable to seize any goods (including standing crop) which are liable to confiscation under this Act, any officer duly authorized, may serve on the owner or person in possession of the goods, an order that he shall not remove, part with or otherwise deal with the goods except with the previous permission of such officer.

Power of attachment of crop illegally cultivated

Any Metropolitan Magistrate, Judicial Magistrate of the First Class or any Magistrate specially empowered in this behalf by the State Government [14][or any officer of a gazetted rank empowered under section 42] may order attachment of any opium poppy, cannabis plant or coca plant which he has reason to believe to have been illegally cultivated and while doing so may pass such order (including an order to destroy the crop) as he thinks fit.

Power to stop and search conveyance

Any officer authorized, may, if he has reason to suspect that any animal or conveyance is, or is about to be, used for the transport of any narcotic drug or psychotropic substance, in respect of which he suspects that any provision of this Act has been, or is being, or is about to be, contravened at any time, stop such animal or conveyance, or, in the case of an aircraft, compel it to land and search.

Disposal of persons arrested and articles seized

1. Any officer arresting a person shall, as soon as may be, inform him of the grounds for such arrest.
2. Every person arrested and article seized under warrant issued, shall be forwarded without unnecessary delay to the Magistrate by whom the warrant was issued and then he shall, with all convenient dispatch, take such measures as may be necessary for the disposal according to law of such person or article.

Disposal of seized narcotic drugs and psychotropic substances

The Central Government may, having regard to the hazardous nature of any narcotic drugs or psychotropic substances, their vulnerability to theft, substitution, constraints of proper storage space or any other relevant considerations, shall, as soon as may be after their seizure, dispose of in notified manner by Government.

Where any narcotic drug or psychotropic substance has been seized and forwarded to the officer-in-charge of the nearest police station or to the officer empowered under section 53, the officer referred to in sub-section (1) shall prepare an inventory of such narcotic drugs or psychotropic substances containing such details relating to their description, quality, quantity, mode of packing, marks, numbers or such other identifying particulars of the narcotic drugs or psychotropic substances.

Immunity from prosecution to addicts volunteering for treatment

Any addict, who is not charged with any offence punishable or who voluntarily seeks to undergo medical treatment for detoxification or de-addiction from a hospital or an institution maintained or recognized by the Government or a local authority and undergoes such treatment, shall not be liable to prosecution once in his lifetime:

Provided that the said immunity from prosecution may be withdrawn if the addict does not undergo the complete treatment for detoxification or deaddiction.

Offences and Penalties

The penalties for various offences under the NDPS Act are given in Table 6.2.

Table 6.2. Penalties for various offences under the NDPS Act

Offences	Penalty	Sections of the Act
Cultivation of opium, cannabis or coca plants without licence	Rigorous imprisonment - up to 10 years + fine up to Rs. 1 lakh	Opium - 18(c) Cannabis - 20 Coca - 16
Embezzlement of opium by licensed farmer	Rigorous imprisonment – 10 to 20 years + fine Rs. 1 to 2 lakhs (regardless of the quantity)	19
Production, manufacture, possession, sale, purchase, transport, import inter-state, export inter-state or use of narcotic drugs and psychotropic substances	Small quantity - Rigorous imprisonment up to 6 months or fine up to Rs. 10,000 or both. More than small quantity but less than commercial quantity – Rigorous imprisonment up to 10 years + fine up to Rs. 1 Lakhs. Commercial quantity – Rigorous imprisonment 10 to 20 years + fine Rs. 1 to 2 Lakhs	Prepared opium – 17 Opium – 18 Cannabis – 20 Manufactured drugs or their preparations – 21 Psychotropic substances – 22
Import, export or transhipment of narcotic drugs and psychotropic substances	Same as above	23
External dealings in NDPS, i.e. engaging in or controlling trade whereby drugs are obtained from outside India and supplied to a person outside India	Rigorous imprisonment 10 to 20 years + fine of Rs. 1 to 2 lakhs (Regardless of the quantity)	24
Knowingly allowing one's premises to be used for committing an offence	Same as for the offence	25
Violations pertaining to controlled substances (precursors)	Rigorous imprisonment up to 10 years + fine Rs. 1 to 2 lakhs	25A
Financing traffic and harboring offenders	Rigorous imprisonment 10 to 20 years + fine Rs. 1 to 2 lakhs	27A
Attempts, abetment and criminal conspiracy	Same as for the offence	Attempts – 28 Abetment and criminal conspiracy – 29
Preparation to commit an offence	Half the punishment for the offence	30

(Contd.)

Offences	Penalty	Sections of the Act
Repeat offence	One and half times the punishment for the offence. Death penalty in some cases.	31 Death – 31A
Consumption of drugs	Cocaine, morphine, heroin – Rigorous imprisonment up to 1 year or fine up to Rs. 20,000 or both. Other drugs – Imprisonment up to 6 months or fine up to Rs. 10,000 or both. Addicts volunteering for treatment enjoy immunity from prosecution	27 Immunity – 64A
Punishment for violations not elsewhere specified	Imprisonment up to six months or fine or both	32

Special Provisions for Use of Narcotic Drugs and Psychotropic Substances for medical and scientific purposes

A narcotic drug and psychotropic substance may be used under following special provisions:

(i) For scientific requirement including analytic requirements of any Government laboratory or any research institution in India or abroad.

(ii) For very limited requirements of a foreigner by a duly authorized person of a hospital or any other establishment of the Government especially approved by that Government.

(iii) For the purpose of de-addition of drug addicts by Government or local body or by an approved charity or local organization or by such other institution as may be approved by the Central Government.

Persons performing medical or scientific functions are required to keep records regarding the acquisition and use of substance in the prescribed form and such records are to be preserved for at least two years.

A narcotic drug and psychotropic substance may be supplied or dispensed for use as to a foreign pursuant to medical prescription only from the authorized licensed pharmacist or other authorized retail distributors, designated by authorities responsible for public health.

QUESTIONS FOR REVISION

1. Discuss briefly the objectives of the Narcotic Drugs and Psychotropic Substances Act, 1985 and how it is achieved?

The Narcotic Drugs and Psychotropic Substances Act, 1985

2. Define the following as per NDPS Act:
   (a) Cannabis or Hemp
   (b) Coca derivatives
   (c) Manufactured drugs
   (d) Opium and opium derivatives
   (e) Narcotic drugs, psychotropic substances.
3. Describe briefly the operations that are prohibited under NDPS Act.
4. Write a note on Narcotic Drugs and Psychotropic Substances Consultative Committee.
5. What are the powers of the Central and State Government in exercising the Narcotic Drugs and Psychotropic Substances Act, 1985.
6. Describe the offences and penalties under the NDPS Act.
7. What are psychotropic substances? Write short notes on Import and Export of Narcotic drugs and Psychotropic substances.
8. Explain in brief the legal procedure for cultivation of poppy plant, extraction opium and its salts.
9. Describe special provisions regarding use of narcotic drugs and psychotropic substance for medical and scientific purposes.

Chapter 7

The Drugs and Magic Remedies (Objectionable Advertisements) Act, 1954

In the present era, advertisements have become an essential part of the competitive life. It has become an essential means by which one introduces his products or services to the buyers and its users. Professionals like lawyers, teachers, doctors, etc. all have to advertise themselves in the present competitive world. No doubt, scientific and ethical advertisements are useful to public but the unethical and misleading ones are highly dangerous to the society.

A lot of difference exists between the common consumer products and the pharmaceuticals. The former are for general people, whereas the latter are for specialized group of people i.e. the doctors and the pharmacists. Prescriptions are written by RMPs and patients should buy only those drugs. So it is the choice of a RMP and not patient and moreover, if drugs are advertised to common public, it may lead to self-medication and other dangers related to it. Hence, it becomes necessary that drugs be advertised only to personnels of the medical profession and not directly to the public as in case of consumer goods. Another problem in India is the advertisement of charms and magic remedies for sexual disorders and venereal diseases which cause serious harm to the ignorant public.

The Drugs and Magic Remedies (Objectionable Advertisements) Act was therefore passed with a view to control and prohibit certain classes of advertisements of drugs in certain cases, which falsely claim to possess magic qualities and remedies. The Act as well as Rules came into force on 1st April, 1955 and was amended in 1963 and it extends to the whole of India except the state of Jammu & Kashmir.

Objectives

The Drugs and Magic Remedies (Objectionable Advertisements) Act was passed on 1st April, 1955 with the following objectives:

(i) To control certain type of advertisements relating to drugs.

(ii) To prohibit certain kind of advertisements relating to magic remedies which make false claims and are likely to mislead the public. The Act read as a whole does not merely prohibit advertisements relating to drugs and medicines connected with diseases specified under the Act but also cover all advertisements which are objectionable or unethical and are used to promote self-medication or self-treatment.

Provisions of the Rules made under the Act, known as Drugs and Magic Remedies (Objectionable Advertisements) Rules are:

(i) Scrutiny of misguiding and misleading advertisements of drugs and the manner in which advertisements can be sent confidentially.

(ii) Steps to be followed and details to be submitted in obtaining the prior sanction of government while publishing an advertisement.

Definitions

(i) **Advertisement** includes all notices, circulars, labels, wrappers or other documents and all announcements, made orally or by means of producing or transmitting light, sound or smoke.

(ii) **Drug** includes:
   (a) A medicine for the internal or external use of human beings or animals;
   (b) Any substance intended to be used for or in the diagnosis, cure, mitigation, treatment or prevention of disease, in human beings or animals;
   (c) Any article, other than food, intended to affect the body of human beings;
   (d) Any article intended for use as a component of any medicine, substance or article referred to above.

(iii) **Magic Remedy** includes talismans, mantras, kavach and any other charm of any kind which is alleged to possess miraculous powers for or in the diagnosis, cure, mitigation, treatment or prevention of any disease in human beings or animals or for affecting, in any way, the structure or any organic function of the body of human beings or animals.

Prohibited Advertisements under Drugs and Magic Remedies Act

The following advertisements are prohibited under this Act:

1. Advertisements, relating to drugs, which are likely to lead to their use in the following ailments or conditions:
   (i) For the procurement of miscarriage or prevention of conception in women.
   (ii) For the correction of menstrual disorders in women.
   (iii) For the maintenance or improvement of the capacity of human beings for sexual pleasure.
   (iv) The diagnosis, cure, mitigation, treatment or prevention of any disease, disorder or condition specified in Schedule J of the Drugs and Cosmetics Rules, 1945.
2. Advertisements which:
   (i) Directly or indirectly give false impression regarding the true character of the drug;
   (ii) Make a false claim for the drug;
   (iii) Are otherwise false or misleading in any material particular.
3. Advertisements relating to magic remedies, claiming their efficacy for any of the conditions outlined in (1) by persons, who purport to carry on the profession of administering magic remedies.

Advertisements whose import and export are prohibited

Import and export of all documents, containing an advertisement of the nature referred to above is prohibited. Any documents containing any such advertisements are deemed to be goods of which import or export has been prohibited under the Sea Customs Act, 1878.

Exempted Advertisements

The following classes of advertisements and displays are exempted from the purview of the Act and hence can be made without any prohibition:
   (i) Sign boards or notices displayed by Registered Medical Practitioner (RMP) indicating that treatment is undertaken for the disease or disorder, advertisements relating to which are otherwise prohibited.
   (ii) Books or treatises relating to the diseases or ailments which are otherwise prohibited to be advertised, provided published from bonafide scientific or social standing.
   (iii) Advertisements sent confidentially, in the prescribed manner, to RMP's. However, such advertisements should bear the following words on top, in a conspicuous manner: For the use only of RMP or a Hospital or a Laboratory.
   (iv) Any advertisement relating to a drug printed or published by the Government or by any person with the prior permission of the Government.
   (v) Advertisements, labels or set of instructions which are permitted under the Drugs and Cosmetics Act or Rules, made thereunder.

The Central Government may also permit the advertisement of any drug, which it feels shall be in the interest of the public.

Type of advertisements that are exempted under this Act

The following classes of advertisements are exempted conditionally (Table 7.1):

Table 7.1. Classes of advertisements exempted conditionally

Class of Advertisement	Conditions
Leaflets or literature accompanying packings of drugs and advertisements of drugs in medical, pharmaceutical, scientific and technical journals	(i) The advertisement contains only such information as is required for the guidance of registered medical practitioner in respect of matters relating to: (a) Therapeutic indications of the drug; (b) Its administration and dosage; (c) Its side effects; (d) The precautions to be observed in the treatment with the drug. (ii) The responsibility to prove that any claim made in the advertisement in respect of the drug is not false, exaggerated or misleading, shall lie on the advertiser.
Price lists or therapeutic indexes published by manufacturers, importers or distributors of drugs duly licensed under the Drugs and Cosmetics Act, 1940 and the Rules thereunder and Medical literature distributed by medical representatives appointed by manufacturers, importers or distributors of drugs, duly licensed under the Drugs and Cosmetics Act, 1940 and the Rules thereunder.	(i) The advertisement contains only such information as is required for the guidance of registered medical practitioner in respect of matters relating to: (a) Therapeutic indications of the drug; (b) Its administration and dosage; (c) Its side effects; (d) The precautions to be observed in the treatment with the drug. (ii) The responsibility to prove that any claim made in the advertisement in respect of the drug is not false, exaggerated or misleading, shall lie on the advertiser. (iii) The distribution of such literature is confined only to the registered medical practitioners, hospitals, dispensaries, medical and research institutions, and chemists and druggists or pharmacies duly licensed under the provisions of the Drugs and Cosmetics Rules.

Offences and Penalties under this Act

Contravention of any provision of the Act is punishable with imprisonment up to six months or fine or both on first conviction, and imprisonment up to one year or fine or both on any subsequent conviction. Any document, article or thing, in respect of which the contravention is made, can also be forfeited.

In case of contravention of the provisions of the Act by a company, every person who, at the time of the commission of the offence, was in charge of the company and was responsible for the conduct of its business, shall be deemed guilty of the offence, unless he can prove that the offence was committed without his knowledge and that he had exercised due diligence to prevent the commission of the offence. Offences under the Act can be tried only in the Courts of the Presidency Magistrates or Magistrates of the First Class.

Diseases which cannot be claimed to be cured – Schedule J (Drugs and Cosmetics Rules, 1945)

Diseases and ailments (by whatever name described) which a drug may not purport to prevent or cure.

AIDS, angina pectoris, appendicitis, arteriosclerosis, baldness, blindness, bronchial asthma, cancer and benign tumour, changes in colour of the hairs and growth of new hairs, change of foetal sex, by drugs, congenital malformations, deafness, diabetes, diseases of heart (in general), diseases and disorders of uterus, epilepsy, fits and psychic disorders, encephalitis, fairness of the skin, female diseases (in general), form structure of breast, gangrene, genetic disorders, glaucoma, goitre, hernia, high/low blood pressure, hydrocele, insanity, increase in brain capacity and improvement in height of children/adult, improvement in size and shape of the sexual organ and duration of sexual performance, improvement in the strength of the natural teeth, improvement in vision, jaundice/hepatitis/liver disorders, leukaemia, leucoderma, maintenance or improvement of the capacity of the human being for sexual pleasure, mental retardation, subnormalities and growth, myocardial infarction, obesity, paralysis, parkinsonism, piles and fistulae, polio, power to rejuvenate, premature ageing, premature greying of hairs, rabies, rheumatic heart diseases, sexual impotence, premature ejaculation and spermatorrhoea, spondylitis, stammering, stones in gall bladder, kidney, bladder, varicose vein.

Any other disease, disorder or condition which requires timely treatment in consultation with a registered medical practitioner or where there is no accepted remedies, may be further included in this list by the Central Government, in consultation with Drugs Technical Advisory Board and any other experts that Government deems fit.

QUESTIONS FOR REVISION

1. Write the mains objectives of Drugs and Magic Remedies Act, 1954.
2. Define the following terms under Drugs and Magic Remedies (Objectionable Advertisements) Act:
   (a) Advertisement
   (b) Drug
   (c) Magic remedy.
3. How do advertisements related to pharmaceutical products differ from other advertisements?
4. What are the advertisements prohibited under the Drugs and Magic Remedies Act, 1954.
5. Write short notes on:
   (a) Exempted advertisements.
   (b) Penalties for those who contravene any provisions of Drugs and Magic Remedies Act and Rules.

Chapter 8

Drugs (Price Control) Order, 2013

Drugs are recognized statutorily as "essential commodity" and they should always be made easily available to each section of community at a reasonable price. This provision has been ensured, under section 3 of the Essential Commodities Act, 1955, by the Central Government, to exercise control over the prices of the bulk drugs as well as formulations.

It was observed and notified by the Department of Pharmaceuticals that the several new essential drugs which were introduced in the country after 1995, and the 348 drugs now covered in the new Drug Prices Control Order (DPCO), were being sold at high prices. With the objective to improvise and endow with the basic health care and availability of basic medicines at an affordable price across the country, the Department of Pharmaceuticals, Ministry of Chemicals and Fertilizers, notified the *Drug Prices Control Order, 2013 ("DPCO, 2013")* in May, 2013 and replaced the *Drugs (Prices Control) Order of 1995*. It has brought 348 essential medicines in the National List of Essential Medicines (NLEM) or 652 medicine packs of various dosages and strengths under direct price control, as against an earlier order of 1995 that regulated prices of only 74 bulk drugs.

The pricing of the drugs as per DPCO, 1995 were fixed on the basis of manufacturing costs declared by the drug manufacturers whereas the DPCO, 2013 clarifies that the retail price ceiling would be a simple average of all brands which have more than a 1% market share, plus a 16% margin for supply chain retailer. Companies selling products above the ceiling will be required to adjust prices downwards, while firms will not be permitted to push up the prices of drugs below the ceiling. Firms will then only be permitted to increase prices each year in line with the wholesale price index. Newly launched medicines will need to be priced at or below the price ceilings. The price ceilings will be fixed until subsequent NLEM revisions, or following set increases or decreases in the number of manufacturers of a given medicine.

Manufacturers of non-essential medicines will be allowed to increase their prices by 10% a year, while new products which are discovered and developed in India, could seek exemption from price controls for five years.

Drugs provisions in the policy also include *promotion of non-branded generic drugs and low-cost drugs by creating a well spread out low-cost pharmacy chain through the Jan Aushadhi Programme*, so that the last mile reach of essential drugs are accessible and affordable to every village in the country.

Objectives

The Drugs (Prices Control) Order, 2013 was passed with the following objectives:

(i) To ensure uninterrupted availability of medicines, since these are essential commodities and to put an end to the arbitrary pricing regime and shift to a market-based price control model which is in favour of consumer.

(ii) Drugs provisions in the policy also include promotion of non-branded generic drugs and low-cost drugs by creating a well spread out low-cost pharmacy chain, through the Jan Aushadhi Programme.

Definitions

(i) **"Active Pharmaceutical Ingredients or Bulk Drug"** means any pharmaceutical, chemical, biological or plant product including its salts, esters, isomers, analogues and derivatives, conforming to standards specified in the Drugs and Cosmetics Act, 1940 (23 of 1940), and which is used as such or as an ingredient in any formulation.

(ii) **"Ceiling price"** means a price fixed by the Government for Scheduled formulations in accordance with the provisions of this Order.

(iii) **"Formulation"** means a medicine processed out of or containing one or more drugs with or without use of any pharmaceutical aids, for internal or external use for or in the diagnosis, treatment, mitigation or prevention of disease and, but shall not include:

(a) any medicine included in any bonafide Ayurvedic (including Siddha) or Unani (Tibb) systems of medicines;

(b) any medicine included in the Homeopathic system of medicine; and

(c) any substance to which the provisions of the Drugs and Cosmetics Act, 1940 (23 of 1940) do not apply.

(iv) **"Generic version of a medicine"** means a formulation sold in pharmacopeial name or the name of the active pharmaceutical ingredient contained in the formulation, without any brand name.

(v) **"Local taxes"** means any tax or levy (except excise or import duty included in retail price) paid or payable to the Government or the State Government, or any local body under any law for the time being in force by the manufacturer or his agent or dealer.

(vi) **"Market share"** means the ratio of domestic sales value (on the basis of moving annual turnover) of a brand, or a generic version of a medicine and the sum of total domestic sales value of the all brands and generic versions of that medicine sold in the domestic market having same strength and dosage form.

(vii) **"Market based data"** means the data of sales related to a drug collected or obtained by the Government as deemed fit, from time to time.

(viii) **"Maximum retail price"** means the ceiling price or the retail price plus local taxes and duties as applicable, at which the drug shall be sold to the ultimate consumer and where such price is mentioned on the pack.

(ix) **"Moving annual turnover"** in a particular month means cumulative sales value for twelve months in domestic market, where the sales value of that month is added and the corresponding sales of the same month in the previous year are subtracted.

(x) **"National List of Essential Medicines"** means National List of Essential Medicines, 2011 published by the Ministry of Health and Family Welfare as updated or revised from time to time and included in the first schedule of this order by the Government through a notification in the Official Gazette.

(xi) **"New drug"** for the purposes of this Order shall mean a formulation launched by an existing manufacturer of a drug of specified dosages and strengths as listed in the National List of Essential Medicines by combining the drug with another drug either listed or not listed in the National List of Essential Medicines or a formulation launched by changing the strength or dosages or both of the same drug of specified dosages and strengths as listed in the National List of Essential Medicines.

(xii) **"Non-scheduled formulation"** means a formulation, the dosage and strengths of which are not specified in the First Schedule.

(xiii) **"Pharmacoeconomics"** means a scientific discipline that compares the therapeutic value of one pharmaceutical drug or drug therapy to another.

(xiv) **"Scheduled formulation"** means any formulation, included in the First Schedule, whether referred to by generic versions or brand name.

(xv) **"Wholesaler"** means a dealer or his agent or a stockist engaged in the sale of drugs to a retailer, hospital, dispensary, medical, educational or research institution or any other agency.

(xvi) **"Wholesale price index"** means annual wholesale price index of all commodities as announced by the Department of Industrial Policy and Promotion, Government of India, from time to time.

The formulations have been divided in category of Scheduled and Non-Scheduled Formulations. The list of medicines in Schedule I (NLEM) is given in Appendix D.

Pricing of Scheduled Formulation

The ceiling price of a scheduled formulation according to DPCO, 2013 can be calculated by the following formula:

Step 1

First the Average Price to Retailer of the scheduled formulation i.e. $P(s)$ shall be calculated as below:

Average Price To Retailer, $P(s)$ = (Sum of prices to retailer of all the brands and generic versions of the medicine having market share more than or equal to one percent of the total market turnover on the basis of moving annual turnover of that medicine) / (Total number of such brands and generic versions of the medicine having market share more than or equal to one percent of total market turnover on the basis of moving annual turnover for that medicine)

Step 2

Thereafter, the ceiling price of the scheduled formulation i.e. $P(c)$ shall be calculated as below:

$$P(c) = P(s) \cdot (1 + M/100)$$

where $P(s)$ = Average Price to Retailer for the same strength and dosage of the medicine as calculated in step 1 above; M = % Margin to retailer and its value = 16.

Calculation of Ceiling Prices of following has also been provided in the DPCO, 2013.

(a) Ceiling price of a scheduled formulation in case of no reduction in price due to absence of competition.
(b) Calculation of Retail price of a new drug for existing manufacturers of scheduled formulations.

Pricing of Non-Scheduled Formulations

Apart from the price fixation of the Scheduled Formulations, the National Pharmaceutical Pricing Authority (NPPA) is also empowered to monitor the maximum retail prices (MRP) of all the drugs, including the non-scheduled formulations and ensure that no manufacturer increases the maximum retail price of a drug more than ten percent of maximum retail price during preceding twelve months and where the increase is beyond ten percent of maximum retail price, it is empowered to reduce the same to the level of ten percent of maximum retail price for next 12 months. The manufacturer shall be liable to deposit the overcharged amount, along with interest thereon, from the date of increase in price in addition to the penalty.

Margin To Retailer & Maximum Retail Price

It is laid down in the Order (Para 7), that while fixing a ceiling price of scheduled formulations and retail prices of new drugs, sixteen percent of price to retailer as a margin to retailer shall be allowed. Para 8 specifies that the maximum retail price of scheduled formulations shall be fixed by the manufacturers on the basis of ceiling price notified by the Government plus local taxes wherever applicable. Even the loose quantities of any formulation shall not be sold at a price which is in excess of pro-rata price of the formulation.

Reference data and source of market based data

1. Initially, the source of market-based data shall be the data available with the pharmaceuticals market data specializing company – IMS Health (IMS) and if the Government deems necessary, it may validate such data by appropriate survey or evaluation.
2. The Government may in the due course of time come out with other appropriate mechanism of collecting or obtaining the market-based data related to drugs and the decision of Government, with respect to collection or obtaining of data shall be final.
3. The market-based data, for fixing the ceiling price of scheduled formulations for the first time, after the notification of this order, shall be the data of May, 2012.
4. The market based data for fixing the retail price of new drugs available in the market shall be the data available for the month, ending

immediately before six months of receipt of application for fixing the price of the new drug.
5. The market-based data for fixing the ceiling price of a scheduled formulation due to a revision in the First Schedule shall be the data, available for the month ending immediately before six month of notification of revision in the First Schedule.
6. Notwithstanding anything contained in this order, the reference date for the formulations which are part of the Drugs (Prices Control) Order, 1995 shall be as per the provisions of paragraph 10 of this Order.

Pricing of the formulations covered under Drugs (Prices Control) Order, 1995

1. The prices of scheduled formulations, which are also specified in the First Schedule to the Drugs (Prices Control) Order, 1995, fixed and notified under the provisions of the said Order, up to 31st May, 2012, shall remain effective for further one year i.e. up to 30th May, 2013 and the manufacturers may revise the prices of such scheduled formulations as per the annual wholesale price index for the previous calendar year announced by Department of Industrial Promotion and Policy and thereafter, the formula as in sub-paragraph (1) of paragraph 4 of this Order shall be applied for fixing the ceiling prices of such formulations.
2. The prices of scheduled formulations, which are also specified in the First Schedule to the Drugs (Prices Control) Order, 1995, fixed and notified under the provisions of Drugs (Prices Control) Order, 1995 after 31st May, 2012, shall remain effective for one year from the date of notification of such prices under Drugs (Prices Control) Order, 1995 and immediately thereafter the manufacturers may revise the prices as per the annual wholesale price index for the previous calendar year announced by Department of Industrial Promotion and Policy and on the 1st April of succeeding financial year, the formula as in sub-paragraph (1) of paragraph 4 of this Order shall be applied for fixing the ceiling prices of such schedule formulations.
3. The prices of scheduled formulations, which are specified in the Drugs (Prices Control) Order, 1995, but not specified in the First Schedule of this Order, fixed and notified under the provisions of the said Order, up to 31st May, 2012, shall remain effective for further one year i.e. up to the 30th May 2013, and thereafter, prices of such formulations shall be regulated as in case of other non-scheduled formulations as stated in Para 20 of this Order.
4. The prices of scheduled formulations, which are specified in the Drugs (Prices Control) Order, 1995 but not specified in the First Schedule of

this Order, fixed and notified under the provisions of the said Order, after 31st May, 2012, shall remain effective for one year from the date of notification of such prices and thereafter, prices of such formulations shall be regulated as in case of other non-scheduled formulations as stated in Para 20 of this Order.

Display of Prices of Scheduled & Non-scheduled Formulations and Price List

DPCO, 2013 (Para 24 and 25) mandate that every manufacturer of a scheduled and non-scheduled formulations, intended for sale, shall display in indelible print mark, on the label of container of the formulation and the minimum pack thereof, offered for retail sale, the maximum retail price of that formulation with the words "Maximum Retail Price" preceding it and the words 'Inclusive of all taxes' succeeding it. The Order (Para 26) lays down that no person shall sell any formulation to any consumer at a price exceeding the price specified in the current price list or price indicated on the label of the container or pack thereof, whichever is less.

Recovery of Overcharged Amount under DPCO, 1987 and 1995

DPCO, 2013 (Para 23) states that notwithstanding anything contained in the Order, the Government shall, by notice, require the manufacturers, importer or distributor or as the case may be, to deposit the amount accrued due to charging of prices higher than those fixed or notified by the Government, under the provisions of Drugs (Prices Control) Order, 1987 and Drugs (Prices Control) Order, 1995, under the provisions of this Order.

Control of sale prices of formulations and Sale of split quantities of formulations

No person shall sell any formulation to any consumer at a price exceeding the price specified in the current price list or price indicated on the label of the container or pack thereof, whichever is less.

No dealer shall sell loose quantity of any formulation at a price which exceeds the pro-rata price of the formulation.

Manufacturer, distributor or dealer not to refuse sale of drug

Subject to the provisions of the Drug and Cosmetics Act, 1940 (23 of 1940) and the Rules made thereunder:
(a) no manufacturer or distributor shall withhold from sale or refuse to sell to a dealer, any drug without good and sufficient reasons;
(b) no dealer shall withhold from sale or refuse to sell any drug available with him to a customer, intending to purchase such drug.

Maintenance of records and production thereof for inspection

Every manufacturer shall maintain records relating to the sales of individual active pharmaceutical ingredients or bulk drugs manufactured or imported and marketed by him, as the case may be, and the sales of formulations units and packs and also such other records as may be directed from time to time by the Government, and the Government shall have the power to call for any record and to inspect such records at the premises of the manufacturer.

Power of entry, search and seizure

1. Any gazetted officer authorised by the Central Government or of a State Government, with a view to securing compliance with the order can
   (a) enter and search any place;
   (b) seize any drug, along with the containers, packages or coverings in which the drug is found and thereafter take all measures necessary for securing production of the drug, containers, packages or coverings, so seized;
   (c) seize any document, such as, cash memo or credit memo books, books of account and records of purchase and sale of the drugs.
2. The provisions of Code of Criminal Procedure, 1973 (2 of 1974), relating to search and seizure shall, so far as may be, apply to searches and seizures under this Order.

Non–application of the provisions of this Order in certain cases

The provisions of this order shall not apply to:

(i) A manufacturer producing a new drug patented under the Indian Patent Act, 1970 (39 of 1970) (product patent) and not produced elsewhere, if developed through indigenous Research and Development, for a period of five years from the date of commencement of its commercial production in the country.

(ii) A manufacturer producing a new drug in the country by a new process developed through indigenous Research and Development and patented under the Indian Patent Act, 1970 (39 of 1970) (process patent) for a period of five years from the date of the commencement of its commercial production in the country.

(iii) A manufacturer producing a new drug involving a new delivery system developed through indigenous Research and Development for a period of five years from the date of its market approval in India.

Provided that the provision of this paragraph shall apply only when a document showing approval of such new drugs from Drugs Controller General (India) is produced before the Government.

NATIONAL PHARMACEUTICAL PRICING AUTHORITY

Under the New Drugs Policy, 1994, the Central Government has constituted an autonomous body – National Pharmaceutical Pricing Authority (NPPA). It had started functioning from September 1st, 1997. The Government has appointed its chairman, secretary and other officials.

All the files and papers, related to the drug industry and which were handled by Bureau of Industrial Cost and Pricing under the Ministry of Chemicals, were transferred to NPPA. With the formation of NPPA, the entire price fixation exercise will be shifted to this body from Department of Chemical Fertilizers. It will lead to great degree of objectivity, transparency as well as speed in drug pricing matters.

Functions of NPPA

(a) To implement and enforce the provisions of Drugs Price Control Order.
(b) To monitor the availability of drugs, identify shortages, if any, and to take remedial steps.
(c) To fix/revise prices of bulk drugs and formulations from time to time.
(d) To monitor prices of the drugs available in the country, including the decontrolled drugs.
(e) To recover dues accrued under the Drugs (Prices Control) Order, 1979 and to deposit the same into the Drug Prices Equalization Account.
(f) To render advice to the Central Government on changes/revisions in the drug policy.
(g) To render assistance to the Central Government in the parliamentary matters relating to drug pricing.

List of Essential Medicines given in Appendix D.

QUESTIONS FOR REVISION

1. Describe the Drugs Prices Control Order and explain the salient features and the objectives of Drugs Prices Control Order.
2. Give a brief account of pricing of scheduled formulations under DPCO.
3. How the maximum price of bulk drugs and formulations is calculated?
4. What is the Ceiling Price and how the price is fixed for it?
5. Define the following as per DPCO:
    (a) Bulk drugs
    (b) Formulations

(c) Dealer
   (d) Distributor
6. How the price of a new drug is fixed?
7. Write short notes on:
   (a) Calculation of retail price of formulation.
   (b) National Pharmaceutical Pricing Authority

Chapter 9

The Poisons Act, 1919

Import, possession and sale of poisons are regulated under this Act. The Poisons Act was passed on 3rd September, 1919 with an object to control the import, possession and sale of poisons. This Act replaced the Poisons Act of 1904, which had certain limitations and the control over the traffic in poisons was inadequate. The Act is applicable to the whole of India except the State of Jammu & Kashmir except to the extent to which the provisions of this Act relate to the import of any specified poisons into India as applicable.

Under this Act, the Central Government has been authorised to regulate the import of poisons across any of the defined frontiers, while the various State Governments have been authorised to make Rules regarding the possession and sale of poisons within their respective territories. For the purposes of the Act, all substances, specified as poisons in notifications issued under the Act, are to be deemed as Poisons.

Import of Poisons

The import of poisons is permitted only by persons who have been granted licence for the purpose by the Central Government. Such persons may import poisons across one of the defined custom frontiers and in accordance with the conditions of the licence. The Central Government may prohibit the import of any specified poison across any defined custom frontiers into India.

Possession and Sale of Poisons

The State Governments may make Rules in order to regulate the possession and sale of poisons, whether wholesale or retail, within whole or specified areas of their territories. Such rules may provide for:

(i) The grant of licences for the possession and sale of any specified class of poisons and fixing of the fees to be paid for grant of such licences.
(ii) The classes of persons to whom the licences for the possession and sale of poisons are to be granted.
(iii) The categories of persons to whom the poisons may be sold.
(iv) The maximum quantity of poison that may be sold to a person.
(v) Maintenance of a sales register by the persons who have been granted licence.
(vi) The safe custody of poisons and labelling of the vessels, packages or coverings, etc., in which poisons are sold or stored for sale.
(vii) Inspection and examination of any such poison possessed by a vendor for sale.

Penalties for the Import, Possession, and Sale of poison prohibited under the Poisons Act, 1919

Any person, who either imports, possesses or sells any poison, except as provided under the Act, is punishable with:

(i) Imprisonment upto 3 months or a fine upto Rs. 500 or both on first conviction.
(ii) Imprisonment upto 6 months or a fine upto Rs. 1000 or both on any subsequent conviction.

Any person, who possesses any poison, whose possession has been forbidden by the State Government, shall be liable to imprisonment, which may extend to one year or with a fine upto Rs. 1000 or both. Any poison in respect of which an offence has been committed together with any vessels, packages, coverings, etc., in which the poison may have been contained, is liable to confiscation.

Issue of Warrants

The District Magistrate, the Sub-Divisional Magistrate and in a presidency town, the Commissioner of Police, may issue a warrant of search of any place in which he has reason to believe that any poison is possessed or sold in contravention of the Act or any Rule thereunder, or that any poison is liable to confiscation under this Act is kept or concealed. The persons to whom this warrant is directed may enter and search the place in accordance with the warrant and provision of the Code of Criminal Procedure.

Rules

The State and the Central Government have the power to make additional Rules to give effect to various provisions of the Act.

QUESTIONS FOR REVISION

1. Write the main objectives of the Poisons Act, 1919.
2. Write short notes on import, possession and sale of poisons.
3. Write briefly on legal control on possession and sale of poisons.
4. Write the penalties for the import, possession, and sale of poison prohibited under the Poisons Act, 1919.

Chapter 10

Medical Termination of Pregnancy Act, 1971

The Medical Termination of Pregnancy (MTP) Act was passed in the Parliament in the year 1971 and Rules in 1975, with a view to provide for termination of pregnancy by Registered Medical Practitioner (RMP) in order to avoid the risks to the mother's health, and for bonafide medical reasons. It was passed to provide for termination of certain pregnancies by registered medical practitioners and for matters connected therewith or incidental thereto.

The Act extends to whole of India except the State of Jammu & Kashmir. It has been divided into eight sections and provides for termination under Section 3 of MTP Act, 1971. The Central Government has power to make Rules and the State Government has the power to make Regulations.

Objectives

(i) When pregnancy arises due to sex crimes such as rape, intercourse with a lunatic woman, etc., where continuance of the pregnancy would involve a serious risk to the life of the pregnant women or grave injury to her physical or mental health, in such cases carrying out abortion legally, under hygienic and safe conditions is important.

(ii) When pregnancy is due to failure of any device or method used by married woman or man for limiting the number of children.

(iii) Eugenic aspects, where the child to be born shall have deformities or serious defect.

(iv) Only Registered Medical Practitioners may terminate pregnancies of women, who are 18 years of age or more with their consent.

(v) When the woman is minor, i.e. below 18 years of age, parents or guardians can give the consent. In all cases of the termination of pregnancy, a written consent is necessary.

Definitions

(i) **"Guardian"** means a person having the care of minor or lunatic.
(ii) **"Lunatic"** means a person as defined in Section 3 of Indian Lunacy Act.
(iii) **"Minor"** means a person who under the provisions of the Indian Majority Act, is to be deemed not to have attained majority.
(iv) **"Registered medical practitioner"** means a persons who possesses any recognized medical qualification as defined under the Indian Medical Council Act and whose name has been entered in a State Medical Register and who has such experience or training in gynaecology and obstetrics as may be prescribed by Rules made under this Act.
(v) **"Approved place"** means a place approved under Rule 4 of the MTP Rules, 1975.
(vi) **"Chief medical officer of the District"** means the chief medical officer of a district, by whatever name called.

Conditions under which Pregnancy can be Terminated

The MTP Act provides that pregnancies may be terminated by Registered Medical Practitioners, possessing experience or training in the gynecology and obstetrics, in accordance with the following provisions:

(i) If the length of pregnancy does not exceed 12 weeks and the medical practitioner is of the opinion, formed in good faith, that continuance of pregnancy involves risk to the life of the woman or poses a grave danger to her mental or physical health or the child to be born is likely to be seriously handicapped due to any physical or mental abnormality.
(ii) The pregnancies caused due to rape or failure of any family planning devices used by the woman or her husband, may be deemed to be posing grave injury to the mental health.
(iii) The pregnancy is terminated with the written consent of the woman if she has attained the age of 18 years. If the woman is less than 18 years of age or is a lunatic (as defined in the Lunacy Act, 1972), the pregnancy can be terminated only with the written consent of her guardian.
(iv) Where the length of pregnancy exceeds 12 weeks, but does not exceed 20 weeks it can be terminated only if at least two medical practitioners are of the opinion that termination is necessary as discussed above.

However, when at least two medical practitioners are of the opinion that termination of pregnancy is immediately necessary to save the life of the woman, pregnancy of any length may be terminated even by medical practitioners, who do not have experience or training in gynecology and obstetrics.

The pregnancies have to be terminated only at a hospital established or maintained by the Government or a place approved by the Government for this purpose.

Conditions for approval of places for Termination of Pregnancy

Places approved for termination of pregnancy should have:
- (i) An operation table with facilities for gynaecological abdominal surgery.
- (ii) Anaesthetic equipment, resuscitation equipment and sterilization equipment.
- (iii) Drugs and parenteral fluids for emergency use.
- (iv) Qualified medical personnel.

The application, for the approval of a place for the termination of pregnancy should be addressed to the Chief Medical Officer of the District concerned, who shall verify or inspect such place and if satisfied, shall recommend the Government to approve the place and issue a certificate of approval. The certificate must be conspicuously displayed at the place so that it is easily visible to persons visiting the place. The certificate can be cancelled or suspended if the prescribed facilities are not maintained and termination of pregnancy at such place cannot be made under safe and hygienic conditions.

Experience or Training for an RMP to Terminate Pregnancy

Any RMP having the following experience/training in the practice of gynaecology and obstetrics can terminate pregnancy under the Act:
- (i) If the RMP was registered in a State Medical Register before the commencement of this Act:
    An experience in the practice of gynaecology and obstetrics for not less than three years.
- (ii) If the RMP was registered on or after the commencement of this Act:
    - (a) Six months of house surgery in gynaecology and obstetrics.
    - (b) In case, he has not done any such house surgery, an experience in the practice of gynaecology and obstetrics, in any hospital for not less than one year.
    - (c) Experience by way of assistance given by the person to a RMP in the performance of twenty-five cases of medical termination of pregnancy in a hospital, established or maintained, or a training institute approved for this purpose, by the Government.

If the RMP holds a post-graduate degree or diploma in gynaecology and obstetrics, the experience or training gained during the course of degree or diploma is sufficient.

Records maintained

Records pertaining to the admissions of women for termination of pregnancy shall be maintained by the Head of the hospital or the owner of the approved place, in special registers kept for this purpose. The entries in the register shall be made serially yearwise.

The *admission register* shall be a *secret document* and the information contained therein shall not be disclosed to any person except as provided under the Act. However, in case of an employed woman, whose pregnancy has been terminated, the RMP shall grant a certificate on demand in order to enable her to obtain leave from her employer. The employer shall however not disclose this information to any other person.

The name or identity of the woman shall not be entered in any case sheet, operation theatre register, follow-up card or any other document or register (*except the admission register*). Any reference to the pregnant woman shall be made on the basis of the serial number assigned to the woman in the admission register. Every *admission register* shall be *destroyed on the lapse of five years* from the date of last entry in the register.

Other papers shall be destroyed on the lapse of three years from the date of termination of the pregnancy concerned, unless otherwise directed.

The consent given by the pregnant woman regarding the termination of her pregnancy together with the certified opinion of the RMP shall be sealed in an envelope by the RMP. The envelope shall bear the serial number assigned to the pregnant woman, the name of the RMP by whom the pregnancy was terminated and shall be marked SECRET. The envelope shall be kept in safe custody by the Head of the hospital or the owner of the approved place.

Offences and Penalties

The termination of a pregnancy by a person, who is not a registered medical practitioner, shall be deemed to be a punishable offence under Indian Penal Code. Anyone who fails to comply with Rules made under the Act or contravenes them, may be fined up to Rs. 1,000.

Rules and Regulations

The Central Government may make Rules to give effect to the provisions of this Act to provide for:

(a) experience and/or training of a registered medical practitioner intending to terminate pregnancies.
(b) such other matters as may be provided by Rules made under this Act.

The State Governments may make regulations to provide for:

(a) Certification of opinion(s) of registered medical practitioners and preservation or disposal of such certificates.
(b) Furnishing of intimation about termination of pregnancies and any matter connected therewith.
(c) Prohibition of disclosure of intimations given under (b) except to specified persons.

No suit or legal action can be instituted against a registered medical practitioner for any damage caused by anything done by him in good faith under the Act.

QUESTIONS FOR REVISION

1. Write aims and objectives of the Medical Termination of Pregnancy Act, 1971.
2. Give a brief account of Legal procedures for termination of pregnancy.
3. Explain the circumstances under which a Registered Medical Practitioner can terminate the pregnancy.
4. Discuss the conditions under which a pregnancy can be terminated.
5. What are the requirements for places to be approved for termination of pregnancy?
6. What qualification and experience is required for a person to perform medical termination of pregnancy at different stages?

Chapter 11

Prevention of Cruelty to Animals Act

Animals are very useful for multiple purposes. Some of them such as cats and dogs are kept as pets that give pleasure and joy to the owners and some act as a source of milk, meat and other dairy products. Animals are also utilized to produce sera, vaccines, hormones, enzymes, etc.

Animal studies play a significant role in development of new drugs. Disease models are induced in animals such as hyperglycemia, hypertension, hyperlipidemia, etc. and any promising new compound tested for its beneficial effect and margin of safety. It is mandatory that a new experiment must be tested in experimental animals before clinical trials are started in humans. Animal testing is done on laboratory animals (dogs, cats, monkeys, rabbits, guinea pigs, rats, mice, etc.). Preclinical or pharmacological screening tests give information about the effect of a new substance on biological system and activity. The studies also include mechanism of action, pharmacokinetics, dose ranges. Toxicity study includes acute, subacute toxicity and long-term toxicity on reproduction, teratogenicity, carcinogenicity. Hence, animal studies indicate efficacy and margin of safety.

No doubt there are limitations on the amount of information obtained through animal studies and so people may think that animal testing is not necessary but it is really not so. By using different species and different routes of administration and properly conducting the toxicity studies, the data do have predictive values.

In all the progressive countries, there are laws to save the animals from infliction of unnecessary pain and sufferings, which prevents the man from behaving cruelly towards them. In our country, there were a variety of such rules in different parts of the country most of them being ineffective in practice. To assess the effectiveness of the existing legislation on the subject and with a view to consolidating various laws into one single Act, the Government of India appointed a Committee to probe into the matter. On the recommendations of this Committee, the 'Prevention of Cruelty to Animals Act', was passed which aimed at preventing unnecessary pain and suffering to animals. This Act is applicable to all parts of the country.

In the Act 'animals' have been defined to include all species of animals (except man) as well as all species of birds. The term 'cruelty' means infliction of unnecessary pain or suffering. However, it has not been defined precisely. The following sections discuss the provisions of the Act which relate to 'Experimentation on Animals'. The other provisions of the Act are of non-pharmaceutical interest.

Objectives

The main objectives of this Act are to:

(a) prevent cruelty to animals;
(b) encourage the considerate treatment of animals; and
(c) improve the level of community awareness about the prevention of cruelty to animals.

Experimentation on Animals

Construction of a Committee

For the experimental testing purposes, the animals which are used, have to be incised and dissected to different degrees and sometimes have to be killed. From an aesthetic point of view, all these manipulations on animals should be so effected that the animals do not suffer any avoidable pain or injuries. A chapter on 'Experimentation on Animals' has been included in the Act and this chapter provides for the constitution of a committee to look after the various aspects of experimentation on animals, such as to supervise and control their use for experimentation thereby saving them from any avoidable pains. The Committee consists of the following members:

(i) Two members each of the Indian Council of Medical Research, Indian Council of Agricultural Research, and Council of Scientific and Industrial Research nominated by the Central Government.
(ii) Two members representing universities granting medical and veterinary degrees nominated by the Central Government.
(iii) One member of the Lok Sabha and one of the Rajya Sabha to be elected by the Houses respectively.

(iv) Five non-official persons actively engaged in the promotion of animal welfare to be nominated by the Central Government.

The Committee is required to ensure that all animals used for scientific experiments are not subjected to unnecessary pain or suffering, before, during or after the experiments. The Committee is authorized to make the Rules to provide for the following matters:

(i) If the experiments are performed in institutions, their heads shall be responsible for compliance with the provisions of the Act and where individuals conduct any experiment on animals, they shall be individually responsible for avoidance of cruelty to the animals.

(ii) The experiments should, as far as possible, be performed while the animal is under the influence of an anesthetic and if the recovery of the animal involves serious suffering, it should be sacrificed while still unconscious.

(iii) If it is possible to use a small animal for an experiment, use of a large animal should be avoided and where it be possible to substitute the use of animals by devices such as models, films, etc., such substitution should be made. Experiments on animals should not be performed merely for acquiring manual skill.

(iv) The animals intended to be used for experiments, should be properly looked after before and after the experiments and records of experiments performed should be maintained.

Inspection

The Committee can authorise any of its officers or any other person to inspect any place where experiments on animals are performed and to check the records required to be maintained under the Act.

Prohibition of experimentation

If the Committee is satisfied that any person or institution is not carrying out experiments on animals in accordance with the Rules, the Committee is empowered to prohibit experimentation on animals by such individual or institution, for definite period of time or indefinitely or impose any special conditions for the performance of experiments.

Penalties

If any person contravenes any conditions imposed by the Committee, he may be punished with a fine extending up to Rs. 200.

Animal Welfare Board of India

The Board is established by the Central Government:

(a) to promote animal welfare generally; and
(b) to protect animals from unnecessary pains and sufferings in particular.

The Board consists of various members. The Central Government nominates one of the members to be its Chairman and another to be its Vice-Chairman. The Central Government may appoint secretary of the Board.

Its main function is to keep the law in force to prevent cruelty to animals and advise the Central Government regarding the amendments in the present Act from time to time. It shall suggest any improvement in design of vehicles or improvisation of facility of sheds, water troughs, veterinary assistance, maintenance of slaughter houses and methods of slaughtering of animals, giving financial assistance, advise method of killing unwanted animals, etc.

Committee for the Control and Supervision of Experiments on Animals (CPCSEA)

The motto of Prevention of Cruelty to Animals (PCA) Act, 1960, as amended in 1982, is to prevent infliction of unnecessary pain or suffering on animals. Under Chapter 4 of the same Act there is provision for the control of experimentation on animals. The Act provides that the Animal Welfare Board constitute a Committee for the Control and Supervision of Experiments on Animals (CPCSEA). This Committee is empowered to take care of the legal and ethical aspects of experimental animals being used in research and enact preventive measures wherever there is violation of the law. For this purpose, the Government has made "Breeding of and Experiments on Animals (Control and Supervision) Rules, 1998", as amended during 2001 and 2006, to regulate the experimentation on animals.

Experimentation on animals in course of medical research and education is covered by provisions of the Prevention of Cruelty to Animals Act, 1960 and Breeding of and Experiments on Animals (Control & Supervision) Rules of 1998, 2001 and 2006 framed under the Act.

Under these provisions, the concerned establishments are required to get themselves registered with CPCSEA, form IAEC, get their Animal House Facilities inspected, and also get specific projects for research cleared by CPCSEA before commencing the research on animals. Further, breeding and trade of animals for such experimentation are also regulated under these Rules. In an amendment brought out in 2006 in the Rules for Breeding of and Experiments on Animals (Control & Supervision), powers to permit experiments on small animals were given to Institutional Animal Ethics Committee (IAEC) of the establishments. Only proposals for conducting experiments on large animals are required to be sent to CPCSEA for approval.

Institutional Animal Ethics Committee (IAEC)

IAEC has been designed to secure the following objectives:

(a) experiments shall be performed in every case by or under the supervision of a person duly qualified in that behalf, that is, Degree or Diploma holders in Veterinary Science or Medicine or Laboratory Animal Science of a University or an Institution recognized by the Government for the purpose and under the responsibility of the person performing the experiment;

(b) that experiments are performed with due care and humanity and that as far as possible experiments involving operations are performed under the influence of some anesthetic of sufficient power to prevent the animals feeling pain;

(c) that animals which, in the course of experiments under the influence of anesthetics, are so injured that their recovery would involve serious suffering, are ordinarily destroyed while still insensible;

(d) that experiments on animals are avoided wherever it is possible to do so; as, for example, in medical schools, hospitals, colleges and the like, if other teaching devices such as books, models, films and the like, may equally suffice;

(e) that experiments on larger animals are avoided when it is possible to achieve the same results by experiments upon small laboratory animals like guinea pigs, rabbits, mice, rats, etc.;

(f) that, as far as possible, experiments are not performed merely for the purpose of acquiring manual skill;

(g) that animals intended for the performance of experiments are properly looked after both before and after experiments;

(h) that suitable records are maintained with respect to experiments performed on animals.

Functions of IAEC

As defined in "Breeding of and Experiments on Animals (Control and Supervision) Rules, 1998":

(i) The primary duty of IAEC is to work for achievement of the objectives, as mentioned above.

(ii) IAEC will review and approve all types of research proposals involving small animal experimentation before the start of the study. For experimentation on large animals, the case is required to be forwarded to CPCSEA in prescribed manner with recommendation of IAEC.

(iii) IAEC is required to monitor the research throughout the study and after completion of study through periodic reports and visit to animal house and laboratory where the experiments are conducted. The Committee has to ensure compliance with all regulatory requirements, applicable Rules, guidelines and laws.

Composition of Institutional Animals Ethics Committee (IAEC)

It shall include eight members as follows:

1. A biological scientist.
2. Two scientists from different biological disciplines.
3. A veterinarian involved in the care of animal.
4. Scientist in charge of animals facility of the establishment concerned.
5. A scientist from outside the institute,
6. A non-scientific socially aware member.
7. A nominee of CPCSEA

Specialist may be co-opted while reviewing special project using hazardous agents such as radioactive substance and deadly microorganisms. The Chairperson of the Committee and Member Secretary would be nominated by the Institution from amongst the eight members. Members against Serial number 5, 6 and 7 will be nominated by CPCSEA, with a provision of a Link nominee for CPCSEA nominee.

QUESTIONS FOR REVISION

1. What are the objectives and salient features of Prevention of Cruelty to Animals Act?
2. Write short notes on:
   (a) Experimentation on animals.
   (b) Prevention of cruelty to animals.
   (c) Constitution and functions of the Committee under Prevention of Cruelty to Animals Act.
3. Give an account of the constitution and functions of Animal Welfare Board of India.
4. Write briefly on constitution and functions of "Committee for Control and Supervision of Experiments on Animals".
5. How are the experimental animals, used for scientific experiments, required to be handled before, during and after the experiments?
6. Discuss briefly the constitution and functions of Institutional Animals Ethics Committee.

Chapter 12

The Insecticides Act, 1968

The Insecticides Act, 1968 was brought into force with effect from August 1971 with a view of regulating the import, manufacture, sale, transport, distribution and use of insecticides, in order to prevent risk to human beings and animals.

During the last 38 years, various provisions of this Act were amended. The Central Government made certain amendments in the Insecticides Act, 1968 and Rules, 1971 through the Insecticides (Amendment) Act, 1999. Further Insecticides (Amendment) Rules, 2006 were enforced in the Act.

Objective

The agricultural crops are liable to be destroyed by insects. Hence, the use of insecticides is necessary to increase the agricultural production. However, the increasing use of insecticides has also opened a gate of various types of diseases due to their toxicity. Some insecticides, such as DDT have a high stability and they pass on from crops to living beings. Also rivers, soils, etc. get polluted due to indiscriminate use of insecticides. Since insecticides are highly toxic chemical compounds, their unsafe handling during manufacture, transportation, distribution, use, etc., can also result in toxicity.

Hence, the Insecticides Act, 1968 was passed with the primary objective of:

(a) protecting human beings and animals from the risks involved in the use of insecticides;

(b) regulating the import, manufacture, sale, transport, distribution and use of insecticides.

The salient features of the Act are as follows:

(i) Establishment of a Central Insecticides Board and the setting up of a Committee called the 'Registration Committee' for the purpose of granting certificates of registration to persons, desiring to import or manufacture insecticides.
(ii) Licensing of persons desiring to manufacture, sell or exhibit for sale or distribution any insecticide.
(iii) Establishment of a Central Laboratory for carrying out certain functions under the Act.
(iv) Prohibition of imports, manufacture, sale, etc., of insecticides in contravention of the provisions of the Act.
(v) Regulation of transport and storage of insecticides, so as to prevent cases of accidental contamination of food with insecticides.
(vi) Provision for taking immediate action by way of prohibition of sale, distribution or use of any insecticide where it is found that the sale, distribution or use of any insecticide is being done in such a way as to involve risk to human beings or vertebrate animals and where immediate action is necessary.

Definitions

(i) **Insecticide** means:
   (a) Any substance specified in the Schedule to the Act, or
   (b) Such other substances (including fungicides and weedicides) as the Central Government may, after consultation with the Board, by notification in the official gazette, include in the schedule from time to time.
   (c) Any preparation containing any one or more of such substances.
(ii) **Manufacture**, in relation to any insecticide, includes:
   (a) Any process or part of the process for making, altering, finishing, packing, labeling, breaking up or otherwise treating or adopting any insecticide with a view to its sale, distribution or use but does not include the packing or breaking up of any insecticide in the ordinary course of retail business.
   (b) Any process by which a preparation containing an insecticide is formulated.
(iii) **Misbranded**: An insecticide shall be deemed to be misbranded:
   (a) If its label contains any statement, design or graphic representation relating thereto which is false or misleading in any material particular, or if its package is otherwise deceptive in respect of its contents.

(b) If it is an imitation of, or is sold under the name of, another insecticide.
(c) If its label does not contain a warning or caution which may be necessary and sufficient, if complied with to prevent risk to human beings or animals.
(d) If any word, statement or other information required by or under this Act to appear on the label is not displayed thereon in the desired conspicuous manner.
(e) If it is not packed or labelled as required by or under this Act.
(f) If it is not registered in the manner required by or under this Act.
(g) If the label contains any reference to registration other than the registration number.
(h) If the insecticide has a toxicity which is higher than the level prescribed or, is mixed or packed with any substance so as to alter its nature or quality or contains any substance which is not included in the registration.

(iv) **Package** means a box, bottle, casket, tin, barrel, case, receptacle, sack, bag, wrapper, or thing in which an insecticide is placed or packed.
(v) **Premises** means any land, shop, stall or place where any insecticide is sold or manufactured or stored or used, and include any vehicle carrying insecticides.

Administrative Agencies

The Act provides for the establishment of the following agencies for the administration of the Act:

1. The Central Insecticides Board.
2. Registration Committee.
3. Other Committees.
4. Central Insecticides Laboratory.
5. Insecticides Analysts.
6. Insecticides Inspectors.

Constitution and Functions of Central Insecticides Board according to Insecticides Act

The Central Government, under the Insecticides Act, constituted a Board to be called as Central Insecticides Board, to advise the Central Government and State Governments on technical matters arising out of the administration of this Act and to carry out other functions assigned to it under this Act.

The matters on which the Board may advise the Central and State Governments include matters relating to:

(i) The risk to human beings and animals involved in the use of insecticides and the safety measures necessary to prevent such risk.
(ii) The manufacture, sale, storage, transport and distribution of insecticides with a view to ensure safety to human beings and animals.

Constitution of the Central Insecticides Board

The Central Insecticides Board consists of the following members:

1. Ex-officio members

(i) The Director General of Health Services, who shall be the Chairman.
(ii) The Drugs Controller, India.
(iii) The Plant Protection Adviser to the Government of India.
(iv) The Director of Storage and Inspection (Department of Food).
(v) The Chief Advisor of Factories.
(vi) The Director, National Institute of Communicable Diseases.
(vii) The Director General, Indian Council of Agricultural Research.
(viii) The Director General, Indian Council of Medical Research.
(ix) The Director, Zoological Survey of India.
(x) The Director General, Indian Standards Institution.
(xi) The Director General of Shipping or, in his absence, the Deputy Director General of Shipping.
(xii) The Joint Director, Traffic (General), Ministry of Railways.
(xiii) The Secretary, Central Committee of Food Standards.
(xiv) The Animal Husbandry Commissioner, Department of Agriculture.
(xv) The Joint Commissioner (Fisheries), Department of Agriculture.
(xvi) The Deputy Inspector General of Forests (Wild Life), Department of Agriculture.
(xvii) The Industrial Adviser (Chemicals), Director General of Technical Development.

2. Nominees of the Central Government

(i) One person to represent the Ministry of Petroleum and Chemicals.
(ii) One Pharmacologist.
(iii) One Medical Toxicologist.
(iv) One person who shall be in charge of the department dealing with public health in a State.
(v) Two persons who shall be Directors of Agriculture in State.
(vi) Four persons, one of whom shall be an expert in industrial health and occupational hazards.
(vii) One person to represent the Council of Scientific and Industrial Research.
(viii) One Ecologist.

The nominated members hold office for three years but are eligible for re-nomination. The Central Government shall appoint a person to be the Secretary of the Board who shall also function as Secretary to the Registration Committee and provide the Board and the Registration Committee with such technical and other staff as it considers necessary.

Functions of the Board

The Board shall, in addition to the functions assigned to it by the Act, carry out the following functions:

(i) Advise the Central Government on the manufacture of insecticides under the Industries (Development and Regulation) Act, 1951.
(ii) Specify the uses of and classification of insecticides on the basis of their toxicity as well as their being suitable for aerial application.
(iii) Advise tolerance limits for insecticides, residues and minimum intervals between the application of insecticides and harvest in respect of various commodities.
(iv) Specify the shelf-life of insecticides.
(v) Suggest colorations, including colouring matter which may be mixed with concentrates of insecticides, particularly those of highly toxic nature.
(vi) Carry out such other functions as are assigned to it by or under this Act.

Registration Committee and Registration of Insecticides

The Central Government constitutes a Registration Committee and it consists of a Chairman and not more than five persons who are Members of the Board (including the Drugs Controller General of India and the Plant Protection Adviser to the Government of India). The main functions of the Committee are:

(i) Registration of insecticides after scrutinizing their formulae and verifying claims made by the importer or the manufacturer, as the case may be, as regards their efficacy and safety to human beings and animals.
(ii) Specify the precautions to be taken against poisoning through the use or handling of insecticides.
(iii) Carry out such other functions as are assigned to it by or under this Act.
(iv) To co-opt such members as members or experts, as are necessary.

Where the Chairman is not a Member of the Board, his term of office and other conditions of service are determined by the Central Government.

A Member of the Registration Committee holds office for so long as he is a Member of the Board. The Registration Committee regulates its own procedure and the conduct of business to be transacted by it.

Other Committees

The Central Insecticides Board may appoint such other Committees as it deems fit with Members not necessarily Members of Board, for such period, and to perform such duties, as it delegates.

Central Insecticides Laboratory and its Functions

The Central Government may establish a Central Insecticides Laboratory and appoint its Director in order to carry out the functions entrusted to it by or under the Act which include the following:

(i) To analyze such samples of insecticides sent to it under the Act by any officer or authority authorized by the Central or State Governments and submission of certificates of the analysis to the concerned authority.

(ii) To analyze samples of materials for insecticide residues under the provisions of the Act.

(iii) To carry out such investigations as may be necessary for the purpose of ensuring the conditions of registration of insecticides.

(iv) To determine the efficacy and toxicity of insecticides.

(v) To carry out such other functions as may be entrusted to it by the Central Government or by a State Government.

The Central Government or the State Government may also appoint persons possessing the prescribed technical and other qualifications as **Insecticide Analysts** for such areas and in respect of such insecticides or class of insecticides as may be specified. No person having any financial interest in the manufacture, import or sale of any insecticide can be appointed as Insecticide Analyst.

Insecticide Inspectors

(i) The Central Government or the State Government may also appoint sufficient number of qualified persons as Insecticide Inspectors for inspecting any establishment licensed for manufacture or sale of insecticides.

(ii) Making such enquiries as may be required to ensure compliance with the provisions of the Act.

(iii) Taking samples of insecticides and sending them to the Insecticide Analyst for analysis.

(iv) Stopping the sale, distribution or use of an insecticide in contravention of the Act.
(v) Seizing stocks of insecticides or records pertaining to it wherever required.
(vi) Taking such other actions as may be deemed necessary for ensuring compliance with the provisions of the Act.

The Insecticide Inspectors are deemed to be public servants within the meaning of Indian Penal Code and may exercise the power of a police officer for the purpose of ascertaining the true name and residence of the person from whom an insecticide has been seized or otherwise taken.

Registration of Insecticides

Any person who desires to import or manufacture any insecticide has to apply to the Registration Committee for the registration of such insecticide and a separate application is required for each insecticide. Every application for registration should be made in such form and should contain such particulars as may be prescribed.

On receipt of any such application for the registration of an insecticide, if the committee is satisfied regarding the safety and efficacy of the insecticide, it may register the same. On payment of the prescribed fees, the Registration Committee shall allot a registration number to the insecticide and issue a certificate of registration. After an insecticide has been registered, any person (other than the original applicant) desiring to import or manufacture that insecticide can be given a registration number and granted the registration certificate on the conditions applicable to the original registration. Where the Registration Committee is of the opinion that the insecticide is being introduced for the first time in India, it may register it provisionally for a period of two years on such conditions as it may specify. The Registration Committee may also refuse to register any insecticide for reasons appearing sufficient to it. Any person aggrieved by the decision of the Registration Committee can appeal to the Central Government within 30 days whose decision shall be final.

Appeal against non-registration or cancellation

Any person aggrieved by a decision of the Registration Committee, within a period of thirty days from the date on which the decision in communicated to him, appeal in the prescribed manner and on payment of the prescribed fee to the Central Government whose decision thereon shall be final.

Grant of Licence

Any person desiring to manufacture or to sell, stock or exhibit for sale or distribute any insecticide, or to undertake commercial pest control operations with the use of any insecticide may make an application to the licensing officer for the grant of a licence.

A licence granted under this Section shall be valid for the period specified therein and may be renewed from time to time for such period and on payment of such fee as may be prescribed.

Conditions under which import, manufacture and sale of insecticides are prohibited

Any person who desires to manufacture, sell, stock or exhibit for sale any insecticide has to obtain a licence for the purpose from the licensing officers appointed in this behalf by the State Governments. No licence is however required for the import of a registered insecticide.

The import and manufacture of the following classes of insecticides is prohibited under the Act:

(i) Any misbranded insecticide.
(ii) Any insecticide, the sale, distribution or use of which is for the time being prohibited.
(iii) Any insecticide, except in accordance with the conditions on which it was registered.
(iv) Any insecticide, in contravention of any other provision of this Act or of any Rule made thereunder.

The sale, distribution, transport or use of the following classes of insecticides is prohibited under the Act:

(i) Any insecticide, which is not registered under this Act.
(ii) Any insecticide, the sale, distribution or use of which is for the time being prohibited.
(iii) Any insecticide in contravention of any other provision of this Act or of any Rule made thereunder.

Offences and Penalties under Insecticides Act, 1968

1. Any person whosoever:
    (i) Imports, manufactures, sells, stocks or exhibits for sale or distributes any insecticide deemed to be misbranded; or
    (ii) Import or manufactures any insecticide without a certificate of registration; or
    (iii) Manufactures, sells, stocks or exhibits for sale or distributes an insecticide without a licence; or
    (iv) Sells or distributes an insecticide prohibited for reasons of public safety; or
    (v) Causes an insecticide, the use of which has been prohibited for reasons of public safety, to be used by any worker; or

(vi) Obstructs an Insecticide Inspector in the exercise of his powers or discharge of his duties under this Act or the rules made thereunder, shall be punishable:
  (a) For the first offence, with imprisonment for a term which may extend to two years, or with fine which may extend to Rs. 2,000, or with both;
  (b) For the second and a subsequent offence, with imprisonment for a term which may extend to three years, or with fine, or with both.
2. Whoever uses an insecticide in contravention of any provision of this Act or any Rule made thereunder shall be punishable with fine which may extend to Rs. 5,000.
3. Whoever contravenes any of the other provisions of this Act or Rule made thereunder or any condition of a certificate of registration or licence granted thereunder, shall be punishable:
  (a) For the first offence, with imprisonment for a term which may extend to six months, or with fine, or with both;
  (b) For the second and a subsequent offence, with imprisonment for a term which may extend to one year, or with fine, or with both.

The stocks of insecticides in respect of which an offence has been committed are liable to be confiscated. The trying court may also order publication of the name, place of residence, offence and the penalty imposed of a person in specified newspapers, if the offender repeats the similar offence a second or a subsequent time.

Offences by Companies

Whenever an offence is committed by a company, every person who at the time of offence, was in charge of, and was responsible to the company for the conduct of its business as well as the company, shall be deemed to be guilty of the offence and shall be liable to be proceeded against and punished accordingly.

However, the person shall not be liable to punishment if he proves that the offence was committed without his knowledge or that he exercised all due diligence to prevent the commission of such offence.

Exemption

Nothing in this Act shall apply to:
(a) the use of any insecticide by any person for his own household purposes or for kitchen, garden or in respect of any land under his cultivation;
(b) any substance specified or included in the Schedule or any preparation containing any one or more such substances, if such substance or

preparation is intended for purposes other than preventing, destroying repelling or mitigating any insects, rodents, fungi, weeds and other forms of plant or animal life not useful to human beings;

(c) the use of any educational, scientific or research organization engaged in carrying out experiments with insecticides.

QUESTIONS FOR REVISION

1. Write the main objectives of Insecticides Act.
2. Define:
   (a) Insecticides.
   (b) Misbranded insecticide.
3. Write the constitution and functions of Central Insecticides Board.
4. Write briefly on Registration Committee and Registration of Insecticides.
5. What are the functions of Central Insecticide Laboratory?
6. Write short notes on:
   (a) Procedure for registration of insecticide prescribed under the Insecticides Act.
   (b) Import, manufacture and sale of insecticides.
   (c) Insecticide Inspectors.
   (d) Central Insecticide Board.

Chapter 13

Shops and Establishment Act

To set up a business, we require not only a business plan, product/service model, financing options, but also a comprehensive list of all the compulsory regulations that the business entity will have to comply with, such as the taxation legislations, licensing requirements, etc. One such important legislation is the Shops and Establishments Act, enacted by every State in India to regulate conditions of work and to provide for statutory obligations of the employers and rights of the employees in unorganized sector of employment and other establishments in their jurisdiction.

The Shops and Establishments Act was passed with a view to ensure fair deals by the employers to their employees. Since the coming of independence in 1947 the numbers and scopes of such Acts have grown rapidly paving way for the social justice in a welfare democratic nation like India. The Act has provisions for the work schedules, environmental conditions, wages, leave, etc. for persons employed in shops and other commercial establishments like hotels, theatres, etc. Almost all the States in the country have their own Shops and Establishments Act which legislate on similar lines, with differences warranted by the situations prevalent in any particular State. The provisions of Delhi Shops and Establishments Act are being discussed in the following sections as a model.

Objectives

(i) To provide for statutory obligations of the employers and rights of the employees in unorganized sector of employment, i.e. shops and establishments.

(ii) To provide for some minimum benefits and relief to the vast unorganized sector of employees employed. This Act is also applicable to the Chemists and Druggists shops.

Registration of Establishments

Under the Act, all shops and commercial establishments to which this Act extends, are required to be registered with the Chief Inspector of Shops within 30 days of the Act, by sending to him the prescribed fee and the following details in the prescribed form:

(i) The name and postal address of the establishment and the name of the employer or the manager, if any.

(ii) The category of the establishment, whether it is a shop, commercial establishment, residential hotel, restaurant, theatre or other place of public entertainment.

(iii) Number of employees working.

The Chief Inspector, on being satisfied about the correctness of the statement, shall register the establishment in the register of establishments and issue a certificate of registration. The registration certificate, issued by the Inspector, has to be prominently displayed in the establishment and should be renewed at prescribed intervals. In case, there is any difference of opinion between the Inspector and the occupier of the establishment regarding its categorization, the matter can be referred to the Government, whose decision is final.

In case the owner of an establishment makes any change in its name, address, managership or category, he shall communicate such change to the Chief Inspector within 15 days of the change. If the Chief Inspector is satisfied as to the correctness of the changes, he may change the entries in his register accordingly and amend the registration certificate or issue a new one if necessary. Likewise, the close down of an establishment must be notified to the Chief Inspector within 15 days of its closure. The Inspector may then remove the name of the establishment from his register. If, however, the Inspector feels that the establishment is likely to restart within six months, he may not remove the name of the establishment and may not cancel its registration certificate.

Work in Establishments

Hours and Timings for Work

Work hours

Adults (18 years and above)	Maximum 9 hours per day, but not more than 5 hours at a stretch and not more than 48 hours (54 hours during stock checking and accounts preparation) a week. Overtime to be paid at double rate per hour, recorded and notified to Chief Inspector 3 days in advance. The period of work, including the time for rest or meals should not be spread over for more than 10.5 hrs on one day.

Young Persons (between 12 and 18 years)	Maximum 6 hours per day (not more than 3.5 hrs at a stretch and maximum spread over per day 8 hours). Not to work between 9 p.m. to 7 a.m. (April to September) and 8 p.m. and 8 a.m. (October to March). The period of work including the time for rest or meals should not be spread over for more than 8 hours on one day. This applies for women as well. *No child, even a member of family, can be made to work as an employee or otherwise.*

Close Day

One day per week. Can be Sunday or any other day. Changeable once a year. In addition to the close day every shop and commercial establishment shall remain closed on three of the National holidays each year as the Government may, by notification in the Official Gazette, specify (it does not apply to pharmacies, and chemists and druggists).

Cleanliness, Ventilation and Lighting

The premises of every establishment shall be kept clean and free from effluvia arising from any drain or privy or other nuisance and shall be cleaned at such times and by such methods, as may be prescribed. These methods may include lime washing, colour washing, painting and disinfecting.

The premises of every establishment shall be kept sufficiently lighted and ventilated during all working hours and suitable arrangements shall be made for supply of drinking water to the employees.

Precautions against fire shall be taken as may be prescribed.

Service Conditions

A. Employment and Dismissals

The employer should furnish a letter of appointment to every employee containing the following particulars:

(i) Name of the employer and the establishment.
(ii) Postal address of the establishment.
(iii) Name, father's name and age of the employee.
(iv) Hours he will be required to work.
(v) Date of appointment.

No employer can dispense with the services of an employee, who has been in his service for three months, without giving him at least one month's notice in writing or in lieu thereof, one month's wages. But such notice is not necessary, if employee is dismissed for misconduct (provided he is given an opportunity to explain the charge or charges against him in writing).

Employees, if they have been in service for more than three months, are also required to give their employers one month's notice or pay a sum equal to their one month's salary, when they want to leave the employment.

If an employee has been dismissed without any reasonable cause or pay in lieu thereof and the magistrate to whom the employee has appealed is so satisfied, the magistrate may award the employee the following compensation, in addition to one month's salary:

- (i) An amount not exceeding one month's salary, if he was in receipt of a salary not exceeding Rs. 100 per month at the time of his dismissal.
- (ii) An amount not exceeding Rs. 100, if the employee's salary, at the time to his dismissal, was more than Rs. 100. No employee can bring a civil suit against the employer, if he has already been awarded the compensation stated above.

B. Wages

Every employer should fix periods, in respect of which the wages shall be payable to the employees. No wage payment period thus fixed should, however, exceed one month. All wages must be paid in cash and should be paid within 7 days of the expiry of the wage day. Where an employment has been terminated, due wages, if any, should be paid within a day of the termination of the employment. Deductions from the wages of an employee can be of one or more of the following kinds, namely:

- (i) Fines.
- (ii) Absence from duty.
- (iii) Loss or damage of goods directly attributable to the employee's default or neglect.
- (iv) House accommodation and other amenities and services provided by the employer.
- (v) Advance or over-payment of wages, provided the advances do not exceed an amount equal to two months wages and the monthly installments of deductions are not more than 1/4 the wages earned in that month.
- (vi) Income tax.
- (vii) Deductions required to be made by an order of the court or other competent authorities.
- (viii) Deductions for payment to a cooperative society or to a scheme of insurance, approved by the Government.

Any employer, desiring to impose a fine on an employed person or to make a deduction for damage or loss caused by him, has to explain him personally and also in writing the act or omission or the damage or loss, in respect of which the fine or deduction is proposed to be imposed or made, and give him an opportunity to offer any explanation in the presence of another person. The amount of the said fine or deduction shall also be intimated to him. All fines and deductions should be recorded in a register maintained for the purpose and should be utilized in accordance with the directions of the Government.

The Government may appoint an officer to hear and decide all claims arising out of delayed payment or non-payment of earned wages of an employee employed in any establishment. Such claims should be made to the authority specified in this behalf by the Government, within six months of the dispute. After the expiry of six months also, the authority may decide to hear the claim, if it is satisfied that there is sufficient reason for delaying such application beyond the normal period of six months. The authority shall hear the applicant and the employer, or give them an opportunity of being heard and after such further enquiry, may direct the payment to the employee of the amount due to him together with the payment of such compensation as the authority may think fit, not exceeding half the amount so due or Rs. 100, whichever is less. In case, the authority decides that the claim of the employee against his employer was a fictitious and a malicious one, it may direct the applicant to pay a penalty up to a maximum of Rs. 100. The decision of the authority shall be considered final. The provisions of Workmen's Compensation Act, 1923, and Rules thereunder apply to employees of shops and establishments.

C. Leave

Every person, employed in the shops and other commercial establishments, shall be entitled to the following kinds of leave:

(i) Privilege leave with full wages for not less than 15 days after 12 months of continuous employment. Privilege leave may be accumulated up to a maximum of 30 days.

(ii) Sickness or casual leave for not more than 12 days in a year with full wages. This leave shall not be accumulated.

When an employee completes a continuous period of 4 months in the service, he shall be entitled to not less than 5 days leave for every such period. Watchmen or caretakers, who have been in service for one year, shall be entitled to at least 30 days privilege leave. If an employee, to whom any leave is due, leaves the employment without having been allowed to avail his leave, he should be paid full wages for the period of leave due to him. The wages, during the leave period, shall be on the basis of the average daily earnings of the employee during the preceding three months, exclusive of any overtime but inclusive of dearness allowance.

Inspection of Establishments

The Government appoints a Chief Inspector and such other Inspectors as may be considered necessary for carrying out the provisions of this Act. The Inspectors, so appointed, shall carry identity cards with them. The Chief Inspectors are empowered, under the Act, to enter at all reasonable times any shop or establishment, with a view to inspect the premises and examine various registers and records required to be maintained under the Act. It shall be the duty of every occupier of a shop or establishment to produce for inspection of an Inspector, all accounts or records required to be kept for the purpose of this Act, and to give any other information in connection therewith as may be required. The Inspector may also make copies of or take extracts from any book, registers or other document maintained and exercise such other powers as may be necessary for the purpose of this Act. The Chief Inspector and every Inspector appointed shall be deemed to be public servant within the meaning of the Indian Penal Code. The Chief Inspector and other Inspectors appointed under this Act are immune from suits, prosecution and legal proceedings, if they do or intend to do anything in good faith.

Offences and Penalties

These are given in Table 13.1.

Table 13.1. Offences and Penalties

A. False entries and omission of entries in records/registers	Imprisonment up to 3 months or/and fine between Rs. 50 and Rs. 250 or both.
B. Obstruction to inspectors	A fine of Rs. 50 to Rs. 250.
C. Failure to keep records	A fine of Rs. 50 for every day on which the contravention occurs or continues.
D. Other offences	Contravention of any other provision of the Act, fine between Rs. 25 and Rs. 250.

Note: No prosecution can be tried in courts, without the previous sanction of the Chief Inspector, not inferior to that of a First Class Magistrate.

When the owner/occupier who is charged with any of the above offences under the Act proves satisfactorily that the offence was committed by his servant/agent without his knowledge and he had used his diligence to comply with the law, the servant or agent shall be liable to prosecution.

Miscellaneous

A. Saving of Other Laws

Any other law, in force for the time being, will be valid and an employee, entitled to any privileges and rights under any other law, contract or custom, before the passage of this Act, shall continue to enjoy such rights and privileges.

Nothing in this Act shall apply to:

Any office of or under the Central Government, or Delhi Administration, banks or any telegraph, telephone or postal service.

B. Exemptions to medical shops.

Shops dealing mainly in medicines or medical or surgical requisites are exempt from the provisions relating to 'opening & closing hours' and 'close day'. The Act also does not apply to establishments for treatment or care of infirm or mentally unfit persons providing indoor treatment or hospitals for the care of the sick.

C. Power to Make Rules

As per the Act, the Government is authorized to make Rules for giving effect to all provisions of the Shop and Establishments Act and to exempt any class of shops from such provisions.

QUESTIONS FOR REVISION

1. Write briefly the objectives and salient features of Shops and Establishment Act of the State.
2. Write short notes on:
   (a) Registration of establishments.
   (b) Hours of working, opening and closing, closing day and cleanliness of shops and establishments.
   (c) Service conditions under Shops and Establishments Act.
3. Outline the provisions of Shops and Establishments Act relating to hours of work and wages.
4. Discuss the following:
   (a) Leave for employees under Shops and Establishments Act.
   (b) Facilities given to women and young persons under Shops and Establishments Act.
   (c) Dismissal of an employee under Shops and Establishments Act.
   (d) Safety measures outlined in the Shops Act and Rules.

Chapter 14

The AICTE Act, 1987

The AICTE was constituted in 1945 as an advisory body in all matters relating to technical education. Even though it had no statutory powers, it played a very important role in the development of technical education in the country. It had four Regional Committees with offices at Chennai, Mumbai, Kanpur and Calcutta. All the new schemes and proposals for starting new Institutions/Programmes were approved by the corresponding Regional Committee and subsequently vetted by the Council.

There was large-scale expansion of technical education in the late fifties and early sixties and again in the eighties. While the expansion in the fifties was done with the approval of the AICTE and the Government of India, the expansion in the eighties was localised mostly in the four States of Karnataka, Maharashtra, Tamil Nadu and Andhra Pradesh and was primarily in the self-financing sector without the approval of the AICTE and Government of India. It was in this period that the National Policy on Education-1986 made a specific mention of the need to make AICTE a statutory body.

In view of the above, AICTE became a statutory body through an Act of Parliament 52, in 1987. The Council, i.e. AICTE was established with a view to the proper planning and coordinated development of the technical education system throughout the country, the promotion of qualitative improvement of such education in relation to planned quantitative growth and the regulation and proper maintenance of norms and standards in the technical education system for matters connected therewith. Technical education was defined as programmes of education, research and training in engineering, technology, architecture, town planning, management, pharmacy and applied arts and crafts and such other programmes or areas as the Central Government may, in consultation with the Council, by notification in the Official Gazette, declare. The Act also laid down the powers, functions and structure of the AICTE.

Pharmacy is an interdisciplinary program utilizing scientific principles of engineering and technology to make various dosage forms. Due to the technical aspect of the course, it was brought within the purview of All India Council for Technical Education (AICTE), after it came into existence as a statutory body in 1987.

The Act has had a profound impact on the qualitative and quantitative growth of pharmaceutical education in India.

Objectives of the AICTE Act, 1987

The main objectives of the Act are:

(i) Proper planning and coordinated development of technical education throughout India.

(ii) The promotion of qualitative improvement in technical education.

(iii) The regulative and proper maintenance of norms and standards in the technical education.

Definitions

(a) Technical Education

Technical education means programmes of education, research and training in engineering, technology, architecture, town planning, management, pharmacy and applied arts and crafts and such other programme or areas as the Central Government may notify.

(b) Technical Institution

Technical institution means an institution, not being a university, which offers courses or programmers of technical education.

Composition and Functions of the Council

The All India Council for Technical Education consists of the following members:

(i) A Chairman and a Vice-chairman, appointed by the Central Government.

(ii) The Secretary to the Government of India in the Ministry of Education, ex-officio.

(iii) The Educational Advisor (General) to the Government of India, ex-officio.

(iv) The Chairmen of the Regional Committees of AICTE, ex-officio.
(v) The Chairmen of all the All India Boards, ex-officio.
(vi) One member to represent the Ministry of Finance.
(vii) One member to represent the Ministry of Science and Technology.
(viii) Four members to represent other ministries.
(ix) Two members of Parliament, one each from Lok Sabha and Rajya Sabha.
(x) Eight members to represent the States and Union territories.
(xi) Four members representing organizations in the fields of industry and commerce.
(xii) Seven members representing:
  (a) The Central Advisory Board of Education
  (b) The Association of Indian Universities.
  (c) The Indian Society for Technical Education.
  (d) The Council of the Indian Institutes of Technology.
  (e) The Pharmacy Council of India.
  (f) The Council of Architecture.
  (g) The National Productivity Council.
(xiii) Four members representing professional bodies in the field of technical and management education.
(xiv) Two members representing interests not included in the above.
(xv) The Chairman, University Grants Commission, ex-officio.
(xvi) The Director, Institutes of Applied Manpower Research, ex-officio.
(xvii) The Director-General, Council of Scientific and Industrial Research, ex-officio.
(xviii) The Director-General, Indian Council for Agricultural Research, ex-officio.
(xix) The Member-Secretary, appointed by the Central Government.

The Council can meet any number of times but shall meet at least once every year. The term of office of a member, other than an ex-officio member, on the first constitution of the Council shall be five years and thereafter three years.

Functions of the Council

The Council is empowered to take such actions which ensure coordinated and integrated development of technical and management education and to maintain their standards. It may:

(i) Lay down norms and standards for courses, curriculum, physical and instructional facilities, staff pattern, staff qualifications, quality instruction, assessment and examinations.
(ii) Fix norms and guidelines for charging tuition and other fees.

(iii) Grant approval for starting new technical institutions and for introduction of new courses and programmes.
(iv) Undertake survey in various fields of technical education and make forecast of the needed growth and development in technical education.
(v) Allocate and disburse grants for technical institutions and universities imparting technical education.
(vi) Promote innovations, research and development.
(vii) Formulate schemes for promoting technical education for women, handicapped and weaker sections of the society.
(viii) Promote linkages between technical education system and industry.
(ix) Evolve suitable performance appraisal systems for mechanical institutions incorporating systems for technical institutions incorporating norms and mechanisms for enforcing accountability.
(x) Formulate schemes for initial, in-service and continuing education of teachers.
(xi) Prevent commercialization of technical education.
(xii) Inspect or cause to inspect any technical education institution.
(xiii) Set up a National Board of Accreditation to periodically conduct evaluation of technical institutions or programmes on the basis of guidelines, norms and standards specified.

Different Bodies of the Council

Following are different bodies of Council:

(i) Executive Committee

The Council shall constitute a Committee, called the Executive Committee, for discharging such functions as may be assigned to it by the Council. The Executive Committee shall consist of the following members:

(i) The Chairman of the Council.
(ii) The Vice-chairman of the Council.
(iii) The Secretary, Ministry of Education, ex-officio.
(iv) Two Chairmen of the Regional Committees.
(v) Three Chairmen of the Board of Studies.
(vi) A member of the Council, representing the Ministry of Finance, ex-officio.
(vii) Four out of eight members of the Council representing the States and the Union Territories.
(viii) Four members with expertise and distinction in areas relevant to technical education to be nominated by the Chairman of the Council.
(ix) The Chairman of the University Grants Commission, ex-officio.

(x) The Director, Institute of Applied Manpower Research, ex-officio.
(xi) The Director-General, Indian Council of Agricultural Research, ex-officio.
(xii) The Member-Secretary of the Council.

The Chairman and the Member-Secretary of the Council shall respectively function as the Chairman and Member-Secretary of the Executive Committee.

(ii) Board of Studies

The Council shall establish the following Boards of Studies:
(i) All India Board of Vocational Education.
(ii) All India Board of Technical Education.
(iii) All India Board of Under-graduate Studies in Engineering and Technology.
(iv) All India Board of Post-graduate Education and Research in Engineering and Technology.
(v) All India Board of Management Studies.
(vi) Such other Boards as it may consider necessary.

Every Board of Studies shall advise the Executive Committee on academic matters falling in its area of concern including norms, standards, model curricula, model facilities and structure of courses.

An All India Board of Pharmaceutical Education (AIB-PE) started functioning since 1994 with Professor J.S. Qadry as its first Chairman. Recently a model syllabus for B.Pharmacy course designed to meet the professional needs by incorporating the recent developments in the field of Pharmaceutical sciences has been made available. Professor C.K. Kokate is the current Chairman of All India Board of Pharmaceutical Education and it is hoped that the model B.Pharmacy syllabus will bring uniformity and enhance the standards of pharmaceutical education. It is likely that in near future, recommendations for post-graduate courses in pharmacy will also be made available.

(iii) Regional Committees

The Council shall establish the following Regional Committees in various parts of the country:
(i) The Northern Regional Committee with its office at Kanpur
(ii) The Southern Regional Committee with its office at Chennai.
(iii) The Western Regional Committee with its office at Mumbai
(iv) The Eastern Regional Committee with its office at Kolkata.
(v) Such other Regional Committees as it may consider necessary.

Additional regional offices at Chandigarh (North Western) and Bhopal, (Central) have also been established and are functioning.

Miscellaneous provisions under AICTE Act

Power to Supersede the Council

If the Central Government is of the opinion that the Council is unable to perform or has persistently failed to perform the duties imposed on it under this Act or has exceeded or abused its powers, it may, by notification in the Official Gazette, supersede the Council for such periods, as may be specified in the notification.

However, before issuing any such notification, the Central Government shall give a reasonable time to the Council to explain its conduct.

Power to Make Rules

The Central Government may, by notification in the Official Gazette, make Rules to carry out the purposes of this Act. Such Rules may provide for all or any of the following matters:

(i) The procedure to be followed by the members in discharge of their functions.
(ii) The inspection of technical institutions and universities.
(iii) The form and manner in which the budget and reports are to be prepared by the Council.
(iv) The manner in which the accounts of the Council are to be maintained.
(v) Any other matter which has to be, or may be, prescribed.

Power to make Regulations

The Council may, by notification in the Official Gazette, make regulation, not inconsistent with the provisions of this Act, in order to carry out the purposes of this Act. Such regulations may provide for all or any of the following matters:

(i) The terms and conditions of service of the officers and employees of the Council.
(ii) Regulating the meetings of the Council and the procedure for conducting business thereat.
(iii) Regulating the meetings of the Executive Committee and the procedure for conducting business thereat.
(iv) The area of concern, the constitution, and powers and functions of the Board of Studies.
(v) The region for which the Regional Committee be established and the constitution and functions of such Committee.

QUESTIONS FOR REVISION

1. Write the main objectives of the AICTE Act and how can they be achieved?
2. What is the constitution of the Council under the AICTE Act?
3. Enumerate the different bodies of the Council. Write the constitution of Executive Committee of the Council.
4. Define technical education and technical institution. Explain the powers and functions of AICTE.

Chapter 15

The Factories Act, 1948

The conditions of the workers, employed in the factories, has usually been pathetic. They are made to work for longer durations, without being paid for the extra time. At times they are not paid regularly and are made to work in unhygienic conditions without providing them the basic amenities. Children are employed for hazardous works. The Factories Act is a social legislation, which has been enacted for occupational safety, health and welfare of workers at work places.

To regulate the working conditions in the factories and to provide them with the basic facilities, benefits, and relief to the workers, the Factories Act, 1948 was passed. The Act was enforced from 1st April, 1949 and it was amended in 1950, 1951, 1954 and 1976. When last amended in June, 1980 it had 120 Sections. It extends to the whole of India. This legislation is being enforced by technical officers i.e. Inspectors of Factories, Dy. Chief Inspectors of Factories who work under the control of the Chief Inspector of Factories and overall control of the Labour Commissioner, Government of National Capital Territory of Delhi.

On the basis of the Central Factories Act, each State has framed its own Factories Rules for the implementation and administration of the Act, like licensing, registration of factories, welfare of workers, etc. It applies to factories covered under the Factories Act, 1948. The industries in which ten (10) or more than ten workers are employed on any day of the preceding twelve months and are engaged in manufacturing process being carried out with the aid of power or twenty or more than twenty workers are employed in manufacturing process being carried out without the aid of power, are covered under the provisions of this Act.

List of Amending Acts and Adaptation Order

1. The Repealing and Amending Act, 1949 (40 of 1949).
2. The Adaptation of Laws Order, 1950.
3. The Repealing and Amending Act, 1950 (35 of 1950).
4. The Part B States (Laws) Act, 1951 (3 of 1951).
5. The Factories (Amendment) Act, 1954 (25 of 1954).
6. The Central Labour Laws (Extension to Jammu & Kashmir) Act, 1970 (51 of 1970).
7. The Factories (Amendment) Act, 1976 (94 of 1976).
8. The Factories (Amendment) Act, 1987 (20 of 1987).

Objectives of the Act

1. To regulate, control and check compliance of provisions of this Act relating to the Safety, Working hours, Employment of young persons and Annual Leave with wages, etc.
2. To provide for healthy and sanitary conditions for workers at their work place.
3. To prevent hazardous growth of the factories through the provisions related to approval of plans before the creation of the factories.

Definitions

1. "**Adult**" means a person who has completed his eighteenth year of age.
2. "**Adolescent**" means a person who has completed his fifteenth year of age but has not completed his eighteenth year.
3. "**Calendar year**" means the period of twelve months beginning with the first day of January in any year.
4. "**Child**" means a person who has not completed his fifteenth year of age.
5. "**Competent person**", in relation to any provision of this Act, means a person or an institution recognized as such by the Chief Inspector for the purposes of carrying out tests, examinations and inspections, required to be done in a factory under the provisions of this Act, having regard to:
    (i) the qualifications and experience of the person and facilities available at his disposal; or
    (ii) the qualifications and experience of the persons employed in such institution and facilities available therein, with regard to the conduct of such tests, examinations and inspections, and more than one person or institution can be recognized as a competent person in relation to a factory.

6. **"Hazardous process"** means any process or activity in relation to an industry specified in the First Schedule where, unless special care is taken, raw materials used therein or the intermediate or finished products, bye-products, wastes, or effluents thereof would:
    (i) cause material impairment to the health of the persons engaged in or connected therewith; or
    (ii) result in the pollution of the general environment.
7. **"Young person"** means a person who is either a child or an adolescent.
8. **"Day"** means a period of twenty-four hours beginning at midnight,
9. **"Week"** means a period of seven days beginning at midnight on Saturday night or such other night as may be approved, in writing for a particular area, by the Chief Inspector of Factories.
10. **"Power"** means electrical energy, or any other form of energy, which is mechanically transmitted and is not generated by human or animal agency.
11. **"Prime mover"** means any engine, motor or other appliance which generates or otherwise provides power.
12. **"Transmission machinery"** means any shaft, wheel, drum, pulley, system of pulleys, coupling, clutch, driving belt or other appliance or device by which the motion of a prime mover is transmitted to or received by any machinery or appliance.
13. **"Machinery"** includes prime movers, transmission machinery and all other appliances whereby power is generated, transformed, transmitted or applied.
14. **"Manufacturing process"** means any process for:
    (i) making, altering, repairing, ornamenting, finishing, packing, oiling, washing, cleaning, breaking up, demolishing, or otherwise treating or adapting any article or substance with a view to its use, sale, transport, delivery or disposal; or
    (ii) pumping oil, water, sewage or any other substance; or
    (iii) generating, transforming or transmitting power; or
    (iv) composing types for printing, by letter press, lithography, photogravure or other similar process or book binding; or
    (v) constructing, reconstructing, repairing, refitting, finishing or breaking up ships or vessels; or
    (vi) preserving or storing any article in cold storage.
15. **"Worker"** means a person [employed, directly or by or through any agency (including a contractor) with or without the knowledge of the principal employer, whether for remuneration or not], in any manufacturing process, or in cleaning any part of the machinery or premises used for a manufacturing process, or in any other kind of work incidental to, or connected with, the manufacturing process, or

the subject of the manufacturing process [but does not include any member of the armed forces of the Union].
16. **"Factory"** means any premises including the precincts thereof:
   (i) whereon ten or more workers are working, or were working on any day of the preceding twelve months, and in any part of which, a manufacturing process is being carried on with the aid of power, or is ordinarily so carried on; or
   (ii) whereon twenty or more workers are working, or were working on any day of the preceding twelve months, and in any part of which, a manufacturing process is being carried on without the aid of power, or is ordinarily so carried on but does not include a mine subject to the operation of [the Mines Act, 1952 (35 of 1952)] or [a mobile unit belonging to the armed forces of the Union, a railway running shed or a hotel, restaurant or eating place].

Approval, Licensing and Registration of Factories

Before starting the operations of a factory, an approval has to be taken from the State Licensing Authority, the Chief Inspector of the Factories (CIF), subsequently the factory is registered.

The State Government may make Rules regarding the submission of plans for approval, the nature and specifications plans for approval, the fees payable for registration and licensing and for the renewal of licences.

Procedure for obtaining the Licence

An application is to be sent to the State Government or Chief Inspectors along with the following:
   (i) Building Plan.
   (ii) Position of the machineries to be described in the plan with the dimensions of the machine.
   (iii) Challan for the payment of the prescribed fees.

If any changes or modifications are suggested by the CIF, they have to be incorporated by the applicant, and if satisfied, the CIF issues the licence.

If no order is communicated to the applicant within three months from the date on which an application for permission accompanied with required documents was sent to State Government by registered post, the permission applied for in the said application shall be deemed to have been granted.

Where a State Government or a Chief Inspector refuses to grant permission to the site, construction or extension of a factory or to the registration and licensing of a factory, the applicant may, within thirty days of the date of such refusal, appeal to the Central Government, if the decision appealed from was of the State Government and to the State Government, in any other case.

Notice by occupier

On obtaining the licence, the occupier of the factory is required to send a written notice, at least fifteen days before he begins to occupy or use any premises as a factory, to the Chief Inspector containing:

  (i) The name and situation of the factory.
  (ii) The name and address of the occupier.
  (iii) The name and address of the owner of the premises or building.
  (iv) The address to which communications relating to the factory may be sent.
  (v) The nature of the manufacturing process.
  (vi) The total rated horse power of electricity installed or to be installed in the factory.
  (vii) The name of the manager of the factory for the purposes of this Act.
  (viii) The number of workers likely to be employed in the factory.
  (ix) The average number of workers per day employed during the last twelve months in the case of a factory, in existence on the date of the commencement of this Act.
  (x) Such other particulars asked by the CIF.

Whenever a new manager is appointed, the occupier shall inform to the CIF, within seven days from the date on which such person takes over charge.

If no person has been designated as manager of a factory, or the person designated does not manage the factory, or if no such person is found, the occupier himself, shall be deemed to be the manager of the factory for the purposes of this Act.

General duties of the occupier

1. Every occupier shall ensure, so far as is reasonably practicable, the health, safety and welfare of all workers while they are at work in the factory.
2. The matters to which such duty extends, shall include:
   (a) maintenance of plant and systems of work in the factory that are safe and without risks to health;
   (b) ensuring safety and absence of risks to health in connection with the use, handling, storage and transport of articles and substances;
   (c) instruction, training and supervision to ensure the health and safety of all workers at work;
   (d) maintenance or monitoring of safe working environment in the factory and provide adequate facilities and arrangements for their welfare at work.

Inspectors and their Powers

The State Government may, by notification in the Official Gazette, appoint Inspectors with prescribed qualification, Chief Inspectors, Joint Chief Inspectors and Deputy Chief Inspectors, as may think necessary.

An Inspector, within the local limits for which he is appointed, may:

(i) enter a factory, make examination of the premises, plant, machinery, article or substance, inquire into any accident or dangerous occurrence, seize, or take copies of any register, record or other document and direct the occupier that the premises shall be left undisturbed as long as it is necessary for the purpose of any examination;

(ii) take measurements and photographs and make such recordings, take with him if necessary any instrument or equipment or exercise such other powers as may be prescribed.

Certifying surgeons

The State Government may appoint qualified medical practitioners to be certifying surgeons for the examination and certification of young persons.

Health and Safety of Workers

1. Cleanliness

Every factory shall be kept clean and free from effluvia arising from any drain, privy or other nuisance, and in particular:

(a) Accumulation of dirt and refuse shall be removed daily from everywhere.
(b) The floor of every workroom shall be cleaned at least once in every week by washing, using disinfectant, or by some other effective method.
(c) Providing effective means of drainage if a floor is liable to become wet.
(d) All inside walls and partitions, all ceilings or tops of rooms and all walls, sides and tops of passages and staircases shall be painted and varnished. All doors and window frames and other wooden or metallic framework and shutters shall be kept painted or varnished and records maintained of the procedures in the prescribed register.

2. Disposal of Wastes and Effluents

It is essential that effective arrangements be made in every factory for the treatment of wastes and effluents, due to the manufacturing process carried on therein, so as to render them innocuous, and for their proper disposal.

3. Ventilation and Temperature

There should be effective and suitable provision in every factory for adequate ventilation by the circulation of fresh air, and such a temperature as will secure to workers therein reasonable conditions of comfort and prevent injury to health.

4. Dust and Fumes

Effective measures shall be taken to prevent its inhalation and accumulation in any workroom, of the dust, fume or other impurity. No stationary internal combustion engine shall be operated unless exhausted properly.

5. Artificial humidification

The State Government may make Rules for prescribing standards of humidification, methods regulating it.

The water used for the purpose shall be taken from a public supply, or other source of drinking water, or shall be effectively purified before it is so used.

6. Overcrowding, Lighting, Drinking Water, Latrines and Spittoons

No room in any factory shall be overcrowded to an extent injurious to the health of the workers employed therein. Sufficient clean latrine and urinal accommodation of prescribed types shall be provided conveniently situated and accessible to workers at all times while they are at the factory and separate enclosed accommodation shall be provided for male and female workers. In every factory there shall be provided a sufficient number of spittoons at convenient places and they shall be maintained in a clean and hygienic condition.

7. Safety

In every factory the machines requiring bolts and grouting shall be fixed accordingly. Fencing of machinery is done, where moving parts may hurt the workers while working. Guards shall be provided to machines with moving belts. Every dangerous part of any other machinery shall be securely fenced by safeguards of substantial construction, while the parts of machinery they are fencing are in motion or in use.

Work on or near machinery in motion

Where in any factory it becomes necessary to examine any part of machinery, while the machinery is in motion, or, to carry out lubrication or other adjusting operation, it shall be made or carried out only by a specially trained adult male worker wearing tight-fitting clothing (which shall be supplied by the occupier).

No woman or young person shall be allowed to clean, lubricate or adjust any part of a prime mover or of any transmission machinery, while the prime mover or transmission machinery is in motion, or to clean, lubricate or adjust any part of any machine if the cleaning, lubrication or adjustment thereof would expose the woman or young person to risk of injury from any moving part, either of that machine or of any adjacent machinery.

Employment of young persons on dangerous machines
No young person shall be required or allowed to work at any machine unless he has received sufficient training in work at the machine, or is under adequate supervision by a person who has a thorough knowledge and experience of the machine.

The speeds indicated in revolving machinery shall not be exceeded.

Prohibition of employment of women and children near cotton-openers
No woman or child shall be employed in any part of a factory for pressing cotton in which a cotton opener is at work.

Pressure plant
If in any factory, any plant or machinery or any part thereof is operated at a pressure above atmospheric pressure, effective measures shall be taken to ensure that the safe working pressure of such plant or machinery or part thereof, is not exceeded.

Protection of eyes
Effective screens or suitable goggles shall be provided for the protection of persons employed, if any such manufacturing process, carried out in any factory, involves risk of injury to the eyes.

Precautions against dangerous fumes, gases, etc.
If in any factory, any gas, fume, vapour or dust is likely to be present to such an extent as to involve risk to persons, no person shall be required or allowed to enter any chamber, tank, vat, pit, pipe, flue or other confined space, unless it is provided with a manhole of adequate size or other effective means of egress and until all practicable measures have been taken to remove any gas, fume, vapour or dust, which may be present so as to bring its level within the permissible limits and to prevent any ingress of such gas, fume, vapour or dust and unless it is provided with a manhole of adequate size or other effective means of egress.

Precautions regarding the use of portable electric light
In any factory, no portable electric light or any other electric appliance of voltage exceeding twenty-four volts shall be permitted for use inside any

chamber, tank, vat, pit, pipe, flue or other confined space, unless provided with adequate safety devices.

Explosive or inflammable dust, gas, etc.

Where in any factory any manufacturing process produces dust, gas, fume or vapour of such character and to such extent as to be likely to explode to ignition, all practicable measures shall be taken to prevent any such explosion by:

(a) Effective enclosure of the plant or machinery used in the process.
(b) Removal or prevention of the accumulation of such dust, gas, fume or vapour.
(c) Exclusion or effective enclosure of all possible sources of ignition.

Precautions in case of fire

In every factory, all practicable measures shall be taken to prevent outbreak of fire and its spread, both internally and externally, and to provide and maintain safe means of escape for all persons in the event of a fire, and the necessary equipment and facilities for extinguishing fire. The workers should be familiar with the means of escape and trained adequately.

Safety of building and machinery and its maintenance

If any building or part of a building or machinery is in such a condition that it is dangerous to human life or safety, the authority may prohibit its use until it has been properly repaired or altered.

Safety officers

In every factory, wherein one thousand or more workers are ordinarily employed, or operation involving any risk of bodily injury, poisoning or disease, or any other hazard to health, to the persons employed in the factory are carried out, the occupier shall employ such number of Safety Officers as may be specified in the notification.

Welfare

In every factory:
(a) adequate and suitable facilities for washing for men and women separately shall be provided;
(b) facilities of first-aid appliances, for changing clothes, keeping clothes not worn, shelters, rest rooms and lunch rooms shall be provided for the use of male and female workers; such facilities shall be conveniently accessible and shall be kept clean;
(c) canteens and crèches for children under the age group of six years shall be provided as per the specifications.

In every factory the occupier shall employ Welfare Officer as may be prescribed by the State Government. The State Government may prescribe the duties, qualifications and conditions of service of officer employed.

Working Hours of Adults and Holidays

Weekly hours and Daily hours

No adult worker shall be required or allowed to work in a factory for more than forty-eight hours in any week. No adult worker shall be required or allowed to work in a factory for more than nine hours in any day.

Weekly holidays

Weekly holidays shall be allowed and where, as a result of the passing of an order, a worker is deprived of any of the weekly holidays, he shall be allowed compensatory holidays, as per the Act of the State.

Shifts and Overtime

In factories, wherever work is carried out by means of and system of shifts, no worker shall be allowed or required to work continuously in two successive shifts.

In a factory, if any worker works for more than nine hours in any day and more than forty-eight hours in any week, he shall be entitled to wages at the rate, as decided by the Act of the State Government for overtime work.

Restriction on double employment and Notice of periods of work

No adult worker shall be required or allowed to work in a factory on any day, on which he has already been working in any other factory, except in such circumstances as may be prescribed.

A display of notice shall be there for periods of work for adults showing clearly for every day the period during which adult workers may be required to work.

Register of adult workers

The manager of every factory shall maintain a register of adult workers, to be available to the Inspector at all times during working hours, or when any work is being carried out in the factory, showing:
  (i) The name of each adult worker in the factory.
  (ii) The nature of his work.
  (iii) The group, if any, in which he is included.
  (iv) Where his group works on shifts, the relay to which he is allotted.
  (v) Such other particulars as may be prescribed.

Employment of Young Persons

Prohibition of employment of young children

No child, who has not completed his fourteenth year, shall be required or allowed to work in a factory.

No female adolescent or a male adolescent, who has not attained the age of seventeen years, shall be required to work in any factory except between 6 a.m. and 7 p.m. The State Government may vary the limits but no female adolescent shall be employed between 10 p.m. and 5 a.m. in any case.

Annual Leave with Wages

Every worker who has worked for a period of 240 days or more in a calendar year, shall be allowed, during the subsequent calendar year, leave with wages for and number of days as per the Act of the State Government.

The State Government may exempt any factory from the provisions of Leave Rules if it is satisfied that Leave Rules applicable to workers are more beneficial to them than those provided under this Act.

Different provisions related to hazardous processes under Factories Act, 1948

Disclosure of information, involving a hazardous process, is compulsory by the occupier. The occupier shall lay down a detailed policy with respect to the health and safety of the workers employed and shall have disaster control measures.

Every occupier of a factory involving any hazardous process is required to maintain health records, appoint persons who possess qualifications and experience in handling hazardous substances and provide medical examination of every worker.

The State Government may appoint a competent person to enquire into the causes of any accident occurring in a factory or where disease, specified in the Third Schedule, has been, or is suspected. It may also appoint one or more persons possessing legal or special knowledge to act as assessors in such inquiry.

General Penalty for Offences

Apart from as otherwise provided, if in any factory there is contravention of any of the provisions of this Act or of Rule made thereunder or of any order in writing given thereunder, the occupier and manager of the factory each be guilty of an offence, punishable with imprisonment for a term as specified in the Act or with fine as per the Rules or with both.

Liability of owner of premises in certain circumstances

Where in any premises separate buildings are leased to different occupiers for use as separate factories, the owner of the premises shall be responsible for the provision and maintenance of common facilities and services, such as approach roads, drainage, water supply, lighting and sanitation.

Where in any premises, independent or self-contained floor or flats are leased to different occupiers for use as separate factories, the owner of the premises shall be liable as if he was the occupier or manager of a factory, for any contravention of the provisions of this Act as specified.

Penalty for Obstructing Inspector

Whoever willfully obstructs an Inspector, in the exercise of any power conferred on him by or under this Act, or fails to produce on demand by an Inspector any registers or other documents in his custody or conceals or prevents any worker in a factory from appearing/being examined by an Inspector, shall be punishable with imprisonment for a term or with fine or with both as per the Act of the State Government.

Offences by Workers

If any worker employed in a factory contravenes any provision of this Act or any Rules or order made thereunder, imposing any duty or liability on workers, he shall be punished with fine as per the Act.

Where a worker is convicted of an offence punishable, the occupier or manager of the factory shall not be deemed to be guilty of that offence, unless it is proved, that he failed to take all reasonable measures for its prevention.

Cognizance of Offences and Limitation of Prosecution

No court shall take cognizance of any offence under this Act except on complaint by, or with the previous sanction in writing of, an Inspector. Further, no Court below that of a Presidency Magistrate or of the Magistrate of the First Class shall try any offence punishable under this Act.

No Court shall take cognizance of any offence punishable under this Act unless complaint thereof is made within three months of the date on which the alleged commission of the offence came to the knowledge of an Inspector.

Appeals

The manager of a factory on whom an order in writing by an Inspector has been served under the provisions of this Act or the occupier of the factory may, within thirty days of the service of the order, appeal against it to the prescribed authority, and such authority may, subject to Rules made in this behalf by the State Government, confirm, modify or reverse the Order.

QUESTIONS FOR REVISION

1. What are the objectives of Factories Act?
2. Explain the procedure to get a factory licence and what are the conditions imposed while issuing the licence.
3. Write a note on the provisions of Factories Act and Rules for safeguarding the health and safety of workers.

Chapter 16

The Legal Metrology Act, 2009

"Legal metrology" means that part of metrology which treats units of weighment and measurement, methods of weighment and measurement and weighing and measuring instruments, in relation to the mandatory technical and legal requirements which have the objects of ensuring public guarantee from the point of view of security and accuracy of the weighments and measurements.

The organization of Weights & Measures was established in 1958 with the object of bringing about the uniformity in Weights & Measures in accordance with the international standards, so as to facilitate trade and commerce. The *Standards of Weights and Measures Act, 1976* providing for establishing Standards of Weights and Measures, regulation of inter-State trade or commerce in weights and measures and other goods which are sold by weight, measure or number was enacted in 1976. In the year 1985, the *Standards of Weights and Measures (Enforcement) Act, 1985* was enacted for enforcement of standards of weights and measures established by or under the 1976 Act. To ensure that all weights or measures used for trade or commerce, for industrial production or for protection of human health and safety are accurate and reliable so that users are guaranteed of their performance and quality as well as the consumer gets the right quantity which he pays for, this Act was enacted to establish standards of weights and measures. With the view to establish the standards of Weights & Measures, regulate, trade and commerce in Weights & Measures and other goods which are sold or distributed by weight, measure or number and for matter connected therewith, the *Legal Metrology Act, 2009* was implemented with effect from 1st April, 2011 and it thereby repealed the Act, the *Standards of Weights and Measures Act, 1976* and the *Standards of Weights and Measures (Enforcement) Act, 1985*.

The Legal Metrology Act, 2009 is "An act to establish and enforce standards of weights and measures, regulate trade and commerce in weights, measures and other goods which are sold or distributed by weights, measure or number and for matters connected therewith or incidental thereto".

Legal Metrology Act, 2009 was enacted as it became essential for the Government to combine the provisions of the existing two Acts to get rid of anomalies and make the provisions simple. It also became necessary to keep the regulation practical so as to protect the interest of consumers.

For the implementation of Legal Metrology Act, 2009 the following Rules have been framed:

(i) The Legal Metrology (Packaged Commodities) Rules, 2011
(ii) The Legal Metrology (Approval of Models) Rules, 2011
(iii) The Legal Metrology (Numeration) Rules, 2010
(iv) The Legal Metrology (General) Rules, 2011
(v) The Legal Metrology (National Standards) Rules, 2011
(vi) The Indian Institute of Legal Metrology Rules, 2011
(vii) The Legal Metrology (Government Approved Test Centre) Rules, 2013.

The State Governments have also framed their State Legal Metrology (Enforcement) Rules for the implementation of the Act, 2009.

There are following zonal offices/institutes/laboratories in the field of Legal Metrology:

(a) **Indian Institute of Legal Metrology Ranchi:** Responsible for providing training in the field of Legal Metrology to the Legal Metrology Officers of Central and State Governments.
(b) **Regional Reference Standard Laboratories situated at Ahmedabad, Bangalore, Bhubaneswar, Faridabad and Guwahati:** These laboratories are working as central agencies between apex laboratory and State Government Laboratories for traceability of standards. These laboratories are also responsible for the testing of models of weights and measures, verification of secondary standards of State Government, calibration of sophisticated weighing and measuring instruments, consumer awareness program, etc.

Definitions

1. **"Legal Metrology"** means that part of metrology which treats units of weighment and measurement, methods of weighment and measurement

and weighing and measuring instruments, in relation to the mandatory technical and legal requirements, which have the object of ensuring public guarantee from the point of view of security and accuracy of the weighments and measurements.

2. "**Legal metrology officer**" means Additional Director, Additional Controller, Joint Director, Joint Controller, Deputy Director, Deputy Controller, Assistant Director, Assistant Controller and Inspector appointed under Sections 13 and 14.

3. "**Label**" means any written, marked, stamped, printed or graphic matter affixed to, or appearing upon, any pre-packaged commodity.

4. "**Premises**" includes:
   (i) a place where any business, industry, production or transaction is carried on by a person, whether by himself or through an agent, by whatever name called, including the person who carries on the business in such premises;
   (ii) a warehouse, godown or other place where any weight or measure or other goods are stored or exhibited;
   (iii) a place where any books of account or other documents pertaining to any trade or transaction are kept;
   (iv) a dwelling house, if any part thereof is used for the purpose of carrying on any business, industry, production or trade;
   (v) a vehicle or vessel or any other mobile device, with the help of which any transaction or business is carried on.

5. "**Prescribed**" means prescribed by Rules made under this Act.

6. "**Protection**" means the utilisation of reading obtained from any weight or measure, for the purpose of determining any step which is required to be taken to safeguard the well-being of any human being or animal, or to protect any commodity, vegetation or thing, whether individually or collectively.

7. "**Pre-packaged commodity**" means a commodity which without the purchaser being present is placed in a package of whatever nature, whether sealed or not, so that the product contained therein has a pre-determined quantity.

8. "**Repairer**" means a person who repairs a weight or measure and includes a person who adjusts, cleans, lubricates or paints any weight or measure or renders any other service to such weight or measure to ensure that such weight or measure conforms to the standards established by or under this Act.

9. "**Sale**", with its grammatical variations and cognate expressions, means transfer of property in any weight, measure or other goods by one person to another for cash or for deferred payment or for any other

valuable consideration and includes a transfer of any weight, measure or other goods on the hire-purchase system or any other system of payment by instalments, but does not include a mortgage or hypothecation of, or a charge or pledge on, such weight, measure or other goods.

10. "**Seal**" means a device or process by which a stamp is made, and includes any wire or other accessory which is used for ensuring the integrity of any stamp.
11. "**Stamp**" means a mark, made by impressing, casting, engraving, etching, branding, affixing pre-stressed paper seal or any other process in relation to any weight or measure with a view to:
    (i) certifying that such weight or measure conforms to the standard specified by or under this Act, or
    (ii) indicating that any mark which was previously made thereon certifying that such weight or measure conforms to the standards specified by or under this Act, has been obliterated.
12. "**Transaction**" means:
    (i) any contract, whether for sale, purchase, exchange or any other purpose, or
    (ii) any assessment of royalty, toll, duty or other dues, or
    (iii) the assessment of any work done, wages due or services rendered.
13. "**Verification**", with its grammatical variations and cognate expressions, includes, in relation to any weight or measure, the process of comparing, checking, testing or adjusting such weight or measure with a view to ensuring that such weight or measure conforms to the standards established by or under this Act and also includes re-verification and calibration.
14. "**Weight**" or "**Measure**" means a weight or measure specified by or under this Act and includes a weighing or measuring instrument.

Objectives

The main objectives of the Legal Metrology Act, 2009 are:

(a) Regulation of weight or measure used in transaction or for protection.
(b) Approval of model of weight or measure.
(c) Verification of prescribed weight or measure by Government approved Test Centre.
(d) Prescribing qualification of Legal Metrology Officers appointed by the Central Government or State Government;
(e) Exempting regulation of weight or measure or other goods meant for export.
(f) Levy of fee for various services.

(g) Nomination of a Director by a company who will be responsible for complying with the provisions of the enactment.
(h) Penalty for offences and compounding of offences.
(i) Appeal against decision of various authorities.
(j) Empowering the Central Government to make Rules for enforcing the provisions of the enactment.

Salient Features

The salient features of the Act are as follows:

1. Every unit of weight or measure shall be in accordance with the metric system based of the international system of units. The base of unit of
     (i) length shall be the metre;
     (ii) mass shall be the kilogram;
     (iii) time shall be the second;
     (iv) electric current shall be the ampere;
     (v) thermodynamic temperature shall be the Kelvin;
     (vi) luminous intensity shall be the candela; and
     (vii) amount of substance shall be the mole.
2. The specification of the base units mentioned in sub-section (1), derived units and other units shall be such as may be prescribed.

Base Unit of Numeration

1. The base unit of numeration shall be the unit of the international form of Indian numeration numerals.
2. Every numeration shall be made in accordance with the decimal system.
3. The decimal multiples and sub-multiples of the numerals shall be of such denominations and be written in such manner as may be prescribed.

Prohibition of quotation, etc., otherwise than in terms of standard units of weight, measure or numeration

No person shall, in relation to any goods, things or service:

(a) quote, or make announcement of, whether by word of mouth or otherwise, any price or charge, or
(b) issue or exhibit any price list, invoice, cash memo or other document, or
(c) prepare or publish any advertisement, poster or other document, or
(d) indicate the net quantity of a pre-packaged commodity, or
(e) express in relation to any transaction or protection, any quantity or dimension, otherwise than in accordance with the standard unit of weight, measure or numeration.

Appointment and Powers of Director, Controller and Legal Metrology Officers

The administrative mechanism of legal metrology in India, in relation to weights and measures, is shared between the Centre and the States. Matters of national policy and other related functions such as uniform laws on weights and measures, technical regulations, training, precision laboratory facilities and implementation of the International Recommendation are the concern of the Central Government. The State Governments and Union Territory Administration are responsible for the day to day enforcement of the laws.

The Central Government may, by notification, appoint a Director of Legal Metrology, Additional Director, Joint Director, Deputy Director, Assistant Director and other employees for exercising the powers and discharging the duties conferred or imposed on them by or under this Act in relation to inter-State trade and commerce. The qualifications of the Director and Legal Metrology Officers appointed shall be such as may be prescribed.

Every Legal Metrology Officer appointed, shall exercise powers and discharge duties under the general superintendence, direction and control of the Director.

At the State level, Directorate of Legal Metrology is essentially a 3-tier organisation comprising of Inspectors of Legal Metrology at the field level, Assistant Controller of Legal Metrology at the district level and Controller of Legal Metrology with Deputy Controllers at the State level. The State Government may, by notification, appoint them and other employees for the State for exercising the powers and discharging the duties conferred or imposed on them by or under this Act in relation to intra-State trade and commerce.

Legal standards of weights and measures of the States and Union Territories are calibrated in the four Regional Reference Standard Laboratories (RRSL) located at Ahmedabad, Bhubaneswar, Bangalore and Faridabad.

Power of inspection and seizure

The Director, Controller or any Legal Metrology Officer may:
(a) enter at any reasonable time into any such premises and search for and inspect any weight, measure or other goods, in relation to which trade and commerce has taken place, or is intended to take place and any record, "register or other document relating thereto;
(b) seize any weight, measure or other goods and any record, register or other document or article which he has reason to believe may furnish

evidence indicating that an offence punishable under this Act has been, or is likely to be, committed in the course of or in relation to, any trade and commerce.

Every search or seizure made under this section shall be carried out in accordance with the provisions of the Code of Criminal Procedure, 1973, relating to searches and seizures.

Every manufacturer, repairer or dealer of weight or measure shall maintain such records and registers as may be prescribed and shall be produced at the time of inspection to the persons authorized.

Declarations on pre-packaged commodities

(i) No person shall manufacture, pack, sell, import, distribute, deliver, offer, expose or possess for sale any pre-packaged commodity unless such package is in such standard quantities or number, and bears thereon, such declarations and particulars in the prescribed manner.

(ii) Any advertisement mentioning the retail sale price of a pre-packaged commodity, shall contain a declaration as to the net quantity or number of the commodity contained in the package in such form and manner as may be prescribed.

Import of Weights and Measures

(i) No person shall import any weight or measure unless he is registered with the Director in such manner and on payment of such fees, as may be prescribed.

(ii) No weight or measure, whether singly or as a part or component of any machine, shall be imported unless it conforms to the standards of weight or measure established by or under this Act.

Prohibition on manufacture, repair or sale of weight or measure without licence

No person shall manufacture, repair or sell, or offer, expose or possess for repair or sale, any weight or measure unless he holds a licence issued by the Controller. No licence to repair shall be required by a manufacturer for repair of his own weight or measure in a State, other than the State of manufacture of the same.

Offences and Penalties

Penal Provisions

The penal provisions for violation of Legal Metrology Act, 2009 and Rules framed thereunder have been detailed in Table 16.1. The penalties mainly

Table 16.1. Penalties for offences under different Sections

Section	Offence	Penalty
Sec. 25	Penalty for use of non-standard weight or measure	Fine up to Rs. 25,000/-; for the second or subsequent offence – imprisonment up to six months and fine
Sec. 26	Penalty for alteration of weight and measure	Fine up to Rs. 25,000/-; for the second or subsequent offence – imprisonment, not less than six months but may extend to one year or fine or both
Sec. 27	Penalty for manufacture or sale of non-standard weight or measure	Fine up to Rs. 25,000/-; second or subsequent offence – imprisonment up to three years or fine or both
Sec. 28	Penalty for making any transaction, deal or contract in contravention of the prescribed standards	Fine up to Rs. 10,000/-; for the second or subsequent offence – imprisonment for a term up to one year or fine or both
Sec. 29	Penalty for quoting or publishing, etc., of non-standard units	Fine up to Rs. 10,000/-; second or subsequent offence – imprisonment up to one year, or fine or both
Sec. 30	Penalty for transactions in contravention of standard weight or measure	Fine up to Rs. 10,000/-; second or subsequent offence – imprisonment up to one year, or fine or both
Sec. 31	Penalty for non-production of documents, etc.	Fine up to Rs. 5,000/-; second or subsequent offence – imprisonment up to one year and also fine
Sec. 32	Penalty for failure to get model approved	Fine up to Rs. 25,000/-; second or subsequent offence – imprisonment up to one year and also fine
Sec. 33	Penalty for use of un-verified weight or measure	Fine up to Rs. 10,000/-; second or subsequent offence – imprisonment up to one year and also fine
Sec. 34	Penalty for sale or delivery of commodities, etc., by non-standard weight or measure	Fine Rs. 2,000 to Rs. 5,000; second or subsequent offence – imprisonment 3 months to one year, or fine, or both
Sec. 35	Penalty for rendering services by non-standard weight, measure or number	Fine Rs. 2,000 to Rs. 5,000; for the second and subsequent offence – imprisonment 3 months to one year, or fine or both
Sec. 36	Penalty for selling, etc., of non-standard packages	Fine up to Rs. 25,000/-; for the second offence – fine up to Rs. 50,000/-; subsequent offence – fine Rs. 50,000 to Rs. 1,00,000 or imprisonment up to one year or both

(Contd.)

Section	Offence	Penalty
Sec. 37	Penalty for contravention by Government approved Test Centre	Fine up to Rs. 1,00,000/-; in case of employee of test centre – imprisonment up to one year or fine up to Rs. 10,000/- or both
Sec. 38	Penalty for non-registration by importer of weight or measure	Fine up to Rs. 25,000/-; for the second and subsequent offence – imprisonment up to six months or fine or both
Sec. 39	Penalty for import of non-standard weight or measure	Fine up to Rs. 50,000/-; for the second and subsequent offence – imprisonment up to one year and also fine
Sec. 40	Penalty for obstructing Director, Controller or Legal Metrology Officer	Imprisonment up to two years; for the second and subsequent offence – imprisonment up to 5 years
Sec. 41	Penalty for giving false information or false return	Fine up to Rs. 5,000/-; for the second or subsequent offence – imprisonment up to six months and also fine
Sec. 42	Vexatious search	Imprisonment up to one year or fine up to Rs. 10,000/- or both
Sec. 43	Penalty for verification in contravention of Act and Rules	Imprisonment up to one year or fine up to Rs. 10,000/- or both
Sec. 44	Penalty for counterfeiting of seals, etc.	Imprisonment 6 months to one year; for the second and subsequent offence – imprisonment 6 months to five years
Sec. 45	Penalty for manufacture of weight and measure without licence	Fine up to Rs. 20,000/-; second or subsequent offence – up to one year or fine or both
Sec. 46	Penalty for repair, sale, etc., of weight and measure without licence	Fine up to Rs. 5,000/-; for the second and subsequent offence – imprisonment up to one year or fine or both
Sec. 47	Penalty for tampering with licence	Fine up to Rs. 25,000/- or with imprisonment up to one year or fine or both

Note: The penalties of the offences are liable to change as per the notifications published by the Government from time to time.

relate with the violation of manufacturing of non-standard Weights & Measures, counterfeiting of seal, short weighment/measurement, use of non-verified weights & measures, not making mandatory declarations on the packaged commodities. The penalty is imposed depending upon the nature of offence committed by the accused. The non-compoundable offences are sent to court of law for trial. The details of major offences and penalties are given in Table 16.1.

Offences by Companies on Nomination

Any company, as per Sec. 49, may, by order in writing, nominate directors to be responsible under Legal Metrology Act for preventing the company of any offence or the company has to give notice to Legal Metrology Director/Controller/Authorized Legal Metrology Office in a prescribed form indicating such director has been nominated along with written consents, and where a company has different establishments /branches/ units, different persons to be responsible can be nominated.

The company so convicted under this Act, for contravention of any of the provisions thereof, the penalty will be to publish an advertisement in newspapers at the expense of the company as the court may direct.

Act not to apply in certain cases

The provisions of this Act, in so far as they relate to verification and stamping of weights and measures, shall not apply to any weight or measure:

- used in any factory exclusively engaged in the manufacture of any arms, ammunition or both, for the use of the Armed Forces of the Union;
- used for scientific investigation or for research;
- manufactured exclusively for export.

The Rules made by a State Government under the Standards of Weights and Measures (Enforcement) Act, 1985 which are in force immediately before the commencement of this Act shall remain in force until the State Government makes Rules in that behalf.

QUESTIONS FOR REVISION

1. What is the objective of Legal Metrology Act, 2009 and how it is achieved?
2. Write short note on Legal Metrology Act, 2009.
3. Write short notes on:
    (a) Appointment and powers of Director, Controller and Legal Metrology Officer.
    (b) Offences and Penalties.

Chapter 17

Minimum Wages Act, 1948

The Minimum Wages Act, 1948 is an Act of Parliament concerning Indian labour law that sets the minimum wages that must be paid to skilled and unskilled labourers. A 'living wage', defined in the Indian Constitution, is the level of income for a worker which will ensure a basic standard of living including good health, dignity, comfort, education and provide for any contingency. The Constitution has also defined a 'fair wage', keeping in mind an industry's capacity to pay. To achieve this, in its First Session during November, 1948, the Central Advisory Council appointed a Tripartite Committee of Fair Wage which came up with the concept of Minimum Wages. A minimum wage is such a wage that it not only guarantees bare subsistence and preserves efficiency but also provides for education, medical requirements and some level of comfort. The Minimum Wages Act was passed in 1948, giving both the Central Government and State Governments jurisdiction in fixing wages. The employments specified in the Schedule are mainly those where sweated labour is more prevalent and where there is a big chance of exploitation of labour. *The Act thus seeks to prevent exploitation of ignorant or less organized or less privileged members of society by the capitalist class.* The Act extends to the whole of India and applies to all persons engaged in scheduled employments in respect of which minimum wages have been fixed.

Objectives of the Minimum Wages Act, 1948

The Minimum Wages Act was passed in 1948 to provide:

(a) for fixing of minimum rates of wages to be paid to workers in certain employments which are included in the Schedule;

(b) For determining the minimum wages in the industry and trade where labour organizations are ineffective or nonexistent;
(c) For revising the minimum wages at regular intervals.

Definitions

1. **Employee:** Any person who is employed for hire or reward to do any work, skilled or unskilled, manual or clerical, in a scheduled employment, in respect of which, minimum rates of wages have been fixed.
2. **Employer:** Any person who employs, whether directly or through another person, or whether on behalf of himself or any other person, one or more employees in any scheduled employment in respect of which minimum rates of wages have been fixed under this Act.
3. **Wages:** All remuneration payable to an employed person on the fulfillment of his contract employment and includes house rent allowance, but does not include:
   (i) The value of:
      (a) any house accommodation, supply of light, water, medical attendance;
      (b) any other amenity or any service excluded by order of the appropriate Government.
   (ii) Any contribution paid by the employer to any Pension Fund or Provident Fund or under any scheme of social insurance.
   (iii) Any travelling allowance or travelling concession.
   (iv) Any special expenses reimbursed to the employee, which had been incurred by him due to the nature of his employment.
   (v) Any gratuity payable on discharge

Provisions for fixing the minimum rates of wages under Minimum Wages Act

The Central Government or State Government has been empowered under the Act to:
   (i) fix the minimum rates of wages payable to employees employed in an employment, specified in Part I or Part II of the Schedule;
   (ii) review at such intervals, as it may think fit, such intervals not exceeding five years, the minimum rates of wages so fixed and revise the minimum rates, when necessary.

Under the Act, the appropriate Government shall fix:
   (i) A "Minimum time rate" that is the minimum rate of wages to be paid for time work.
   (ii) A "minimum piece rate" that is the minimum rate of wages to be paid for piece work.

(iii) A "guaranteed time rate" that is the minimum rate of remuneration to apply in the case of employees employed on piece work for the purpose of securing to such employees a minimum rate of wages on a time work basis.
(iv) An "overtime rate" that is the minimum rate (whether a time rate or a piece rate) to apply in respect of an overtime work done by employees.

Under the Act, the Government may fix or revise different minimum rates of wages for:

(i) Different scheduled employments.
(ii) Different classes of work in the same scheduled employment.
(iii) Adult, adolescents, children and apprentices.
(iv) Different localities.

The minimum rates of wages may be fixed by any one or more of the following wage-periods, namely:

(i) by the hour.
(ii) by the day.
(iii) by the month.
(iv) by such other larger wage-period as may be prescribed.

Minimum Rates of Wages

The minimum rate of wages fixed or revised by the Government in respect of scheduled employments shall consist of:

(i) Basic rate of wages and a special allowance (dearness also referred to as cost of living allowance) to be revised at appropriate intervals based on the variation in the cost of living index number applicable to such workers; or
(ii) A basic rate of wages with or without the cost of living allowance, and the cash value of the concessions in respect of supplies of essential commodities at concession rates, where so authorized; or
(iii) An all-inclusive rate allowing for the basic rate, the cost of living allowance and the cash value of the concessions, if any.

The cost of living allowance and the cash value of the concessions in respect of supplies of essential commodities at concession rates shall be computed by a competent authority appointed by the appropriate Government.

Procedure for fixing and revising minimum wages

In fixing minimum rates of wages in respect of any scheduled employment for the first time under this Act or in revising minimum rates of wages so fixed, the appropriate government shall either:

Appoint committees and sub-committees and advise it in respect of such fixation or revision as the case may be or after considering the advice of the committee or committee appointed, it may revise the minimum rates of wages in respect of each scheduled employment.

Wages in Kind

Although the minimum wages payable under this Act shall be paid in cash, the Government may authorize the payment of minimum wages either wholly or partly in kind. The Government may also make provision for the supply of essential commodities at confessional rates.

The value of wages in kind and of concessions in respect of supplies of essential commodities at concessional rates shall be estimated by the competent authority appointed by the Government, in the prescribed manner.

Payment of Minimum Rates of Wages

Where in respect of any scheduled employment, the employer shall pay to every employee engaged in a scheduled employment under him, wages at a rate not less than the minimum rate of wages fixed by such notification for that class of employees in that employment, without any deductions except as may be authorized within such time and subject to such conditions as may be prescribed.

Provision affixing hours of work in a factory

Under this Act the Government may:
  (i) Fix the number of hours of work in a normal working day, inclusive of specified intervals.
  (ii) Provide for a day of rest in every period of seven days and for the payment of remuneration in respect of such days of rest.
  (iii) Provide for payment of work on a day of rest at a rate not less than the overtime rate.

Wages of Worker who works for less than Normal Working Day

If an employee, whose minimum rate of wages have been fixed under this Act by the day, is employed for a period less than that fixed for a normal working day, he is entitled to receive wages for a full normal working day. However, he shall not be entitled to receive wages for a full normal working day:

(i) In any case where his failure to work is caused by his unwillingness to work and not due to the failure of the employer to provide him with work.

(ii) In such other cases and circumstances as may be prescribed.

Wages for Two or More Classes of Work

Where an employee does two or more classes of work to each of which a different minimum rate of wages is applicable the employer shall pay, to such employee in respect of the time respectively occupied in each such class of work, wages at not less than the minimum rate in force in respect of each such class.

Minimum time rate wages for piece work

Where an employee is employed on piece work for which minimum time rate and not a minimum piece rate has been fixed under this Act, the employer shall pay to such employee wages at not less than the minimum time rate.

Maintenance of registers and records

1. Every employer shall maintain such registers and records giving such particulars of employees as:
   (a) the work performed by them;
   (b) the wages paid to them;
   (c) the receipts given.
2. Every employer shall keep exhibited notices in the prescribed form containing prescribed particulars.
3. Entries shall be made and authenticated in wage books or wage slips by the employer or his agent.

Powers and duties of Inspectors appointed as per the provisions of Minimum Wages Act

The appropriate government may, by notification in the Official Gazette, appoint such persons as it thinks fit, to be Inspectors for the purposes of this Act and define the local limits within which they shall exercise their functions.

(i) Enter, at all reasonable hours, any premises or place where employees are employed or work is given out to out-workers in any scheduled employment, for the purpose of examining any register, record of wages or notices required to be kept or exhibited under this Act.

(ii) Examine any person whom he finds in any such premises or place and who, he has reasonable cause to believe, is an employee employed therein or an employee to whom work is given out therein.
(iii) Require any person giving out work and any out-workers, to give information regarding the names and addresses of the persons to, for and from whom the work is given out or received, and with respect to the payments to be made for the work.
(iv) Seize or take copies of any register, record of wages or notices, if he has reason to believe, that an offence has been committed by an employer.
(v) Exercise such other powers as may be prescribed.

Every Inspector is deemed to be a public servant within the meaning of the Indian Penal Code and any person required to produce any document or thing or to give any information by an Inspector is deemed to be legally bound to do so.

Claim

The appropriate Government may, by notification in the Official Gazette, appoint a suitable authority to hear and decide for any specified area, all claims arising out of payment of less than the minimum rates of wages or in respect of the payment of remuneration for days of rest or for work done on such days.

The authority shall hear the applicant and the employer or give them an opportunity of being heard and after such further inquiry if any as it may consider necessary, may without prejudice to any other penalty to which the employer may be liable under this Act.

If the authority hearing any application under this Section is satisfied that it was either malicious or vexatious it may direct that a penalty be paid to the employer by the person presenting the application.

Penalty and offences prescribed under the Minimum Wages Act

Any employer who:
(i) pays to any employee less than the minimum rates of wages fixed for that employee's class of work, or less than the amount due to him under the provisions of this Act; or
(ii) contravenes any Rule or Order made regarding the working hours, etc.

shall be punishable with imprisonment for a term which may extend to six months, or with fine which may extend to five hundred rupees, or with both.

General Provision for Punishment of other Offences

Any employer who contravenes any provision of this Act, for which no other penalty has been provided, shall be punishable with fine which may extend to five hundred rupees.

Cognizance of offences

No court shall take cognizance of a complaint against any person for an offence:

Unless an application in respect of the facts constituting such offence has been presented under Sections prescribed in Act, and has been granted wholly or in part and the appropriate Government or an officer authorized by it, in his behalf, has sanctioned the making of the complaint.

Offences by Companies

If an offence is committed by a company, every person who at the time of offence, was incharge of, and was responsible to the company for the conduct of its business as well as the company, shall be deemed to be guilty of the offence and shall be liable to be proceeded against and punished accordingly. However, the person shall not be liable to punishment if he proves that the offence was committed without his knowledge or that he exercised all due diligence to prevent the commission of such offence.

Where it is proved that the offence has been committed with the consent of, or is attributable to any neglect on the part of, any director, manager, secretary or other officer of the company, such director, manager, secretary or other officer of the company, shall also be deemed to be guilty of that offence and shall be liable to be punished accordingly.

Payment of undisbursed amounts due to employees

All amounts payable by an employer to an employee as the amount of minimum wages of the employee under this Act or otherwise due to the employee under this Act or any Rule or Order made thereunder, shall, if such amounts could not or cannot be paid to the employee on account of his death before payment or on account of his whereabouts not being known, be deposited with the prescribed authority who shall deal with the money so deposited in such manner as may be prescribed.

Protection against attachment of assets of employer with Government

Any amount deposited with the appropriate Government by an employer to secure the due performance of a contract with that Government and any other amount due to such employer from that Government in respect of such contract shall not be liable to attachment under any decree or order of any court in respect of any debt or liability incurred by the employer other than any debt or liability incurred by the employer towards any employee employed in connection with the contract aforesaid.

Exemption and exceptions

The appropriate Government may subject to such conditions if any as it may think fit to impose direct that the provisions of this Act shall not apply in relation to:

(a) the wages payable to disabled employees;
(b) all or any class of employees employed in any scheduled employment or to any locality where there is carried on a scheduled employment.

Nothing in this Act shall apply to the wages payable by an employer to a member of his family who is living with him and is dependent on him.

QUESTIONS FOR REVISION

1. Write the main objectives of the Minimum Wages Act, 1948.
2. Explain the provisions for fixing the minimum wages rates of wages under the Minimum Wages Act.
3. Write notes on:
    (a) Powers and duties of Inspectors appointed.
    (b) Penalties and offences prescribed under the Minimum Wages Act.

Chapter 18

Intellectual Property Rights

Intellectual property rights are defined as the rights given to persons over the creations of their minds. They usually give the creator an exclusive right over the use of his/her creation for a certain period of time.

There was a time when, property of any individual or organization was measured in terms of physical tangible assets like land, buildings, valuables like cars, gold machinery, etc. But with passage of time, intangible assets also got recognition and now we know these intangible assets as intellectual property or IP. Now, in modern concept of ownership, we count both intangible and tangible property as property associated with an organization. Intellectual Property is the property, which has been created by exercise of Intellectual Faculty. It is the result of person's Intellectual Activities. Thus Intellectual Property refers to creation of mind such as inventions, designs for industrial articles, literary, artistic work, symbols which are ultimately used in commerce. Intellectual Property rights allow the creators or owners to have the benefits from their works when these are exploited commercially. These rights are statutory rights governed in accordance with the provisions of corresponding legislations.

Intellectual Property rights reward creativity and human endeavour, which fuel the progress of humankind. Intellectual property rights are mainly concerned with the following two areas:

(i) Copyright and rights related to copyright

The rights of authors of literary and artistic works (such as books and other writings, musical compositions, paintings, sculpture, computer programs and films) are protected by copyright, for a minimum period of

50 years after the death of the author. Also protected through copyright and related (sometimes referred to as "neighbouring") rights are the rights of performers (e.g. actors, singers and musicians), producers of phonograms (sound recordings) and broadcasting organizations. The main social purpose of protection of copyright and related rights is to encourage and reward creative work.

(ii) Industrial property

Industrial Property can usefully be divided into two main areas:

1. One area can be characterized as the protection of distinctive signs, in particular trademarks (which distinguish the goods or services of one undertaking from those of other undertakings) and geographical indications (which identify a good as originating in a place where a given characteristic of the good is essentially attributable to its geographical origin). The protection of such distinctive signs *aims to stimulate and ensure fair competition and to protect consumers, by enabling them to make informed choices between various goods and services. The protection may last indefinitely, provided the sign in question continues to be distinctive.*
2. Other types of industrial property are protected primarily to stimulate innovation, design and the creation of technology. In this category fall inventions (protected by patents), industrial designs and trade secrets. The social purpose is to provide protection for the results of investment in the development of new technology, thus giving the incentive and means to finance research and development activities.

A functioning intellectual property regime should also facilitate the transfer of technology in the form of foreign direct investment, joint ventures and licensing. *The protection is usually given for a finite term (typically 20 years in the case of patents).* While the basic social objectives of intellectual property protection are as outlined above, it should also be noted that the exclusive rights given are generally subject to a number of limitations and exceptions, aimed at fine-tuning the balance that has to be found between the legitimate interests of right holders and of users.

This innovative and creative capacity is protected under the intellectual property system of WTO. Recognizing this fact, India as a founder member of WTO, has ratified the Agreement on Trade Related Intellectual Property Rights (TRIPs). As per the agreement, all member countries, including India are to abide by the mutually negotiated norms and standards within the stipulated timeframe. *Accordingly, India has set up an Intellectual Property Right (IPR) regime, which is WTO compatible and is well established at all levels whether statutory, administrative or judicial.*

For complementing the administrative set-up, several legislative initiatives have been taken. It includes, the Trade Marks Act, 1999; the Geographical Indications of Goods (Registration and Protection) Act, 1999; the Designs Act, 2000; the Patents Act, 1970 and its subsequent amendments in 2002 and 2005; Indian Copyright Act, 1957 and its amendment Copyright (Amendment) Act, 1999; Semiconductor Integrated Circuit Layout Design Act, 2000; as well as the Protection of Plant varieties and Farmer's Rights Act, 2001.

Classification of Intellectual Property Rights

The intellectual property rights are classified into the following seven categories i.e.
1. Patent
2. Industrial Design
3. Trade Marks
4. Copyright
5. Geographical Indications
6. Layout designs of integrated circuits
7. Protection of undisclosed information/Trade Secret according to TRIPs agreements.

First of all an idea is generated in mind and this is converted in some form of property. For instance, an idea is either converted into an innovation or invention; some literary or artistic work; some aesthetic or decorative feature of article; brand name, trade dress or packaging style, etc. All forms of property are protected by various legal instruments. The analogy can be better understood with the following (Table 18.1).

Table 18.1

Intellect	Property	Right	Examples
Idea	Invention and innovations	Patent	Lipitor drug of Pfizer (cholesterol lowering medication), sitagliptin of MSD
Idea	Expression (fixed on a medium)	Copyright	Advertising material, Manuals, Pamphlets, Brochures, Packaging style, etc.
Idea	Aesthetic look, new shape and configuration	Industrial design	Shape of digital audio player, shape of printer, shape of tractor, Look of Titan wrist watches, shape of car, etc.
Idea	Source identifier	Trademark	BSNL, Bata, Coca Cola, Swaraj, Preet Agro
Idea	Source identifier	Trade dress	Packaging style – Kurkure, Odonil, Dettol Soap packaging

They strategically manage and maintain SMEs need to identify and protect the Intellectual Property available with their organization. With the registration of the Intellectual Property Rights, the organizations are required to strategically manage and maintain this exclusive rights, the organization must take measures to protect their rights as well as against the infringers to create and protect value created and added with the growing goodwill in the market. Securing rights in Intellectual Property entitles the right holder to commercialize its Intellectual Property. The right holder may transfer or sell its Intellectual Property by way of assignment, licensing or franchising. In return for such transfers, the right holder may receive a lump sum payment, a royalty or a combination of both. The protective measures taken by the organizations will enable the organizations to exploit their rights fully by licensing them at the time of expansion of the business and negotiating the deals and thereby improving profits of the organization and bringing a healthy competitiveness.

Patents

A patent is a statutory right for an invention granted for a limited period of time to the patentee by the Government, in exchange of full disclosure of his invention for excluding others, from making, using, selling, importing the patented product or process for producing that product for those purposes without his consent. Patent protection is territorial right and therefore it is effective only within the territory of India. However, filing an application in India enables the applicant to file a corresponding application for same invention in convention countries, within or before expiry of twelve months from the filing date in India. Therefore, separate patents should be obtained in each country where the applicant requires protection of his invention in those countries. There is no patent valid worldwide. An invention relating either to a product or process that is new, involving inventive step and capable of industrial application can be patented. However, it must not fall into the categories of inventions that are non-patentable under Sections 3 and 4 of the Act. It is basically a monopoly right for 20 years, FROM DATE OF PRIORITY, granted for your invention. It is granted for invention, provided invention must be novel, technically advanced or economically significant and industrially useful. It may be solution to an existing problem.

An invention to become patentable subject matter must meet the following criteria:

(i) It should be novel.
(ii) It should have inventive step or it must be non-obvious.
(iii) It should be capable of industrial application.
(iv) It should not fall within the provisions of Sections 3 and 4 of the Patents Act, 1970.

For example, now-a-days with increasing crowd and vehicles, parking is a big problem. We also know that conventional bicycle stands requires more space and the cycles will occupy space equal to its length when parked in these stands. Vertical Bicycle Parking (Bike Racks) is a solution to this problem which saves more than 50% of space comparing with conventional bicycle parking. Such solutions have been patented by respective inventor. In another instance, sticking property of burr was recognized by George de Mestral, a Swiss engineer, as potential for a practical new fastener and developed Velcro and later patented it. Now-a-day, we frequently read in newspaper that a pharmaceutical company has been granted patent on a drug. So, a solution may be hidden in problem itself. Remember, patents protect only functional aspect of the invention.

Trademarks

Trade marks are an important tool for communicating the value of a product or service to the market. Trade mark protection is the cornerstone of a variety of brand strategies based on product differentiation and market segmentation, which are very important when managing competition, creating customer demand, and securing market share. In light of that, it is clear that trademarks are crucial to your industry. In many instances, for example, it is the trade mark that determines, which product a customer will buy.

Types of Trademarks that can be registered are listed in Table 18.2.

Table 18.2

Category of Mark	Function	Example
Trade Marks	To distinguish goods	HMT, ERKA, VETA
Service Marks	To distinguish service	BSNL, DFDC
Collective Marks	To distinguish goods or services by members of an association	ISI, AGMARK
Certification Marks	To distinguish goods or services certified by a certifying authority	
Well Known Marks	Very famous in the market and as a result benefit from stronger protection	Philips, Whirlpool

It is a mark capable of being represented graphically and which is capable of distinguishing the goods or services of one person from those of others. It may be word like Nokia, abbreviation like VIP, combination of letters like BMW, arbitrary word like Apple for computers, numerals like 555 washing cakes, etc. Trademarks are registered as per classes like Class 1 Chemicals used in Industry, Class 5 Pharmaceuticals Preparation, Class 9 Electronic Components, Class 30 Food Items, Class 35 Trading, Class 41 Educational Services, Class 43 Restaurants, and so on. There are 45 classes in all i.e. class 1 to 34 for products and class 35 to 45 for services.

Duration: 10 years and can be renewed unlimited.

Industrial Design

"When companies are competing at equal price and functionality, design is the only differential that matters" – Mark Dziersk, Renowned Industrial Designer. Industrial designs refer to creative activity which result in the ornamental or formal appearance of a product and design right refers to a novel or original design that is accorded to the proprietor of a validly registered design. Industrial designs are an element of intellectual property. Under the TRIPs Agreement, minimum standards of protection of industrial designs have been provided for. As a developing country, India has already amended its national legislation to provide for these minimal standards.

The essential purpose of design law is to promote and protect the design element of industrial production. It is also intended to promote innovative activity in the field of industries. The existing legislation on industrial designs in India is contained in the New Designs Act, 2000 and this Act will serve its purpose well in the rapid changes in technology and international developments. India has also achieved a mature status in the field of industrial designs and in view of globalization of the economy, the present legislation is aligned with the changed technical and commercial scenario and made to conform to international trends in design administration.

"Design" means only the features of shape, configuration, pattern or ornament or composition of lines or colour or combination thereof applied to any article whether two-dimensional or three-dimensional or in both forms, by any industrial process or means, whether manual, mechanical or chemical, separate or combined, which in the finished article appeal to and are judged solely by the eye, but does not include any mode or principle or construction or any thing which is in substance a mere mechanical device, and does not include any trade mark, as define in clause (v) of sub-section of Section 2 of the Trade and Merchandise Marks Act, 1958, property mark or artistic works as defined under Section 2(c) of the Copyright Act, 1957.

It protects shape, configuration and outer appearance of an article. Today, consumer market is driven by pleasant look of an article. We can see designer dresses, trendy bicycles, eye appealing LCDs, etc. When we compare two products having almost equal functionality and price, the design is the feature which helps us to select the product to be bought. Design registration is also done as per classification scheme.

Essential requirements for the registration of 'design' under the Designs Act, 2000

1. The design should be new or original, not previously published or used in any country before the date of application for registration. The novelty may reside in the application of a known shape or pattern to new subject matter. Practical example: The known shape of "Kutub Minar" when applied to a cigarette holder the same is registrable. However, if the design for which application is made does not involve any real mental activity for conception, then registration may not be considered.
2. The design should relate to features of shape, configuration, pattern or ornamentation applied or applicable to an article. Thus, designs of industrial plans, layouts and installations are not registrable under the Act.
3. The design should be applied or applicable to any article by any industrial process. Normally, designs of artistic nature like painting, sculptures and the like which are not produced in bulk by any industrial process are excluded from registration under the Act.
4. The features of the design in the finished article should appeal to and are judged solely by the eye. This implies that the design must appear and should be visible on the finished article, for which it is meant. Thus, any design in the inside arrangement of a box, money purse or almirah may not be considered for showing such articles in the open state, as those articles are generally put in the market in the closed state.
5. Any mode or principle of construction or operation or any thing which is in substance a mere mechanical device, would not be registrable design. For instance, a key having its novelty only in the shape of its corrugation or bend at the portion intended to engage with levers inside the lock associated with cannot be registered as a design under the Act. However, when any design suggests any mode or principle of construction or mechanical or other action of a mechanism, a suitable disclaimer in respect there of is required to be inserted on its representation, provided there are other registrable features in the design.
6. The design should not include any Trade Mark or property mark or artistic works as define under the Copyright Act, 1957. Once you produced and sold more than fifty articles and did not file design application you will lose all the rights in design. The law of Design in India provides for 32 classes of articles for registration. India follows international classification of design i.e. Locarno Agreement.

Copyright

Advertising material, manuals, pamphlets, brochures, packaging style, etc. of an article can be copyrighted. These packaging styles are also termed as get up or trade dress of the product. Example – Packing style of chips, biscuits, detergents, washing powder packets, etc. Today, as numerous products by different companies are launched in the market, it is essential to protect our packaging to avoid duplicity by competitor.

Copyright plays a crucial role in the textile and clothing, leather, furniture and footwear industries since it is free of charge, easy and fast to obtain and does not require any formalities (self-executing right). A work is considered protected by copyright as soon as it comes into creation. This protection may, for example, cover reference works, newspapers, computer programs, databases, artistic works (designs, paintings, shapes and colours) architecture and advertisements, maps and technical drawings. You just have to be able to prove a certain date of creation and the originality or novelty of your creation. *The original creators of works protected by copyright have the exclusive right to use or authorize others to use the work under certain terms. The creator of a work can prohibit or authorise its:*

- reproduction in various forms, such as printed publication;
- initial distribution to the public through sale and other transfer of ownership in tangible copies;
- rental of copies to the public;
- translations into other languages or adaptation.

Many creative works protected by copyright require mass distribution, communication and financial investment for their dissemination. Therefore, creators often license the rights to their works to the individuals or companies best able to market the works in return for payment. These payments are often made according to the actual use of the work and are then referred to as royalties.

Geographical Indications

Geographical indication can be described as an indication which originates from a definite geographical territory. It is used to identify agricultural, natural or manufactured goods. The manufactured goods should be produced or processed or prepared in that territory. It should have a special quality or reputation or other characteristics. Some major examples of possible Indian Geographical Indications are:

Basmati Rice, Darjeeling Tea, Kanchipuram Silk Saree, Alphonso Mango, Phulkari, Nagpur Orange, Kolhapuri Chappal, Bikaneri Bhujia, Agra Petha.

Benefits of registration of geographical indications are:
- It confers legal protection to Geographical Indications in India.
- Prevents unauthorized use of a Registered Geographical Indication by others.
- It provides legal protection to Indian Geographical Indications which in turn boost exports.
- It promotes economic prosperity of producers of goods produced in a geographical territory.

A feature of industrial property that is mentioning geographical indication referring to a country or place of origin of that product is termed as Geographical Indication of goods. Geographical Indications are covered as an element of Intellectual Property under the Paris Convention for the Protection of Industrial Property. The TRIPs provides protection to Geographical Indications. In India, Geographical Indications are recognized and protected under the Geographical Indications of Goods (Registration & Protection) Act, 1999. To remember

- Apply for Patent before disclosing it (publication in document or selling or public use).
- Adopt Trademark that is not similar to other in same business line.
- File Trademark as soon as possible as competitor may file before you file.
- File Design Application before marketing the product or file before you sell 50 pieces of article.

Jurisdiction for filing

For filing Patent Application, the respective metro cities have Patent Office and accordingly they have regional jurisdiction. Patent Office Delhi has jurisdiction over States of Haryana, Himachal Pradesh, Jammu & Kashmir, Punjab, Rajasthan, Uttar Pradesh, Uttaranchal, Delhi and the Union Territory of Chandigarh. Likewise Trademark Registry Delhi has jurisdiction over northern States. In case of Copyright we have one copyright office at New Delhi under Ministry of HRD. In case of Industrial Design, the application can be filed either at corresponding regional Patent Office or directly to Patent Office, Kolkata.

Where any offence under this Act has been committed by a company, every person who at the time, the offence was committed was in charge of, and was responsible to the company for, the conduct of the business of the company, as well as the company, shall be deemed to be guilty of such offence and shall be liable to be proceeded against and punished accordingly.

QUESTIONS FOR REVISION

1. What are Intellectual Property Rights? Explain the objectives of IPR.
2. Classify Intellectual Property Rights. Write notes on:
   (a) Trademarks
   (b) Copyrights.

Chapter 19

The Patents Act, 1970

The word Patent originated from the Latin word "**Patene**", which means "**to open**". A patent is a monopoly right granted to a person who has invented a new and useful article or a new process of making an article. The history of Patent law in India starts from 1911, when the Indian Patents and Designs Act, 1911, was enacted. Then, due to substantial changes in the political and economic conditions of the country, the urge was felt to enact a comprehensive law on the subject which would protect interests of both, the inventor as well as consumer The present Patents Act, 1970 came into force in the year 1972, amending and consolidating the existing law relating to patents in India. The Patents Act, 1970, was again amended by the Patents (Amendment) Act, 2005, wherein product patent was extended to all fields of technology including food, drugs, chemicals and micro-organisms. After the amendment, the provisions relating to Exclusive Marketing Rights (EMRs) have been repealed, and a provision for enabling grant of compulsory licence has been introduced. The provisions relating to pre-grant and post-grant opposition have been also introduced. The Act extends to the whole of India.

A patent is a statutory right for an invention granted for a limited period of time, to the patentee by the Government, in exchange of full disclosure of his invention for excluding others, from making, using, selling, importing the patented product for those purposes without his consent. Patent protection is a territorial right and therefore it is effective only within the territory of India. However, filing an application in India enables the applicant to file a corresponding application for the same invention in convention countries within or before expiry of twelve months from the filing date in India. It is basically *a monopoly right for twenty years granted for your invention. It is granted for invention provided it is novel, technically advanced or economically significant and industrially useful.* It may be a solution to an existing problem. In India, a patent application can be filed, either alone or jointly, by true and first inventor or his assignee.

Definitions

1. **Assignee** includes the legal representative of a deceased assignee, and references to the assignee of any person include references to the assignee of the legal representative or assignee of that person.
2. **Exclusive licence** means a licence from a patentee which confers on the licensee, or on the licensee and persons authorized by him, to the exclusion of all other persons (including the patentee), any right in respect of the patented invention, and "exclusive licensee" shall be construed accordingly.
3. **Invention** means any new and useful:
    (i) Art, process, method or manner of manufacture.
    (ii) Machine, apparatus or other article.
    (iii) Substance produced by manufacture and includes any new and useful improvement of any of them, and an alleged invention.
4. **Medicine** or **Drug** includes:
    (i) All medicines for internal or external use of human beings or animals.
    (ii) All substances intended to be used for or in the diagnosis, treatment, mitigation or prevention of diseases in human beings or animals.
    (iii) All substances intended to be used for or in the maintenance of public health, or the prevention or control of any epidemic disease among human beings or animals.
    (iv) Insecticides, germicides, fungicides, weedicides and all other substances intended to be used for the protection or preservation of plants.
    (v) All chemical substances which are ordinarily used as intermediates in the preparation or manufacture of any of the medicines or substances above referred to.
5. **Patent** means a patent granted under this Act.
6. **Patent agent** means a person for the time being registered under this Act as a patent agent.
7. **Patented article** and **Patented process** means respectively an article or process in respect of which a patent is in force.

8. **Patentee** means the person for the time being entered on the register as the grantee or the proprietor of the patent.
9. **Patent of addition** means a patent granted in accordance with prescribed section in the Act.
10. **Patent office** means the patent office referred to in Section in the Act.

Inventions which are non patentable under Patents Act

The following are not inventions, within the meaning of this Act, and hence are not patentable:

(i) An invention which is frivolous or which claims anything obviously contrary to well established natural laws.

(ii) An invention the primary or intended use of which would be contrary to laws or morality or injurious to public health.

(iii) The mere discovery of a scientific principle or the formulation of an abstract theory.

(iv) The mere discovery of any new property or new use for a known substance or of the mere use of known process, machine or apparatus, unless such known process results in a new product or at least one new reactant.

(v) A substance obtained by a mere admixture resulting only in the aggregation of the properties of the components thereof or a process for producing such substance.

(vi) The mere arrangement or rearrangement or duplication of known devices each functioning independently of one another in a known way.

(vii) A method or process of testing applicable during the process of manufacture for rendering the machine, apparatus or other equipment more efficient or for the improvement or restoration of the existing machine, apparatus or other equipment or for the improvement or control of manufacture.

(viii) A method of agriculture or horticulture.

(ix) Any process for the medicinal, surgical, curative, prophylactic or other treatment of human beings or any process for a similar treatment of animals or plants to render them free of disease or to increase their economic value or that of their products.

Inventions relating to atomic energy not patentable

No patent shall be granted in respect of any invention relating to atomic energy falling under the Atomic Energy Act, 1962.

Inventions where only methods or processes of manufacture are patentable

1. In the case of inventions:
   (i) claiming substances intended for use, or capable of being used, as food or as medicine or as drug, or
   (ii) relating to substances prepared or produced by chemical processes (including alloys, optical glass, semiconductors and inter-metallic compounds).

   No patent shall be granted in respect of claims for the substances themselves, but for the claims for the methods or processes of manufacture shall be patentable.
2. Notwithstanding anything contained in sub-section (1) above, a claim for patent of an invention for a substance itself intended for use, or capable of being used, as medicine or drug may be made and shall be dealt in the manner as provided by the Patents (Amendment) Act, 1999.

Persons entitled to apply for patents

1. Person should be citizen of India, above 21 years of age and graduate from any Indian university.
2. An application for a patent for an invention may be made by any of the following persons, that is to say:
   (a) by any person claiming to be the true and first investor of the invention;
   (b) by any person being the assignee of the person claiming to be the true and first inventor in respect of the right to make such an application;
   (c) by the legal representative of any deceased person who immediately before his death was entitled to make such an application.
3. An application may be made by any of the persons referred to therein either alone or jointly with any other person.

Types of patents and the procedure for obtaining a patent

Following types of patents are granted under the Act:
   (i) An ordinary patent.
   (ii) A patent of addition for improvement in or modification of an invention for which a patent has already been applied for or granted.
   (iii) A patent granted in respect of a convention application filed under Section 135 of the Act.
   (iv) A product patent for a medicine or drug as provided by the Patents (Amendment) Act, 1999.

Procedure for getting a Patent

An application for an ordinary patent including that for a product patent may be made by the person claiming to be the first or true inventor, his legal representative, or his assignee, either alone or jointly with any other person. An application for a patent of addition may be made only by the applicant for original patent.

Every application for a patent should be for one invention only and should be made in the prescribed form and filed in the Patent Office (Head Office at Kolkata and Branch Offices at Chennai, Mumbai and Delhi). If the application is made by virtue of an assignment, then the proof of the right to make an application should be furnished. It must be stated in the application that the applicant is in possession of the invention and the name of the owner claiming to be the true and first inventor must also be stated.

Every application must be accompanied by a provisional or a complete specification. A provisional specification is a document in a prescribed form containing a description of the essential features of the invention. A complete specification is a document drawn in a prescribed form and contains the following:

(i) A full description of the invention and its operation or use and the method of performance.
(ii) Disclosure of the best method of performing the invention known to the applicant and for which he is entitled to claim protection.
(iii) A statement of claim or claims defining the scope of the invention for which protection is sought.

Every specification, whether provisional or complete shall describe the invention and begin with a title sufficiently indicating the subject-matter to which the invention relates. Where an application is accompanied by a provisional specification, a complete specification must be filed within 12 months from the date of filing of the application.

On receiving the application for a patent along with complete specification, the Controller shall refer it to an examiner for making a report to him in respect of:

(i) Whether the application and specification are in accordance with the requirements of this Act and of any Rules made thereunder.
(ii) Whether there is any lawful ground of objection to the grant of patent under the Act in pursuance of the applications.
(iii) The result of investigation made by him regarding anticipation of the invention by virtue of a previous publication or prior claim.
(iv) Any other matter which may be prescribed.

The examiner to whom the application and specification relating thereto has been referred to should ordinarily make the report to the Controller within a period of eighteen months from the date of such reference. If the report is adverse to the applicant or requires any amendment of application, the Controller shall communicate the gist of the objections to the applicant and give him an opportunity of being heard. The Controller is also empowered to refuse to proceed with the application or require the application, specification or drawings to be amended to his satisfaction. On the acceptance of the complete specification, the Controller shall notify the applicant and advertise in the Official Gazette that the specification has been accepted and thereupon the application and specification with the drawings, if any shall be open to public inspection. On and from the date of advertisement of the acceptance of a complete specification till the date of sealing of a patent, the applicant shall have the like privileges and rights as if the patent for the invention had been sealed on the date of advertisement of acceptance of the complete specification. However, the applicant shall not be entitled to institute any proceedings for infringement until the patent has been sealed.

Grounds on which the grant of patent can be opposed

Any person may oppose the grant of patent within a period of four months from the date of advertisement of the acceptance, on any of the following grounds:

(i) That the invention or part thereof has been obtained by the applicant wrongfully from him or from a person under or through whom he claims.

(ii) That the invention in question has been published before the priority date of the claim:
   (a) In any specification filed in pursuance of an application for a patent made in India on or after the 1st January, 1912.
   (b) In India or elsewhere, in any other document.

(iii) That the invention so far as claimed in any claim of the complete specification is claimed in a claim of a complete specification published on or after the priority date of the applicant's claim and filed in pursuance of an application for a patent in India, being a claim of which the priority date is earlier than that of the applicant's claim.

(iv) That the invention in question was publicly known or used in India before the priority date of that claim.

(v) That the invention in question is obvious and clearly does not involve any inventive step.

(vi) That the subject of any claim of the complete specification is not an invention within the meaning of this Act or is not patentable under this Act.
(vii) That the complete specification does not sufficiently and clearly describe the invention or the method by which it is to be performed.
(viii) That the applicant has failed to disclose sufficient information to the Controller or has furnished the information which in any material particular was false to his knowledge.
(ix) That in case of a convention application, the application was not made within twelve months from the date of first application for protection of the invention made in a Convention country by the applicant or a person from whom he derives title.

On receiving any such notice of opposition, the Controller shall notify the applicant and give him and the opponent an opportunity to be heard before deciding the case. If at any time after the acceptance of the complete specification and before the grant of a patent it comes to the notice of the Controller that the invention, so far as claimed in any claim of the complete specification, has been published before the priority date of the claim:

(i) In any specification filed in pursuance of an application for patent made in India on or after 1st January, 1912.
(ii) In any other document in India or elsewhere.

The Controller may refuse to grant the patent unless the complete specification is amended to his satisfaction within the time as may be prescribed.

If a person claims to be the inventor of an invention, or a substantial part of it, in respect of which an application for the grant of a patent is pending, the Controller may permit his name to be mentioned as an inventor in the patent granted in pursuance of the application. However, the mention of any person as inventor under this Section shall not confer or derogate from any rights under the patent.

Once a patent is granted, the Controller shall cause it to be sealed with the seal of the patent office and the date of sealing shall be entered in the register. Date of patent is the date on which the complete specification is filed. In case of death of the applicant whose patent has been sealed or in case of a body corporate which ceases to exist before the patent is sealed, the Controller may suitably amend the patent.

Procedure for surrender and revocation of patents

Surrender of Patents

A patentee may at any time offer to surrender his patent by giving notice in the prescribed manner to the Controller. The Controller shall then advertise the offer of surrender in the prescribed manner and also notify every person whose name appears in the register as having an interest in the patent. After hearing the patentee and any opponent, if the Controller is satisfied that the patent may be surrendered, he may accept the offer and by order, revoke the Patent.

Revocation of Patents

A patent may be revoked by the High Court on any of the following grounds:

(i) That the invention, so far as claimed in any claim of the complete specification, was claimed in a valid claim of earlier priority date contained in the complete specification of another patent granted in India.

(ii) That the patent was granted on the application of a person not entitled under the provisions of this Act to apply there for.

(iii) That the patent was granted wrongfully in contravention of the rights of the petitioner or any person under or through whom he claims.

(iv) That the subject of any claim of the complete specification is:
 (a) not an invention within the meaning of the Act;
 (b) is not new;
 (c) is obvious or does not involve any inventive step;
 (d) is not useful;
 (e) is not patentable under this Act.

(v) That the complete specification does not sufficiently and fairly describe the invention and the method by which it is to be performed.

(vi) That the scope of any claim of the complete specification is not sufficiently and clearly defined or that any claim of the complete specification is not fairly based on the matter disclosed in the specification.

(vii) That the applicant has failed to disclose to the Controller the information required by him or has furnished information which in any material was false to his knowledge.

(viii) That the patent was obtained on a false suggestion or representation.

(ix) That the applicant contravened any direction for secrecy.

(x) That leave to amend complete specification was obtained by fraud.

A patent may be revoked by the High Court on the petition of the Central Government, if the High Court is satisfied that the patentee has, without reasonable cause, failed to comply with the request of the Central Government to make use or exercise the patented invention for the purposes of Government upon reasonable terms.

Where the Central Government is of opinion that a patent or the mode in which it is exercised is mischievous to the State or generally prejudicial to the public, it may, after giving the patentee an opportunity to be heard, make a declaration to that effect in the Official Gazette and thereupon the patent shall be deemed to be revoked.

Revocation of patent in public interest

Where the Central Government is of opinion that a patent or the mode in which it is exercised is mischievous to the State or generally prejudicial to the public, it may, after giving the patentee an opportunity to be heard, make a declaration to that effect in the Official Gazette and thereupon the patent shall be deemed to be revoked.

Register of patents and removal from Register

A register of patents is kept at the patent office which contains the names, addresses of grantees of patents, notifications of assignments and of transmissions of patents and other such required particulars which affects the validity or proprietorship of patents.

The register is kept under the control and management of the Controller. At all convenient times, the register shall be open to inspection by the public and certified copies duly sealed, of any entry in register, shall be given to any person on payment of the prescribed fee. The register shall be prima facie evidence of any matters required or authorized by or under this Act to be entered therein.

The Central Government may remove the name of any person from the register on giving reasonable opportunity of being heard but after the enquiry thinks fit to remove or has been convicted of any professional misconduct

Use of Inventions for the Purpose of Government

At any time after an application for a patent has been filed at the patent office or a patent has been granted, the Central Government and any person authorized in writing by it, may use the invention for the purpose of Government in accordance with the provisions of this Chapter.

Moreover, if the Central Government is satisfied that it is necessary to acquire a patent from the applicant or the patentee for a public purpose, publish a notification to that effect in the Official Gazette, and thereupon the invention or patent and all rights in respect of the invention or patent shall, by force of this Section, stand transferred to and be vested in the Central Government. The Central Government shall pay to the applicant or, as the case may be, the patentee and other persons appearing on the register as having an interest in the patent such compensation as may be agreed upon between the Central Government and the applicant, or the patentee and other persons.

Offences and Penalties under the Patents Act, 1970

Contravention of secrecy provisions relating to certain inventions

If any person fails to comply with any secrecy directions given for defence purposes, he shall be punishable with imprisonment for a term upto two years, or with fine, or with both.

Falsification of entries in register, etc.

If any person makes, or causes to be made, a false entry in any register kept under this Act, or produces any such false entry as an evidence, he shall be punishable with imprisonment for a term which may extend to two years, or with fine, or with both.

Unauthorized claim of Patent rights

If any person falsely represents that any article sold by him is patented in India or is the subject of an application for a patent in India, he shall be punishable with fine which may extend to five hundred rupees.

Wrongful use of words "Patent office"

If any person uses on his place of business or any document issued by him or otherwise the words "Patent office" or any other words which would reasonably lead to the belief that place of business is, or is officially connected with, the patent office, he shall be punishable with imprisonment for a term which may extend to six months, or with fine, or with both.

Refusal or failure to supply information

(i) If any person refuses or fails to furnish to the Central Government or to the Controller, any information which he is required to furnish, lie shall be punishable with fine which may extend to one thousand rupees.

(ii) If any person, being required to furnish any such information furnishes information or statement which is false, and which he either knows or has reason to believe to be false or does not believe to be true, he shall be punishable with imprisonment which may extend to six months, or with fine, or with both.

Practice by non-registered Patent Agents

If a person who is not registered as a Patent agent describes himself or practices as a Patent Agent, he shall be punishable with fine which may extend to five hundred rupees in the case of a first offence and two thousand rupees in case of a second or subsequent offence.

Offences by Companies

If the person committing an offence under this Act is a company, the company as well as every person in charge of and responsible to the company for the conduct of its business at the time of commission of the offence shall be deemed to be guilty of the offence and shall be liable to be proceeded against and punished accordingly: However, the person shall not be liable to any punishment if he proves that the offence was committed without his knowledge or that he exercised all due diligence to prevent the commission of such offence.

Where an offence under this Act has been committed by a company and it is proved that the offence has been committed with the consent or connivance of, or that the commission of the offence is attributable to any neglect on the part of any director, manager, secretary or other officer of the company, such director, manager, secretary or other officer shall also be deemed to be guilty of that offence and shall be liable to be proceeded against and punished accordingly.

Restrictions upon publication of specifications

An application for a patent, and any specification filed in pursuance thereof, shall not, except with the consent of the applicant, be published by the Controller or be open to public inspection at any time before the date of advertisement of acceptance of the application in pursuance of applicable section.

Few important abbreviations and their expansion connected with patents

GATT	General Agreement on Trade and Tariffs
WTO	World Trade Organization
TRIPs	Trade Related Intellectual Property Rights
EMR	Exclusive Marketing Rights
IPR	Intellectual Property Rights
DST	Department of Science and Technology
TIFAC	Technology Information Forecasting and Assessment Council
CITIES	Convention on International Trade In Endangered Species
GRAIN	Genetic Resources Action International
ICAR	Indian Council for Agricultural Research
IJIRA	Indian Jute Industries Research Association
TSKP	Tamarind Seed Kernel Power
CSIR	Council for Scientific and Industrial Research
CLRI	Central Leather Research Institute
CRRI	Central Road Research Institute
AIMS	Ayurvedic Indian Medical System
ICMR	Indian Council for Medical Research
NIV	National Institute of Virology
GI	Geographical Indications
GATS	General Agreement Trade in Services

QUESTIONS FOR REVISION

1. What are the requirements for applying to a patent?
2. What are the various types of patents and explain the procedure for obtaining a patent.
3. Write a note on grounds on which patent can be opposed.
4. Explain the following:
   (a) Product Patent
   (b) Procedure for surrender and revocation of patents.
5. Discuss the offences and penalties under the Patents Act.

Chapter 20

Right to Information Act, 2005

The Right to Information Act, 2005 (RTI) is a comprehensive legislation that would confer statutory rights on citizens for seeking information from public authorities and replaced the Freedom of Information Act, 2002. Under the provisions of the Act any citizen may request information from a "public authority" (a body of Government or "instrumentality of State") which is required to reply expeditiously or within thirty days. The Act also requires every public authority to computerise their records for wide dissemination and to proactively provide certain categories of information so that the citizens need minimum recourse to request for information formally. This law was passed by Parliament on 15 June, 2005 and came fully into force on 12 October, 2005. The Act applies to all States and Union Territories of India except Jammu & Kashmir. The Act is expected to bring good governance and promote more transparency and accountability.

Objectives of the Right to Information Act, 2005

The main objectives of the Right to Information Act are:

(a) To empower the citizens, promote transparency and accountability in the working of the Government.
(b) To control corruption, and make our democracy work for the people in real sense.
(c) To make the government more accountable to the citizens and making the citizens informed about the activities of the Government.

Right to Information

Right to Information means the right to information, accessible under this Act, which is held by or under the control of any public authority and includes the right to:

(i) Inspection of work, documents, records.
(ii) Taking notes, extracts, or certified copies of documents or records.
(iii) Taking certified samples of material.
(iv) Obtaining information in the form of diskettes, floppies, tapes, video cassettes or in any other electronic mode or through printouts, where such information is shared in a computer or in any other device.

Subject to the provisions of the Act, all citizens have right to information.

Information

Information means any material in any form, including records, documents, memos, e-mail, opinions, advices, press releases, circulars, orders, log books, contacts, reports, papers, samples, models, data material held in any electronic form and information relating to any private body which can be accessed by a public authority under any law for the time being in force.

In common practice, information refers to a thing told, knowledge or items of knowledge. In relation to electronic forms, 'information' as per Information Technology Act, 2000 includes data, text, images, sound, voice, codes, computer programs, software and databases or microfilm or computer generated microfiche. Information may be of facts or of law. It may come from external sources or even from material already on records or may be derived from the discovery of new and important matter of fresh facts.

Records

Records includes:

(i) Any document, manuscript and file;
(ii) Any microfilm, microfiche and facsimile copy of a document;
(iii) Any reproduction of image or images embodied in such microfilm (whether enlarged or not); and
(iv) Any other material produced by a computer or any other device.

Request for Information

Any person, who desires to obtain any information, shall make a request in writing or through electronic means, in English or Hindi or in the official language of the area in which the application is being made to the Central

Public Information Officer (or the Assistant PIO) of the public authority concerned. The request should specify the particulars of the information sought by the applicant and should be accompanied by the requisite fee.

If an applicant cannot make a request in writing, the Public Information Officer shall provide all possible assistance to the applicant making the request orally to reduce same in writing.

The applicant need not to give any reason for requisitioning the information or any other personal details except those that may be necessary for contacting him. Where a request is made to a public authority for an information:

(i) which is held by another public authority; or
(ii) which is subject matter of or is more closely connected with the functions of another public authority

then the public authority, which received the request, shall transfer the request (or an appropriate part thereof) to such other public authority, as fast as practicable but not later than 5 days from the receipt of the application. The applicant shall be informed about such transfer.

The Central Information Commission

1. The Central Government shall, by notification in the Official Gazette, constitute a body to be known as the Central Information Commission to exercise the powers and to perform the functions assigned under this Act.
2. The Central Information Commission shall consist of:
   (a) the Chief Information Commissioner; and
   (b) such number of Central Information Commissioners, not exceeding ten, as may be deemed necessary.
3. The Chief Information Commissioner and Information Commissioners shall be appointed by the President on the recommendation of a committee consisting of:
   (a) the Prime Minister, who shall be the Chairperson of the committee;
   (b) the Leader of Opposition in the Lok Sabha; and
   (c) a Union Cabinet Minister to be nominated by the Prime Minister.

The State Information Commission

Every State Government shall, by notification in the Official Gazette, constitute a State Information Commission to exercise the powers conferred on, and to perform the functions assigned to it, under this Act.

The State Information Commission shall consist of the State Chief Information Commissioner, and such number of State Information Commissioners, not exceeding ten, as may be deemed necessary.

The State Chief Information Commissioner and the State Information Commissioners shall be appointed by the Governor on the recommendation of a Committee consisting of the Chief Minister, the Leader of Opposition in the Legislative Assembly and a Cabinet Minister to be nominated by the Chief Minister.

Powers and functions of the Information Commissions, appeal and penalties

1. As per the provisions of this Act, it shall be the duty of the Central Information Commission or State Information Commission, as the case may be, to receive and inquire into a complaint from any person—
   (a) who has been unable to submit a request to a Central Public Information Officer or State Public Information Officer, as the case may be, either by reason that no such officer has been appointed under this Act, or because the Central Assistant Public Information Officer or State Assistant Public Information Officer, as the case may be, has refused to accept his or her application for information or appeal under this Act for forwarding the same to the Central Public Information Officer or State Public Information Officer;
   (b) who has been refused access to any information requested under this Act;
   (c) who has not been given a response to a request for information or access to information within the time limit specified under this Act;
   (d) who has been required to pay an amount of fee which he or she considers unreasonable;
   (e) who believes that he or she has been given incomplete, misleading or false information under this Act; and
   (f) in respect of any other matter relating to requesting or obtaining access to records under this Act.
2. Where the Central Information Commission or State Information Commission, as the case may be, is satisfied that there are reasonable grounds to inquire into the matter, it may initiate an inquiry in respect thereof.
3. The Central Information Commission or State Information Commission, as the case may be, shall, while inquiring into any matter under this section, have the same powers as are vested in a civil court.

Public Information Officers and their Role

As per the Act, every public authority shall designate as many Public Information Officers (PIOs) in all administrative units or offices under it, as may be necessary to provide information to persons requesting for it.

A PIO has been assigned following functions:
(a) To deal with requests from persons seeking information and reasonable assistance to the persons seeking such information.
(b) To render all reasonable assistance to the person making the request orally to reduce the same in writing.
(c) To dispose a request for information expeditiously.

Processing of Request

The PIO refers the concerned office and the other officer to whom the request is referred by PIO for supply of information, shall supply the complete information to the PIO at the earliest, but not later than 10 days and if it is getting delayed due to any reason, the reasons are to be communicated to the PIO as an interim reply. Once the information is received, the PIO will supply the same to the applicant within thirty days of the receipt of request or reject the request for any of reasons specified in Act. However, where the information sought for concerns the life or liberty of a person, the same shall be provided within 48 hours of the receipt of request. If the concerned officer fails to provide the information, he/she will be liable for neglect of duty.

On receipt of a request for information, the PIO shall provide the information on payment of prescribed fee. The PIO shall send an intimation to the applicant, stating:

(a) The details of fees, towards cost of providing the information, together with the calculation details, and requesting him to deposit fees.
(b) The applicant can seek review of the decision on fees charged by him or the form of access.

Disposal of Request for Information Partly Exempted

When a part of the information which is desired is exempted from disclosure, then the applicant shall be provided information of only part which is not so exempted and can be provided. In such cases, for allowing access to a part of the record, the PIO shall give a notice to the applicant informing:

(a) That only part of the record requested is being provided.
(b) The reasons for the decision and the name and designation of the person giving the decision.
(c) The amount of fees required to be deposited by the applicant and calculation details thereof.

If PIO fails to give a decision on a request within the specified time limit, the request shall be deemed to have been refused. The following shall be communicated to the applicant:

(a) The reasons for such rejection.
(b) The period within which an appeal against such rejection may be preferred.

Fee for Providing the Information

The information shall be provided to the applicant on payment of requisite fee. In relation to public authorities falling under the jurisdiction of Central Government, the applicant shall be required to pay the following fee:

(a) Request for obtaining information – Rs 10 per request under Sec 6 of the Act.
(b) For large size paper – Actual charge or cost price.
(c) For samples or models – Actual cost or price.
(d) For inspection or records:
   (i) For the first hour – Nil
   (ii) For each subsequent hour – Rs 5/- (or part thereof)
(e) For information provided in diskette – Rs 50/- per diskette or floppy.
(f) For information provided in printed – Price fixed for the form publication.
(g) For extracts from a publication – Rs 2/- per page of photocopy.

Exemption

Certain information as mentioned in Sections 8 and 9 of the Act may not be provided due to the sensitive nature of the information. The information, disclosure of which will prejudicially affect the sovereignty and integrity of India, the security, strategic, scientific or economic interests of the state, relation with foreign state or lead to incitement of an offence.

In addition any information which relates to personal information, the disclosure of which has no relationship to any public activity or interest, or which could cause unwarranted invasion of the privacy of the individual may also not be disclosed unless the PIO/Appellate Authority is satisfied that the larger public interest justifies the disclosure of such information.

Information which may appear innocuous when seen in isolation but may give away sensitive information when collated by different sources is also to be exempted. The PIO shall see all requests keeping the above points in view.

Information Not Exempt from Disclosure

The exemption from disclosure shall not apply in the following cases:

(a) Information which cannot be denied to the Parliament or a State Legislature.

(b) When the public interest in disclosure outweighs the harm to the protected interest.
(c) Any information relating to any occurrence, event or matter which has taken place, occurred or happened twenty years before the date of request for such information, except when information is covered under Sec 8(1)(a)(e) or (i).
(d) Information pertaining to the allegations of corruption and human rights violation relating to the intelligence and security.

Penalties

If the Central Information Commission at the time of deciding any complaint or appeal finds that PIO has, without any reasonable cause, has refused to receive an application for information, has not furnished the information within the time specified, has malafidely denied the request for information, knowingly has given incorrect, incomplete or misleading information, destroyed the information which is the subject of the request, obstructed in any manner in furnishing the information, and PIO is found persistently committing any of the aforesaid defaults, CIC may:

(a) Impose a penalty of Rs 250/- for each day till application is received or information is furnished, subject to maximum of Rs 25,000/-.
(b) Recommendation for disciplinary action as applicable.

QUESTIONS FOR REVISION

1. What are the objectives and salient features of Right to Information Act, 2005?
2. Write notes on:
   (a) Powers and functions of the Information Commissions.
   (b) Exemptions and information not exempt from disclosure.
   (c) Penalties.

Appendices

APPENDIX A

BANNED DRUGS

List of Drugs Prohibited for Manufacture and Sale through Gazette Notifications under Section 26A of Drugs & Cosmetics Act, 1940 by the Ministry of Health and Family Welfare, Govt. of India

1. Amidopyrine.
2. Fixed dose combinations of vitamins with anti-inflammatory agents and tranquilizers.
3. Fixed dose combinations of Atropine in Analgesics and Antipyretics.
4. Fixed dose combinations of Strychnine and Caffeine in tonics.
5. Fixed dose combinations of Yohimbine and Strychnine with Testosterone and Vitamins.
6. Fixed dose combinations of Iron with Strychnine, Arsenic and Yohimbine.
7. Fixed dose combinations of Sodium Bromide/Chloral Hydrate with other drugs.
8. Phenacetin.
9. Fixed dose combinations of Antihistaminic with Anti-diarrhoeals.
10. Fixed dose combinations of Penicillin with Sulphonamides.
11. Fixed dose combinations of Vitamins with Analgesics.
12. Fixed dose combinations of any other Tetracycline with Vitamin C.

13. Fixed dose combinations of Hydroxyquinoline group of drugs with any other drug except for preparations meant for external use.
14. Fixed dose combinations of Corticosteroids with any other drug for internal use.
15. Fixed dose combinations of Chloramphenicol with any other drug for internal use.
16. Fixed dose combinations of crude Ergot preparations except those containing Ergotamine, Caffeine, Analgesics, Antihistamines for the treatment of migraine, headaches.
17. Fixed dose combinations of Vitamins with Anti-TB drugs except combination of Isoniazid with Pyridoxine Hydrochloride (Vitamin B_6).
18. Penicillin skin/eye ointment.
19. Tetracycline liquid oral preparations.
20. Nialamide.
21. Practolol.
22. Methapyrilene, its salts.
23. Methaqualone.
24. Oxytetracycline liquid oral preparations.
25. Demeclocycline liquid oral preparations.
26. Combination of Anabolic Steroids with other drugs.
27. Fixed dose combination of Oestrogen and Progestin (other than oral contraceptive) containing per tablet Estrogen content of more than 50 mcg (equivalent to Ethinyl Estradiol) and Progestin content of more than 3 mg (equivalent to Norethisterone Acetate) and all fixed dose combination injectable preparations containing synthetic Oestrogen and Progesterone (Subs. by Noti. No. 743 (E) dt. 10-08-1989).
28. Fixed dose combination of Sedatives/Hypnotics/Anxiolytics with analgesics-antipyretics.
29. Fixed dose combination of Rifampicin, Isoniazid and Pyrazinamide, except those which provide daily adult dose given below:

Drugs	Minimum	Maximum
Rifampicin	450 mg	600 mg
Isoniazid	300 mg	400 mg
Pyrazinamide	1000 mg	1500 mg

30. Fixed dose combination of Histamine H-2 receptor antagonists with antacids except for those combinations approved by Drugs Controller, India.
31. The patent and proprietary medicines of fixed dose combinations of essential oils with alcohol having percentage higher than 20% proof except preparations given in the Indian Pharmacopoeia.

32. All pharmaceutical preparations containing Chloroform exceeding 0.5% w/w or v/v whichever is appropriate.
33. Fixed dose combination of Ethambutol with INH other than the following: INH Ethambutol 200 mg, 600 mg, 300 mg, 800 mg.
34. Fixed dose combination containing more than one antihistamine.
35. Fixed dose combination of any anthelmintic with cathartic/purgative except for Piperazine/Santonin.
36. Fixed dose combination of Salbutamol or any other drug having primarily bronchodilatory activity with centrally acting anti-tussive and/or antihistamine.
37. Fixed dose combination of laxatives and/or anti-spasmodic drugs in enzyme preparations.
38. Fixed dose combination of Metoclopramide with systemically absorbed drugs except fixed dose combination of metoclopramide with Aspirin/Paracetamol.
39. Fixed dose combination of centrally acting, antitussive with antihistamine, having high atropine-like activity in expectorants.
40. Preparations claiming to combat cough associated with asthma containing centrally acting antitussive and/or an antihistamine.
41. Liquid oral tonic preparations containing glycerophosphates and/or other phosphates and/or central nervous system stimulant and such preparations containing alcohol more than 20% proof.
42. Fixed dose combination containing Pectin and/or Kaolin with any drug which is systemically absorbed from GI tract except for combinations of Pectin and/or Kaolin with drugs not systemically absorbed.
43. Chloral Hydrate as a drug.
44. Dover's Powder I.P.
45. Powder Tablets I.P.
46. Antidiarrhoeal formulations containing Kaolin or Pectin or Attapulgite or Activated Charcoal.
47. Antidiarrhoeal formulations containing Phthalyl Sulphathiazole or Sulphaguanidine or Succinyl Sulphathiazole.
48. Antidiarrhoeal formulations containing Neomycin or Streptomycin or Dihydrostreptomycin including their respective salts or esters.
49. Liquid oral antidiarrhoeals or any other dosage form for paediatric use containing Diphenoxylate Loperamide or Atropine or Belladona including their salts or esters or metabolites Hyoscyamine or their extracts or their alkaloids.
50. Liquid oral antidiarrhoeals or any other dosage form for paediatric use containing halogenated hydroxyquinolines.
51. Fixed dose combination of antidiarrhoeals with electrolytes.

52. Patent and Proprietary Oral Rehydration Salts other than those conforming to the following parameters:
    (a) Patent and Proprietary Oral Rehydration Salts on reconstitution to one litre shall contain:

Sodium	50–90 millimoles
Total osmolarity	240–290 millimoles
Dextrose : Sodium molar ratio	Not less than 1 : 1 and not more than 3 : 1

    (b) Patent and Proprietary Cereal-based Oral Rehydration Salts on reconstitution to one litre shall contain:

Sodium	50–90 millimoles
Total osmolarity	Not more than 290 milliosmoles
Precooked rice	Equivalent to not less than 50 gm and not more than 80 gm as total replacement of Dextrose

    (c) Patent and Proprietary Oral Rehydration Salts (ORS) may contain parameters specified above and labelled with the indication for "Adult Choleretic Diarrhoea only".
    (d) Patent and Proprietary Oral Rehydration Salts shall not contain Mono- or Polysaccharides or Saccharine sweetening agent.
53. Fixed dose combination of Oxyphenbutazone or Phenylbutazone with any other drug.
54. Fixed dose combination of Analgin with any other drug.
55. Fixed dose combination of Dextropropoxyphene with any other drug other than anti-spasmodic and/or non-steroidal anti-inflammatory drugs (NSAIDs).
56. Fixed dose combination of a drug, standards of which are prescribed in the Second Schedule to the said Act with an Ayurvedic, Siddha or Unani drug.
57. Mepacrine Hydrochloride (Quinacrine and its salts) in any dosage form for use for female sterilization or contraception.
58. Fenfluramine and Dexfenfluramine.
59. Fixed dose combination of Diazepam and Diphenhydramine Hydrochloride.
60. Rimonabant.
61. Rosiglitazone.
62. Nimesulide formulations for human use in children below 12 years of age.
63. Cisapride and its formulations for human use.
64. Phenylpropanolamine and its formulation for human use.
65. (*)Human Placental Extract and its formulations for human use.

66. Sibutramine and its formulations for human use.
67. R-Sibutramine and its formulations for human use.
68. Gatifloxacin formulations for systemic use in humans by any route including oral and injectable.
69. Tegaserod and its formulations for human use.

---

*Prohibition revoked vide Gazette Notification GSR No. 418(E) dated 30 May, 2011.

LIST OF DRUGS PROHIBITED FOR IMPORT

1. Nialamide
2. Practolol
3. Amidopyrine
4. Phenacetin
5. Methapyrilene and its salts
6. Methaqualone

Drug Formulation	Effective	Notification
Analgin and all formulations containing Analgin for human use	With immediate effect	GSR 378(E) dt: 18-06-2013
Fixed dose combination of Flupenthixol + Malitrecin for human use	With immediate effect	GSR 377(E) dt: 18-06-2013
Pioglitazone and all formulations containing Pioglitazone for human use	With immediate effect	GSR 379(E) dt: 18-06-2013
Dextyropropoxyphene and formulations containing Dextyropropoxyphene for human use	With immediate effect	GSR 332(E) dt: 23-05-2013

APPENDIX B

SCHEME OF TESTING AND INSPECTION FOR CERTIFICATION OF DISINFECTANT FLUID, PHENOLIC TYPE ACCORDING TO IS 1061:1997
(With Amendment No. 1)

1.0 **LABORATORY:** A laboratory shall be maintained which shall be suitably equipped and staffed where different tests given in the specification shall be carried out in accordance with the method given in the Table 1.

1.1. All testing apparatus shall be periodically checked and calibrated and records of such checks/calibration shall be maintained.

2.0 **TEST RECORDS:** All records of tests and inspection shall be kept in suitable forms approved by the Bureau.

2.1. Copies of any record and other connected papers that may be required by the Bureau shall be made available at any time on request.

3:0 **QUALITY CONTROL:** It is recommended that, as far as possible, Statistical Quality Control (SQC) methods may be used for controlling the quality during production as envisaged in the scheme. See IS 397 (Part 1):1972, IS 397 (Part 2):1975 and IS 397 (Part 3):1980.

4.0 In addition efforts shall be made to gradually introduce the Quality Management System as per IS/ISO 9001 as appropriate to the activities of the organization.

5.0 **STANDARD MARK:** The Standard Mark as given in column (1) of the First Schedule of the licence shall be stencilled on each container of Disinfectant Fluids, Phenolic type or printed on the label applied to the container as the case may be, provided always that the material in the container to which this Mark is thus applied conforms to every requirement of the specification. In case of 25 litres tins the Standard Mark may also be incorporated in the lead seal.

6.0 **MARKETING:** In addition, the following information shall be given on each container or printed on the label applied to it:

  (a) Name of the product
  (b) Manufacturer's name, initials or trade mark
  (c) Class, Grade and Type of the material and phenol coefficient (Rideal Walker or Rideal Walker and staphylococcal)
  (d) Batch number/Control Unit

(e) Month and year of manufacture
(f) Net volume in ml or l
(g) Any specific instructions for use
(h) A statement that mercury compounds have not been added to the product
(i) Date of expiry
(j) Any other marking required under the Weights and Measure (Packaged Commodities) Rules and Drugs and Cosmetic Rules, 1956
(k) CM/L

7.0 **PACKING:** The material shall be packed as per Cl. 5 of IS 1061: 1997.

8.0 **CONTROL UNIT:** For the purpose of this scheme, the entire quantity of disinfectant fluids, phenolic type homogenized at a time in one tank shall be considered as a Control Unit.

9.0 **LEVELS OF CONTROL:** The tests, as indicated in Table 1 and at the levels of control specified therein, shall be carried out on the whole production of the factory covered by this Scheme and appropriate records and charts maintained in accordance with Paragraph 2 above. All the production which conform to the Indian Standard and covered by this licence shall be marked with the Standard Mark.

9.1 A sample of the material shall be drawn from each C.U. and tested for all the requirements of the specification except for stability on storage. If the sample fails in any of the requirements, the batch shall be rejected. The rejected material could, however, be reprocessed and the defects rectified. Such reprocessed material when tested again shall conform to all the requirements of the specification for the relevant grade before it is used for making.

9.2 The sample of each type shall be kept for stability on storage every month and shall be tested just before the expiry period declared by the manufacturer. If it fails, a thorough check shall be made of the process of manufacture, as also of the raw materials used in the manufacture of the materials.

9.3 Mercury compounds shall be strictly excluded from all grades of disinfectant fluids.

10.0 In respect of all other clauses of the specification and at all stages of production appropriate controls and checks shall be maintained by the factory so as to ensure that the product conforms to the various requirements of the specification.

11.0 **RAW MATERIALS:** It is recommended that routine analysis of various raw materials used in the manufacture of disinfectant fluid shall be made on each lot received in the factory and appropriate records to be maintained.

12.0 **REJECTION:** A separate record shall be maintained giving information relating to the rejection of the production not conforming to the requirements of the specification and the method of its disposal. Such material in no case be stored together with those conforming to the requirements of the specification.

13.0 **SAMPLE:** The licensee shall supply, free of charge, the samples required in accordance with the Bureau of Indian Standard (Certification) Regulations, 1988, as subsequently amended, from his factory or godown. The Bureau shall pay for the samples taken by it from the open market.

14.0 **REPLACEMENT:** Whenever a complaint is received soon after the goods with Standard Marks have been purchased and used and if there is adequate evidence that the goods have not been misused, defective goods are replaced free of cost by the licensee in case the complaint is proved to be genuine and the warranty period (when applicable) has not expired. The final authority to judge the conformity of the product to the Indian Standard shall be with the Bureau.

14.1 In the event of any damages caused by the goods bearing the Standard Mark or claim being filed by the consumers against BIS Standard Mark and not 'conforming to' the relevant Indian standard, entire liability arising out of such non-conforming product shall be of licensee and BIS shall not in any way be responsible in such cases.

15.0 **STOP MARKING:** The marking of the product shall be stopped under intimation to the Bureau if, at any time, there is some difficulty in maintaining the conformity of the product to the specification, or the testing equipment goes out of order the marking may be resumed as soon as the defects are removed under intimation to BIS.

15.1 The marking of the product shall be stopped immediately if directed to do so by BIS for any reason. The marking may then be resumed only after permission by BIS. The information regarding resumption of markings shall also be sent to the Bureau.

16.0 **PRODUCTION DATA:** The licensee shall send to the Bureau as per the enclosed Proforma, to be authenticated by a Chartered Accountant a statement of quantity produced, marked and exported by them and the trade value thereof at the end of each operative year of the licence.

IS 1061: 1997
DISINFECTANT FLUIDS, BLACK AND WHITE
TABLE 1 LEVELS OF CONTROL
(Clause 9.0.5 of Scheme of Testing and Inspection)

		TEST DETAILS		LEVELS OF CONTROL		Remarks
		Test Method				
Clause	Requirements	Clause	Reference	No. of Samples	Frequency	
4.1	Composition and Description	4.1.1 or 4.1.2	IS 1061:1997	One	Each Control Unit	
4.2	Stability after dilution	Annex-A	-do-	One	-do-	
4.3	Germicidal Value	Annex-B & C	-do-	One	-do-	
4.4	Mercury Compound	Annex-D	-do-	One	Once in a month	
4.5	Stability on storage	4.2, 4.3 & 4.5	-do-	One	Once in a month	

APPENDIX C

THE SCHEDULE
List of Psychotropic Substances

No.	International Non-proprietary Names	Other Non-proprietary Names
1.		DET
2.		DMHP
3.		DMT
4.	(+)-Lysergide	LSD, LSD-25
5.		Mescaline
6.		Parahexyl
7.	Eticyclidine	Pce
8.	Rolicyclidine	Php, pcpy
9.		Psilocine, psilotsin
10.	Psilocybine	
11.		STP, DOM
12.	Tenocyclidine	Tcp
13.		THC
14.		DOB
15.		MDA
16.	Amphetamine	
17.	Dexamphetamine	
18.	Mecloqualon	
19.	Methamphetamine	
20.	Methaqualone	
21.	Methylphenidate	
22.	Phencyclidine	Pcp
23.	Phenmetrazine	
24.	Amobarbital	
25.	Cyclobarbital	
26.	Glutethimide	
27.	Pentazocine	
28.	Pentobarbital	
29.	Secobarbital	
30.	Alprazolam	
31.	Amfepramone	
32.	Barbital	
33.	Benzphetamine	

No.	International Non-proprietary Names	Other Non-proprietary Names
34.	Bromazepam	
35.	Camazepam	
36.	Chlordiazepoxide	
37.	Clobazam	
38.	Clonazepam	
39.	Clorazepate	
40.	Clotiazepam	
41.	Cloxazolam	
42.	Delorazepam	
43.	Diazepam	
44.	Estazolam	
45.	Ethchlorvynol	
46.	Ethinamate	
47.	Ethylloflazepate	
48.	Fludiazepam	
49.	Flunitrazepam	
50.	Flurazepam	
51.	Halazepam	
52.	Haloxazolam	
53.	Ketazolam	
54.	Lefetamine	Spa
55.	Loprazolam	
56.	Lorazepam	
57.	Lormetazepam	
58.	Mazindol	
59.	Medazepam	
60.	Meprobamate	
61.	Methylphenobarbital	
62.	Methypylon	
63.	Nimetazepam	
64.	Nitrazepam	
65.	Nordazepam	
66.	Oxazepam	
67.	Oxazolam	
68.	Phendimetrazine	
69.	Phenobarbital	
70.	Phentermine	
71.	Pinazepam	
72.	Pipradrol	
73.	Prazepam	

No.	International Non-proprietary Names	Other Non-proprietary Names
74.	Temazepam	
75.	Tetrazepam	
76.	Triazolam	
77.	Cathione	
78.		DMA
79.		DOET
80.		MDMA
81.		4-Ethylaminorex
82.		MMDA
83.		N-ethyl MDA
84.		N-hydroxy MDA
85.		PMA
86.		TMA
87.	Fenetyline	
88.	Levamfetamine	Levamphetamine, Lovemethamphetamine
89.		
90.	Metamfetamine racemate	Methamphetamine mecnate
91.		delta-9-***tetrahydrocannabinol & stereochemical variants
92.	Buprenorphine	
93.	Butalbital	
94.	Cathine	(+)-norpseudo-Ephedrine
95.	Allobarbital	Mefenorex
96.	Etilamfetamine	N-ethylamphetamine
97.	Fencamefamin	
98.	Fenproporex	
99.	Mefenorex	
100.	Midazolam	
101.	Pemoline	
102.	Pyrov aerone	
103.	Secbutabarbital	
104.	Vinylbital	
105.		Rutobarbital
105A.	Etryptamine	
105B.	Methcathinone	
105C.	Zipeprol	
105D.	Aminorex	
105E.	Brotizolam	
105F.	Mesocarb	
110.	Salts and preparations of above	

APPENDIX D

LIST OF ESSENTIAL MEDICINES

Medicine/Drug	Category
Acetazolamide	Miotics and anti-glaucoma medicines
Acetyl salicylic acid	• Analgesics, antipyretics, nonsteroidal anti-inflammatory medicines • Medicines used to treat gout and disease modifying agents used in rheumatoid disorders • Non-opioid analgesics, antipyretics and non-steroidal anti-inflammatory medicines
Acetyl salicylic acid	• Antimigraine medicines • For treatment of acute attack
Acetyl salicylic acid	• Cardiovascular medicines • Antianginal medicines
Acetyl salicylic acid	• Antithrombotic medicines
Acriflavin + Glycerin	• Disinfectants and antiseptics • Antiseptics
Actinomycin D	• Cytotoxic medicines
Activated Charcoal	• Antidotes and other substances used in poisonings • Nonspecific
Acyclovir	• Antiviral medicines • Antiherpes medicines • Antiinfective medicines
Acyclovir	• Antiinfective medicines
Adenosine	• Antiarrhythmic medicines
Adrenaline bitartrate	• Antiallergics and medicines used in anaphylaxis
Albendazole	• Anti-infective medicines • Anthelminthics • Intestinal anthelminthics
Albumin	• Plasma fractions for specific use
Allopurinol	• Medicines used to treat gout • Medicines used in palliative care

(Contd.)

Medicine/Drug	Category
Alpha Interferon	• Cytotoxic medicines
Alprazolam	• Medicines used for generalized anxiety and sleep disorders
Aluminium hydroxide + Magnesium hydroxide	• Gastrointestinal medicines • Antacids and other antiulcer medicines
5-Amino salicylic acid (5-ASA)	• Antiinflammatory medicines
Amikacin	• Other antibacterials
Amiodarone	• Antiarrhythmic medicines
Amitriptyline	• Medicines used in mood disorders • Medicines used in depressive disorders
Amlodipine	• Antihypertensive medicines
Amoxicillin	• Antibacterials beta lactam medicines
Amoxicillin + Clavulinic acid	• Antibacterials beta lactam medicines
Amphotericin B	• Antifungal medicines • Antileishmaniasis medicines
Ampicillin	• Antibacterials beta lactam medicines
Anti-D immunoglobin (Human)	• Sera and immunoglobins
Antitetanus human immunoglobin	• Sera and immunoglobins
Artesunate (To be used only in combination with Sulfadoxine + Pyrimethamine)	• Antimalarial medicines for curative treatment
Ascorbic acid	• Vitamins and minerals
Atenolol	• Antihypertensive medicines
Atorvastatin	• Hypolipidemic medicines
Atracurium besylate	• Muscle relaxants (peripherally acting)
Atropine sulphate	• Preoperative medication and sedation for short-term procedures
Atropine sulphate	• Antidotes and other substances used in poisonings – Specific

(Contd.)

Medicine/Drug	Category
Atropine sulphate	• Mydriatics
Azathioprine	• Disease modifying agents used in rheumatoid disorders • Antineoplastic, immunosuppressives and medicines used in palliative care • Immunosuppressive medicines
Azithromycin	• Other antibacterials
B.C.G. vaccine	• Vaccines for universal immunisation
Barium sulphate	• Radiocontrast media
Beclomethasone dipropionate	• Medicines acting on the respiratory tract • Antiasthmatic medicines
Benzathine benzylpenicillin	• Antibacterials beta lactam medicines
Benzoin compound	• Disinfectants and antiseptics • Antiseptics
Benzyl benzoate	• Scabicides and pediculicides
Betamethasone dipropionate	• Antiinflammatory and antipruritic medicines
Betamethasone	• Antioxytocics
Betaxolol hydrochloride	• Miotics and anti-glaucoma medicines
Bisacodyl	• Laxatives
Bleaching powder	• Disinfectants
Bleomycin	• Cytotoxic medicines
Bromocriptine mesylate	• Antiparkinsonism medicines
Bupivacaine hydrochloride	• Local anesthetics
Busulphan	• Cytotoxic medicines
Calamine	• Antiinflammatory and antipruritic medicines
Calcium gluconate	• Antidotes and other substances used in poisonings – Specific • Vitamins and minerals
Calcium ipodate	• Radiocontrast media
Carbamazepine	• Anticonvulsants/antiepileptics
Carbimazole	• Thyroid and antithyroid medicines

(Contd.)

Medicine/Drug	Category
Carboplatin	• Cytotoxic medicines
Cefixime	• Antibacterials beta lactam medicines
Cefotaxime	• Antibacterials beta lactam medicines
Ceftazidime	• Antibacterials beta lactam medicines
Ceftriaxone	• Antibacterials beta lactam medicines
Cephalexin	• Antibacterials beta lactam medicines
Cetrimide	• Disinfectants and antiseptics • Antiseptics
Cetrizine	• Antiallergics and medicines used in anaphylaxis
Chlorambucil	• Cytotoxic medicines
Chloramphenicol	• Ophthalmological preparations, anti-infective agents
Chlorhexidine	• Disinfectants and antiseptics • Antiseptics
Chloroquine phosphate	• Antimalarial medicines for curative treatment
Chlorpheniramine maleate	• Antiallergics and medicines used in anaphylaxis
Chlorpromazine hydrochloride	• Psychotherapeutic medicines • Medicines used in psychotic disorders
Ciprofloxacin hydrochloride	• Other antibacterials • Ophthalmological preparations • Anti-infective agents
Cisplatin	• Cytotoxic medicines
Clindamycin	• For prophylaxis • Antimalarial medicines for curative treatment
Clofazimine	• Antileprosy medicines
Clomiphene citrate	• Ovulation inducers
Clopidogrel	• Cardiovascular medicines • Antianginal medicines
Clotrimazole	• Antifungal medicines
Cloxacillin	• Antibacterials beta lactam medicines
Coal tar	• Medicines affecting skin differentiation and proliferation

(Contd.)

Medicine/Drug	Category
Codeine phosphate	• Antitussives
Colchicine	• Medicines used to treat gout
Condoms	• Barrier methods
Co-Trimoxazole (Trimethoprim + Sulphamethoxazole)	• Other antibacterials • Antipneumocystosis and antitoxoplasmosis medicines
Cryoprecipitate	• Plasma fractions for specific use
Cyanocobalamin	• Medicines affecting the blood • Antianaemia medicines
Cyclophosphamide	• Cytotoxic medicines
Cyclosporins	• Antineoplastic, immunosuppressives and medicines used in palliative care • Immunosuppressive medicines
Cytosine arabinoside	• Cytotoxic medicines
D.P.T. vaccine	• Vaccines for universal immunisation
Dacarbazine	• Cytotoxic medicines
Danazol	• Cytotoxic medicines
Dapsone	• Antileprosy medicines
Daunorubicin	• Cytotoxic medicines
Desferrioxamine mesylate	• Antidotes and other substances used in poisonings – Specific
Dexamethasone	• Antiallergics and medicines used in anaphylaxis • Hormones, other endocrine medicines and contraceptives • Adrenal hormones and synthetic substitutes
Dexchlorpheniramine maleate	• Antiallergics and medicines used in anaphylaxis
25% Dextrose	• Medicines used to treat hypoglycemia
Dextran-40	• Blood products and plasma substitutes • Plasma substitutes
Dextran-70	• Blood products and plasma substitutes • Plasma substitutes
Dextromethorphan	• Antitussives

(Contd.)

Medicine/Drug	Category
Diazepam	• Preoperative medication and sedation for short-term procedures
Diazepam	• Anticonvulsants/antiepileptics
Diazepam	• Medicines used for generalized anxiety and sleep disorders
Diclofenac	• Analgesics, antipyretics, nonsteroidal anti-inflammatory medicines • Medicines used to treat gout and disease modifying agents used in rheumatoid disorders • Non-opioid analgesics, antipyretics and non-steroidal anti-inflammatory medicines
Dicyclomine hydrochloride	• Antispasmodic medicines
Didanosine	• Antiretroviral medicines • Nucleoside reverse transcriptase inhibitors
Diethylcarbamazine citrate	• Antifilarials
Digoxin	• Medicines used in heart failure
Dihydroergotamine	• Antimigraine medicines • For treatment of acute attack
Diloxanide furoate	• Antiprotozoal medicines • Antiamoebic and antigiardiasis medicines
Diltiazem	• Cardiovascular medicines • Antianginal medicines
Diltiazem	• Antiarrhythmic medicines
Dimercaprol	• Antidotes and other substances used in poisonings – Specific
Diphtheria	• Antitoxin sera and immunoglobins
Dithranol	• Medicines affecting skin differentiation and proliferation
Dobutamine	• Medicines used in heart failure
Domperidone	• Antiemetics
Dopamine hydrochloride	• Medicines used in heart failure
Doxorubicin	• Cytotoxic medicines
Doxycycline	• Other antibacterials

(Contd.)

Medicine/Drug	Category
Efavirenz	• Non-nucleoside reverse transcriptase inhibitors
EMLA cream	• Local anesthetics
Enalapril maleate	• Antihypertensive medicines
Enoxaparin	• Medicines affecting coagulation
Erythromycin estolate	• Other antibacterials
Esmolol	• Antiarrhythmic medicines
Ethambutol	• Antituberculosis medicines
Ether	• General anesthetics and oxygen
Ethinylestradiol	• Estrogens
Ethinylestradiol + Levonorgesterol	• Contraceptives • Hormonal contraceptives
Ethinylestradiol + Norethisterone	• Contraceptives • Hormonal contraceptives
Ethyl alcohol 70%	• Disinfectants and antiseptics • Antiseptics
Etoposide	• Cytotoxic medicines
Factor IX complex (Coagulation Factors II, VII, IX, X)	• Plasma fractions for specific use
Factor VIII concentrate	• Plasma fractions for specific use
Famotidine	• Gastrointestinal medicines, antacids and other antiulcer medicines
Fentanyl	• Opioid analgesics
Ferrous sulphate/fumarate	• Medicines affecting the blood • Antianaemia medicines
Filgrastim	• Medicines used in palliative care
Fluconazole	• Antifungal medicines
Flumazenil	• Antidotes and other substances used in poisonings – Specific
Fluorescein	• Diagnostic agents, ophthalmic medicines
5-Fluorouracil	• Cytotoxic medicines

(Contd.)

Medicine/Drug	Category
Fluoxetine hydrochloride	• Medicines used in mood disorders • Medicines used in depressive disorders • Medicines used for obsessive compulsive disorders and panic attacks
Flutamide	• Cytotoxic medicines
Folic acid	• Medicines affecting the blood • Antianaemia medicines
Folinic acid	• Cytotoxic medicines
Formaldehyde solution	• Disinfectants
Framycetin sulphate	• Antiinfective medicines
Fresh frozen plasma	• Blood products and plasma substitutes • Plasma substitutes
Furosemide	• Diuretics
Gemcitabine hydrochloride	• Cytotoxic medicines
Gentamicin	• Other antibacterials • Ophthalmological preparations • Anti-infective agents
Gentian violet	• Disinfectants and antiseptics • Antiseptics
Glibenclamide	• Medicines used in diabetes mellitus, insulins and other antidiabetic agents
Glucagon	• Medicines used to treat hypoglycemia
Glucose	• Solutions correcting water, electrolyte and acid-base disturbances – Parenteral
Glucose with sodium chloride	• Solutions correcting water, electrolyte and acid-base disturbances – Parenteral
Glutaraldehyde	• Disinfectants
Glycerin	• Medicines affecting skin differentiation and proliferation
Glyceryl trinitrate	• Cardiovascular medicines • Antianginal medicines
Griseofulvin	• Antifungal medicines
Haloperidol	• Psychotherapeutic medicines • Medicines used in psychotic disorders

(Contd.)

Medicine/Drug	Category
Halothane with vaporizer	• General anesthetics and oxygen
Heparin sodium	• Medicines affecting coagulation • Antithrombotic medicines
Hepatitis B vaccine	• Vaccines for universal immunisation
Homatropine	• Mydriatics
Hormone releasing IUD	• Contraceptives • Hormonal contraceptives
Hydrochlorothiazide	• Diuretics • Antihypertensive medicines
Hydrocortisone sodium succinate	• Antiallergics and medicines used in anaphylaxis • Hormones, other endocrine medicines and contraceptives • Adrenal hormones and synthetic substitutes • Medicines acting on the respiratory tract • Antiasthmatic medicines
Hydrogen peroxide	• Disinfectants and antiseptics • Antiseptics
Hydroxychloroquine phosphate	• Disease modifying agents used in rheumatoid disorders
Hydroxyethyl starch (Hetastarch)	• Blood products and plasma substitutes • Plasma substitutes
Hyoscine butyl bromide	• Antispasmodic medicines
Ibuprofen	• Analgesics, antipyretics, nonsteroidal anti-inflammatory medicines • Medicines used to treat gout and disease modifying agents used in rheumatoid disorders • Non-opioid analgesics, antipyretics and non-steroidal anti-inflammatory medicines
Ifosfamide	• Cytotoxic medicines
Imatinib	• Cytotoxic medicines
Imipramine	• Medicines used in mood disorders • Medicines used in depressive disorders
Indinavir	• Protease inhibitors
Insulin injection (Soluble)	• Medicines used in diabetes mellitus, insulins and other antidiabetic agents

(Contd.)

Medicine/Drug	Category
Intermediate-acting (Lente/NPH Insulin)	• Medicines used in diabetes mellitus, insulins and other antidiabetic agents
Intraperitoneal dialysis solution	• Peritoneal dialysis solution
Iodine	• Thyroid and antithyroid medicines
Iopanoic acid	• Radiocontrast media
Ipratropium bromide	• Medicines acting on the respiratory tract • Antiasthmatic medicines
Iron dextran	• Medicines affecting the blood • Antianaemia medicines
Isoflurane	• General anesthetics and oxygen
Isoniazid	• Antituberculosis medicines
Isosorbide 5 mononitrate/ dinitrate	• Cardiovascular medicines • Antianginal medicines
Ispaghula	• Laxatives
IUD containing copper	• Intrauterine devices
Ketamine hydrochloride	• General anesthetics and oxygen
L-Asparaginase	• Cytotoxic medicines
Lamivudine	• Antiretroviral medicines • Nucleoside reverse transcriptase inhibitors
Lamivudine + Nevirapine + Stavudine	• Antiretroviral medicines • Nucleoside reverse transcriptase inhibitors
Lamivudine + Zidovudine	• Antiretroviral medicines • Nucleoside reverse transcriptase inhibitors
Leflunomide	• Disease modifying agents used in rheumatoid disorders
Levodopa + Carbidopa	• Antiparkinsonism medicines
Levonorgesterol releasing contraceptives	• Hormonal contraceptives
Levothyroxine	• Thyroid and antithyroid medicines
Lignocaine	• Diagnostic agents • Ophthalmic medicines
Lignocaine hydrochloride	• Local anesthetics • Antiarrhythmic medicines

(Contd.)

Medicine/Drug	Category
Lignocaine hydrochloride + Adrenaline	• Local anesthetics
Lithium carbonate	• Medicines used in bipolar disorders
Lorazepam	• Anticonvulsants/antiepileptics
Losartan potassium	• Antihypertensive medicines
Magnesium sulphate	• Anticonvulsants/antiepileptics
Mannitol	• Diuretics
Measles vaccine	• Vaccines for universal immunisation
Medroxy progesterone acetate	• Progestogens
Mefloquine	• For prophylaxis • Antimalarial • Medicines for curative treatment
Meglumine iothalamate	• Radiocontrast media
Meglumine iotroxate	• Radiocontrast media
Melphalan	• Cytotoxic medicines
Mercaptopurine	• Cytotoxic medicines
Mesna	• Cytotoxic medicines
Metformin	• Medicines used in diabetes mellitus, insulins and other antidiabetic agents
Methotrexate	• Disease modifying agents used in rheumatoid disorders
Methotrexate	• Cytotoxic medicines
Methyl cellulose	• Ophthalmic surgical aids
Methyl ergometrine	• Oxytocics and antioxytocics • Oxytocics
Methyl prednisolone	• Hormones, other endocrine medicines and contraceptives • Adrenal hormones and synthetic substitutes
Methyldopa	• Antihypertensive medicines
Methylrosanilinium chloride (Gentian violet)	• Antiinfective medicines
Methylthioninium chloride (Methylene blue)	• Antidotes and other substances used in poisonings – Specific

(Contd.)

Medicine/Drug	Category
Metoclopramide	• Antiemetics
Metoprolol	• Cardiovascular medicines • Antianginal medicines
Metronidazole	• Other antibacterials • Antiprotozoal medicines • Antiamoebic and antigiardiasis medicines
Miconazole	• Dermatological medicines (Topical) • Antifungal medicines • Ophthalmological preparations • Anti-infective agents
Midazolam	• Preoperative medication and sedation for short-term procedures
Mifepristone	• Oxytocics and antioxytocics • Oxytocics
Misoprostol	• Oxytocics and antioxytocics • Oxytocics
Mitomycin-C	• Cytotoxic medicines
Morphine sulphate	• Preoperative medication and sedation for short-term procedures
Morphine sulphate	• Opioid analgesics
Morphine sulphate	• Medicines used in palliative care
Multivitamins (As per Schedule V of Drugs and Cosmetics Rules)	• Vitamins and minerals
N/2 Saline	• Solutions correcting water, electrolyte and acid-base disturbances – Parenteral
N/5 Saline	• Solutions correcting water, electrolyte and acid-base disturbances – Parenteral
N-acetylcysteine	• Antidotes and other substances used in poisonings – Specific
Naloxone	• Antidotes and other substances used in poisonings – Specific
Nelfinavir	• Protease inhibitors
Neomycin + Bacitracin	• Antiinfective medicines
Neostigmine	• Muscle relaxants (Peripherally acting)

(Contd.)

Medicine/Drug	Category
Nevirapine	• Non-nucleoside reverse transcriptase inhibitors
Nicotinamide	• Vitamins and minerals
Nifedipine	• Antihypertensive medicines • Antioxytocics
Nitrofurantoin	• Other antibacterials
Nitrous oxide	• General anesthetics and oxygen
Norethisterone	• Progestogens
Normal saline	• Solutions correcting water, electrolyte and acid-base disturbances – Parenteral
Nystatin	• Antifungal medicines
Ofloxacin	• Antituberculosis medicines
Olanzapine	• Psychotherapeutic medicines • Medicines used in psychotic disorders
Omeprazole	• Gastrointestinal medicines, antacids and other antiulcer medicines
Ondansetron	• Medicines used in palliative care • Antiemetics
Oral poliomyelitis vaccine (LA)	• Vaccines for universal immunisation
Oral Rehydration Salts	• Medicines used in diarrhoea, oral dehydration salts • Solutions correcting water, electrolyte and acid-base disturbances – Oral
Oxaliplatin	• Cytotoxic medicines
Oxygen	• General anesthetics and oxygen
Oxytocin	• Oxytocics and antioxytocics Oxytocics
Paclitaxel	• Cytotoxic medicines
Pantoprazole	• Gastrointestinal medicines, antacids and other antiulcer medicines
Paracetamol	• Analgesics, antipyretics, nonsteroidal anti-inflammatory medicines • Medicines used to treat gout and disease modifying agents used in rheumatoid disorders • Non-opioid analgesics, antipyretics and non-steroidal anti-inflammatory medicines • Antimigraine medicines • For treatment of acute attack

(Contd.)

Medicine/Drug	Category
Penicillamine	• Antidotes and other substances used in poisonings – Specific
Pentamidine isothionate	• Antileishmaniasis medicines • Antipneumocystosis and antitoxoplasmosis medicines
Permethrin	• Scabicides and pediculicides
Pheniramine maleate	• Antiallergics and medicines used in anaphylaxis
Phenobarbitone	• Anticonvulsants/antiepileptics
Phenylephrine	• Mydriatics
Phenytoin sodium	• Anticonvulsants/antiepileptics
Phytomenadione	• Medicines affecting coagulation
Pilocarpine	• Miotics and anti-glaucoma medicines
Piperazine	• Anti-infective medicines • Anthelminthics • Intestinal anthelminthics
Platelet Rich Plasma	• Plasma fractions for specific use
Polygeline	• Blood products and plasma substitutes • Plasma substitutes
Polyvalent antisnake venom	• Sera and immunoglobins
Potassium chloride	• Solutions correcting water, electrolyte and acid-base disturbances – Parenteral
Potassium permanganate	• Disinfectants
Povidone iodine	• Antiinfective medicines • Disinfectants and antiseptics • Antiseptics • Ophthalmological preparations • Anti-infective agents
Pralidoxime chloride (2-PAM)	• Antidotes and other substances used in poisonings – Specific
Praziquantel	• Antischistosomals and antitrematode medicines
Prednisolone	• Antiallergics and medicines used in anaphylaxis • Hormones and antihormones • Hormones, other endocrine medicines and contraceptives • Adrenal hormones and synthetic substitutes

(Contd.)

Medicine/Drug	Category
Prednisolone acetate	• Anti-inflammaory agents
Prednisolone sodium phosphate	• Anti-inflammaory agents
Premix Insulin 30 : 70 injection	• Medicines used in diabetes mellitus, insulins and other antidiabetic agents
Primaquine	• Antimalarial medicines for curative treatment
Procainamide hydrochloride	• Antiarrhythmic medicines
Procarbazine	• Cytotoxic medicines
Promethazine	• Preoperative medication and sedation for short-term procedures • Antiallergics and medicines used in anaphylaxis • Antiemetics
Propofol	• General anesthetics and oxygen
Propranolol hydrochloride	• Antimigraine medicines for treatment of acute attack
Propyliodone	• Radiocontrast media
Protamine sulphate	• Medicines affecting coagulation
Pyrazinamide	• Antituberculosis medicines
Pyridostigmine	• Muscle relaxants (Peripherally acting) and
Pyridoxine	• Medicines affecting the blood • Antianaemia medicines • Vitamins and minerals
Pyrimethamine	• Antimalarial medicines for curative treatment
Quinine sulphate	• Antimalarial medicines for curative treatment
Rabbies immunoglobin	• Sera and immunoglobins
Rabies vaccine	• Vaccines for universal immunisation
Raloxifene	• Hormones and antihormones
Ranitidine	• Gastrointestinal medicines, antacids and other antiulcer medicines
Riboflavin	• Vitamins and minerals
Rifampicin	• Antileprosy medicines • Antituberculosis medicines

(Contd.)

Medicine/Drug	Category
Ringer lactate	• Solutions correcting water, electrolyte and acid-base disturbances –Parenteral
Ritonavir	• Protease inhibitors
Salbutamol sulphate	• Medicines acting on the respiratory tract • Antiasthmatic medicines
Salicylic acid	• Medicines affecting skin differentiation and proliferation
Saquinavir	• Protease inhibitors
Sevoflurane	• General anesthetics and oxygen
Silver sulphadiazine	• Antiinfective medicines
Sodium bicarbonate	• Solutions correcting water, electrolyte and acid-base disturbances – Parenteral
Sodium iothalamate	• Radiocontrast media
Sodium meglumine diatrizoate	• Radiocontrast media
Sodium nitrite	• Antidotes and other substances used in poisonings – Specific
Sodium nitroprusside	• Antihypertensive medicines
Sodium stibogluconate	• Antileishmaniasis medicines
Sodium thiosulphate	• Antidotes and other substances used in poisonings – Specific
Sodium valproate	• Anticonvulsants/antiepileptics • Medicines used in bipolar disorders
Specific antisnake venom	• Antidotes and other substances used in poisonings – Specific
Spironolactone	• Diuretics
Stavudine	• Antiretroviral medicines • Nucleoside reverse transcriptase inhibitors
Stavudine + Lamivudine	• Antiretroviral medicines • Nucleoside reverse transcriptase inhibitors
Streptokinase	• Antithrombotic medicines
Streptomycin sulphate	• Antituberculosis medicines
Succinyl choline chloride	• Muscle relaxants (Peripherally acting)

(Contd.)

Medicine/Drug	Category
Sulfadoxine + Pyrimethamine	• Antimalarial medicines for curative treatment
Sulfasalazine	• Disease modifying agents used in rheumatoid disorders
Sulphacetamide sodium	• Ophthalmological preparations • Anti-infective agents
Sulphadiazine	• Other antibacterials
Tamoxifen citrate	• Hormones and antihormones
Terbutaline sulphate	• Antioxytocics
Testosterone	• Androgens
Tetanus toxoid vaccines	• For universal immunisation
Tetracaine hydrochloride	• Local anaesthetics
Thiamine	• Vitamins and minerals
Thiopentone sodium	• General anesthetics and oxygen
Timolol maleate	• Miotics and anti-glaucoma medicines
Tramadol	• Opioid analgesics
Trihexyphenidyl hydrochloride	• Antiparkinsonism medicines
Tropicamide	• Diagnostic agents, ophthalmic medicines
Tuberculin, purified protein derivative	• Immunologicals • Diagnostic agents
Urokinase	• Antithrombotic medicines
Vancomycin hydrochloride	• Other antibacterials
Vecuronium	• Muscle relaxants (Peripherally acting)
Verapamil	• Antiarrhythmic medicines
Vinblastine sulphate	• Cytotoxic medicines
Vincristine	• Cytotoxic medicines
Vitamin A	• Vitamins and minerals
Vitamin D (Ergocalciferol)	• Vitamins and minerals
Warfarin sodium	• Medicines affecting coagulation
Water for injection	• Miscellaneous

(Contd.)

Medicine/Drug	Category
Zidovudine	• Antiretroviral medicines • Nucleoside reverse transcriptase inhibitors
Zidovudine + Lamivudine + Nevirapine	• Antiretroviral medicines • Nucleoside reverse transcriptase inhibitors
Zinc oxide	• Astringent medicines
Zinc sulfate	• Antidiarrhoeal medicines

List of Abbreviations

IP	Indian Pharmacopoeia
USP	United States Pharmacopoeia
NFI	National Formulary of India
NFUSA	National Formulary of United States of America
BP	British Pharmacopoeia
BPC	British Pharmaceutical codex
RP	Russian Pharmacopoeia
SP	Swiss Pharmacopoeia
FP	French Pharmacopoeia
DTAB	Drugs Technical Advisory Board
DPCO	Drug Price Control Order
NLEM	National List of Essential Medicines
NPPA	National Pharmaceutical Pricing Authority
MTP	Medical Termination of Pregnancy
RMP	Registered Medical Practitioner
PCA	Prevention of Cruelty to Animal
CPCSEA	Committee for Control and Supervision of Experiments on Animals
IAEC	Institutional Animals Ethics Committee
AICTE	All India Council for Technical Education
AIVPE	All India Board of Pharmaceutical Education
PIO	Public Information Officer
CIC	Central Information Commission
EMR	Exclusive Marketing Rights
WTO	World Trade Organization

TRIPS	Trade Related Intellectual Right
IPR	Intellectual Property Rights
RRSL	Regional Reference Standard Laboratory
CBN	Central Bureau of Narcotics
NDPS	Narcotic Drugs and Pharmacopoeial Substances
GOAW	Government Opium and Alkaloidal Works
CCF	Chief Controller of Factories
NCD	Narcotic Control Division
DTL	Drugs Testing Laboratory
CDL	Central Drugs Laboratory
DCO	Drugs Control Officer
LA	Licensing Authority
BPC	British Pharmaceutical Codex
GMP	Good Manufacturing Practices
GLP	Good Laboratory Practices
LVP	Large Volume Parentrals
DCC	Drugs Consultative Committee

Index

A

Adulterated drug, 31
Advertisement, 169
  whose import and export are prohibited, 170
AICTE Act, 1987, 215
  Composition and functions of the Council, 216
  Different bodies of the Council, 218
  Functions of the Council, 217
  Objectives, 216
All India Pharmaceutical Congress Association, 2
Animal Welfare Board of India, 194
Ayurvedic preparations, 140
Ayurvedic, Siddha and Unani drugs, 32
  Drug Inspector, 112
  Labelling and packaging of, 114
  Manufacture of, 113
  Provisions applicable to, 109
  Sale of, 115
  Standards, 115
Ayurvedic, Siddha and Unani Drugs Consultative Committee, 111
Ayurvedic, Siddha and Unani Drugs Technical Advisory Board, 110

B

Bachelor of Pharmacy (Practice) Regulations, 2014, 24
Banned drugs, 283
Base unit of numeration, 239
Bhatia Committee, 3
Bhore Committee, 3
Bonded laboratory
  Plan of a typical laboratory, 134
Bonded manufactory, 131

C

Cannabis (hemp), 149, 151
  Plant, 151
Ceiling price, 175
Central Bureau of Narcotics (CBN), 150
Central Drugs Laboratory (CDL), 2, 35
Central Factories Act, 222
Central Information Commission, 277
Central Insecticides Board, 200
  Constitution and functions of, 200, 201
Central Insecticides Laboratory and its functions, 203
Chief Medical Officer of the district, 188

Chopra Committee, 2
   Recommendations of, 2
Classification of Intellectual Property Rights, 255
Code of ethics
   Objectives, 7
Code of pharmaceutical ethics, 6
Committee for the control and supervision of experiments on animals (CPCSEA), 195
Convention on Illicit Traffic in Narcotic Drugs and Psychotropic Substances, 1988, 150
Convention on Psychotropic Substances, 1971, 150
Copyright, 260
   Rights related to copyright, 253
Cosmetics, 32, 120
   Labelling and packaging of, 123, 124
   List of colours, dyes and pigments used in soaps, 129
   Misbranded cosmetics, 32
   Provisions applicable to, 120
   Spurious, 32
   Sale of, 122
   Standards, 123

D

Dangerous Drugs Act, 1930, 1, 149
Deaddiction centers and National Fund for Control of Drug Abuse, 155
Department of Ayush, 115
Department of Pharmaceuticals, Ministry of Chemicals and Fertilizers, 174
Dhanvantari Nighantu, 149
Director, Controller and Legal Metrology Officer
   Appointment and powers of, 237, 240
Disinfectant fluids, black and white (Levels of control), 291
Drugs, 30, 169, 264
   Adulterated, 31

Definitions, 90
Labelling of, 102, 119
   General requirements of, 102
   List of colours permitted to be used, 126
List of drugs prohibited for import, 287
List of drugs prohibited for manufacture and sale, 283
List of essential medicines, 295
Misbranded, 31
Sale of, 90
Spurious, 31
Standards used in different classes of, 127
Wholesale of, 95
Drug Prices Control Order (DPCO), 174
Drugs and cosmetics
   Import of, 64
   Manufacture of, 72
   Sale of drugs, 90
      Definitions, 90
   Offences and penalties, 99, 100
Drugs and Cosmetics Act, 1940, 2, 29
   Administration of the Act, 33
   Categories of drugs and cosmetics prohibited to be imported in India, 64
   Classes of drugs exempted from the provisions of Chapter IV of the Act, 49
   Definitions, 30
   Directions of Central Governments to State Governments, 125
   Dispensing and compounding of drugs
      Particulars to be recorded, 61
   Drug Inspector (Drugs Control Officer), 39
   Drugs and cosmetics prohibited to be manufactured and sold under the Act, 75
   Drugs which can be imported under licence or permit, 65
   Good Manufacturing Practices, 49
   Government Analyst
      Duties of, 38

Index

Qualifications of, 36
Grant of licence
  Conditions for, 58, 75, 79
  to testing institutions, 58
Grant of general licences for retail sale
  Conditions for, 93
Grant of restricted licence for retail sale
  Conditions for, 94
Import, 113, 117, 120
Import licence
  Conditions for getting, 66
Import of drugs
  by Govt. hospital/autonomous medical institution for treatment of patients, 69
  for examination, test or analysis, 67
  for personal use, 68
  Offences and penalties relating to, 72
  Places through which drugs may be imported into India, 70
  Power of Central Government to prohibit import in public interest, 71
  Procedure for, 69
  Substances exempted from provisions relating to, 70
Import of new drugs, 68
Import of Schedules C, C1 and X drugs, 67
Inspection
  Procedure of, 42
Inspectors
  Duties of, 40
  Qualifications for the appointment of, 40
Labelling, 102, 119
  General requirements of, 102
Labelling and packaging, 114, 123
  of cosmetics, 124
  of drugs, 102
Labels for products extemporaneously prepared and dispensed in pharmacy shops, 106

Licensing Authority, 39, 112
  Qualification of, 39
List of colours, dyes and pigments used in soaps, 129
List of colours permitted to be used in drugs, 126
Loan licence
  for manufacture of Ayurvedic, Siddha and Unani medicines, 115
  Manufacture on, 85
  Types of, 85
Manufacture of drugs for examination, test or analysis, 84
Manufacture of drugs other than those specified in Schedules C, C1 and X, 75
Manufacture of drugs specified in Schedule X, 83
Manufacture of drugs those are specified in Schedules C and C1 excluding Part X-B and Schedule X drugs, 79
Manufacture of new drugs, 87
Manufacture on loan licences, 85
Manufacturing licences
  General procedure for getting, 73
Manufacturing of drugs and cosmetics
  Application form No. and licence and inspection fee, 74
Objectives, 29
Offences and penalties, 99, 100, 116
  related to import of drug, 71
Packing of drugs, 106
  specified in Schedule X, 109
Patent or proprietary medicines, 32
Procedure for import of cosmetics, 121
Prohibited in the labelling, 106
Records of purchases of drugs, 99
Retail sale of drugs, 93
Sale application form, licence form and fees for renewal, 92
Schedules to the Act, 44

Significant labelling requirements of drugs, 103
Special provisions related to biological and other special products, 88
Standards used in different classes of drugs, 127
Storage of Schedule X drugs and drugs with expiry dates, 99
Storage of veterinary medicines, 99
Summary trials of offences, 126
Supply of Schedules C and C1 drugs, 98
Supply of Schedules H and X drugs, 98
Suspension and cancellation of licences, 100
Drugs and Cosmetics Rules, 1945, 29
    Schedules to the Rules, 44
        Schedule A, 44
        Schedule B, 44
        Schedule C, 44
        Schedule C1, 45
        Schedule D, 45, 47
        Schedule D-I, 45
        Schedule D-II, 45
        Schedule E, 45
        Schedule E-I, 45
        Schedule F, 45
        Schedule F(I), 45
        Schedule F(II), 45
        Schedule F(III), 45
        Schedule FF, 45
        Schedule G, 45
        Schedule H, 45
        Schedule H-1, 45
        Schedule I, 46
        Schedule J, 46, 47
        Schedule K, 46, 49
        Schedule L, 46
        Schedule L-1, 46
        Schedule M, 46, 49
        Schedule M1, 46
        Schedule M2, 46
        Schedule M3, 46
        Schedule N, 46, 59
        Schedule O, 46, 62
        Schedule P, 46, 62
        Schedule P-I, 46
        Schedule Q, 46
        Schedule R, 46
        Schedule R-I, 46
        Schedule S, 46
        Schedule T, 46
        Schedule T-A, 46
        Schedule U, 46, 62
        Schedule U-I, 47
        Schedule V, 47, 63
        Schedule W, 47
        Schedule X, 47
        Schedule Y, 47
Drugs and Magic Remedies (Objectionable Advertisements) Act, 1954, 3, 168
    Diseases and ailments, 172
    Exempted advertisements, 170, 171
    Objectives, 169
    Offences and penalties, 172
    Prohibited advertisements under the Act, 169
Drugs Consultative Committee (DCC), 35
Drugs Enquiry Committee (DEC), 2
Drugs Inspector (Drugs Control Officer), 39
Drugs (Price Control) Order, 2013, 174
    Average price to retailer, 177
    Active pharmaceutical ingredients or bulk drug, 175
    Control of sale prices of formulations, 180
    Display of prices of scheduled and non-scheduled formulations and price list, 180
    Objectives, 175
    Pricing of non-scheduled formulations, 178
    Pricing of scheduled formulation, 177
Drugs Technical Advisory Board (DTAB), 2, 33
    Constitution, 33
Dutiable goods, 131

E

Education Regulations, 23
Essential Commodities Act, 1955, 29, 174
Ethics for Indian pharmacists, 6
Excise duty, 115
Excise Officer, 131
   Regulatory powers of, 145
Experience or training for an RMP to terminate pregnancy, 189
Experimentation on animals, 193
Export of alcoholic preparations, 143

F

Factories Act, 1948, 222
   Annual leave with wages, 232
   Appeals, 233
   Approval, licensing and registration of factories, 225
   Cognizance of offences and limitation of prosecution, 233
   Hazardous process, 224
      Different provisions related to, 232
   General penalty for offences, 232
   Health and safety of workers, 227
   Inspectors and their powers, 227
   Liability of owner of premises in certain circumstances, 233
   List of Amending Acts and Adaptation Order, 223
   Objectives, 223
   Offences by workers, 233
   Penalty for obstructing Inspector, 233
   Procedure for obtaining the licence, 225
   Shifts and overtime, 231
   Working hours of adults and holidays, 231
Factories Rules, 222
Freedom of Information Act, 2002, 275
Functions of IAEC, 196
Functions of NPPA, 182

G

Generic version of a medicine, 176
Good Manufacturing Practices, 49

H

Hathi Committee, 4
Hemp (cannabis), 149, 151
Homeopathic medicine, 33
   Provisions applicable to, 116
   Sale of, 118

I

Import of drugs by Govt. hospital/autonomous medical institution for treatment of patients, 69
Import of drugs for examination, test or analysis, 67
Import of drugs for personal use, 68
Import of poisons, 184
Indian Institute of Legal Metrology, Ranchi, 236
Indian Journal of Pharmacy, 2
Indian Pharmaceutical Association, 2
Indian Pharmacopoeial Committee, 3
Industrial design, 258
Industrial property, 254
Insecticide, 199
Insecticide analysts, 203
Insecticide inspectors, 203
Insecticides (Amendment) Act, 1999, 198
Insecticides (Amendment) Rules, 2006, 198
Insecticides Act, 1968 and Rules, 1971, 198
   Administrative agencies, 200
   Appeal against non-registration or cancellation, 204
   Conditions under which import, manufacture and sale of insecticides are prohibited, 205
   Exemption, 206
   Grant of licence, 204
   Objective, 198
   Offences and penalties, 196, 205
   Offences by companies, 206
   Salient features, 199

Institutional Animal Ethics
    Committee (IAEC), 196
Intellectual Property Rights, 253
    Classification of, 255
    Copyright and rights related to
        copyright, 253
    Designs Act, 2000, 259
    Geographical indications, 260
    Industrial design, 258
    Industrial property, 254
    Jurisdiction for filing patent
        application, 261
    Types of trademarks that can be
        registered, 257

J

Joint State Pharmacy Council, 17
    Constitution of, 18
    Functions of, 19

L

Legal metrology, 235, 236
Legal Metrology Act, 2009, 235
    Act not to apply in certain cases, 244
    Declarations on pre-packaged
        commodities, 241
    Import of weights and measures, 241
    Objectives, 238
    Offences and penalties, 241
    Offences by companies on
        nomination, 244
    Penalties for offences under
        different Sections, 242
    Power of inspection and seizure, 240
    Regional Reference Standard
        Laboratories, 236
    Rules, 236
    Salient features, 239

M

Magic remedy, 169
Manufacture of
    Alcoholic preparations
        in bond (bonded laboratory), 133
        outside bond (non-bonded
            laboratory), 138

Ayurvedic, Homoeopathic
    preparations and patent and
    proprietary preparations, 140
Master of Pharmacy (M. Pharm)
    course Regulations, 2, 24
Medical Termination of Pregnancy
    Act, 1971, 187
    Approved place, 188
    Conditions for approval of places
        for termination of pregnancy,
        189
    Conditions under which pregnancy
        can be terminated, 188
    Experience or training for an RMP
        to terminate pregnancy, 189
    Objectives, 187
    Offences and penalties, 190
    Records maintained, 190
    Rules and Regulations, 190
Medicinal and Toilet Preparations
    (Excise Duties) Act, 1955 and
    Rules, 1956, 3, 130
    Bonded manufactory, 131
    Bonded laboratory
        Plan of a typical laboratory, 134
    Definitions, 131
    Denatured spirit, 132
    Denoted alcohol, 132
    Disposal of recovered alcohol, 137
    Disposal of sub-standard
        preparations, 137
    Dutiable goods, 131
    Excise Officer, 131
    Export of alcoholic preparations,
        143
    Homoeopathic preparations, 141
    Non-bonded manufactory, 131
    Non-bonded laboratory
        General description, 138
    Objectives, 130
    Offences and penalties, 147
    Patent and proprietary preparations,
        141
    Prosecutions, 147
    Restricted preparation, 132
    Standard preparation, 132
    Sub-standard preparation, 132
    Toilet preparation, 131

Unrestricted preparation, 132
Transport of alcoholic goods, 143
Medicinal cannabis, 153
Minimum Wages Act, 1948, 245
   Cognizance of offences, 251
   Exemption and exceptions, 252
   General provision for punishment of other offences, 251
   Maintenance of registers and records, 249
   Minimum rates of wages, 247
   Minimum time rate wages for piece work, 249
   Objectives, 245
   Offences by companies, 251
   Payment of minimum rates of wages, 248
   Payment of undisbursed amounts due to employees, 251
   Penalty and offences, 250
   Powers and duties of Inspectors appointed as per the provisions of the Act, 249
   Procedure for fixing and revising minimum wages, 247
   Provision affixing hours of work in a factory, 248
Mudaliyar Committee, 4

N

Narcotic Commissioner, 153
Narcotic drug, 131, 153
   List of psychotropic substances, 292
Narcotic Drugs and Psychotropic Substances Act, 1985, 149, 151
   Amending Act, 150
   Commercial quantity, 152
   Conditions for issue of licence for the manufacture of synthetic manufactured drugs, 160
   Cultivation, production, sale, etc. of opium, 156
   Import, export, transshipment of narcotic drugs and psychotropic substances, 160
   Manufacture, 152
   Manufactured drug, 152
   Manufacture of
      Cocaine, morphine, etc., 158
      Manufactured drugs and psychotropic substances, 158, 159
      Medicinal hemp, 158
      Opium, 158
      Other narcotic drugs, 159
   Objectives, 151
   Offences and penalties, 164, 165
   Officers and administrative agencies, 154
   Production of opium, 157
   Prohibition of certain operations under the Act, 154
   Sale of opium, 158
   Schedules, 161, 162
   Transshipment, 161
Narcotic Drugs and Psychotropic Substances Consultative Committee, 155
National List of Essential Medicines (NLEM), 174, 176
National Pharmaceutical Pricing Authority, 182
Non-scheduled formulation, 176

O

Opium, 149, 153
   Cultivation of, 156
   Manufacture of, 158
   Production of, 157
   Sale of, 158
Opium Act, 1878, 1, 149
Opium crop cycle, 157
Opium derivative, 153
Opium poppy, 153

P

Patent, 256, 263, 264
   Agent, 264
   Abbreviations and their expansion, 273
   of addition, 265
   office, 265
   Procedure for getting, 266, 267

Procedure for surrender and revocation, 269
Types of, 266
Patents Act, 1970, 263
   Assignee, 264
   Definitions, 264
   Drug, 264
   Exclusive licence, 264
   Invention, 264
   Inventions which are non-patentable under Patents Act, 265
   Medicine, 264
   Offences and penalties, 272
   Patented article, 264
   Patented process, 264
   Patentee, 265
   Use of inventions for the purpose of Government, 271
Patents (Amendment) Act, 2005, 263
Pharmaceutical legislation in India, 1
   Objectives of, 1
   History of, 1
Pharmacist
   Evolution as an integral part of the healthcare system, 4
   Qualification for registration, 25
Pharmacist's Oath, 10
Pharmacoeconomics, 177
Pharmacopoeia of India (IP), 3
Pharmacy Act, 1948, 12, 13
   Objectives, 13
Pharmacy Council of India (PCI), 3, 13
   Constitution of, 13
   Functions of, 15
Pharmacy education
   Regulation under the Pharmacy Act, 25
Pharmacy Practice Regulations, 2015, 4, 24
   Objectives, 24
Pharmacy profession
   Regulation under the Pharmacy Act, 26
Poisons Act, 1904, 184
Poisons Act, 1919, 1, 184
   Issue of warrants, 185

Penalties for the import, possession, and sale of poison prohibited under the Act, 185
Possession and sale of poisons, 184
Prevention of Cruelty to Animals Act, 192
   Committee for the control and supervision of experiments on animals (CPCSEA), 195
   Composition of Institutional Animals Ethics Committee (IAEC), 197
   Experimentation on animals, 193
   Objectives, 193
Psychotropic substance, 154
   Import, export, transshipment of, 160
Public Information Officers and their role, 278

R

Regional Reference Standard Laboratories, 236
Registered Medical Practitioner (RMP), 188
Registered pharmacist
   Offences and penalties, 27
Registration Committee and Registration of Insecticides, 202, 204
Registration of establishments, 209
Right to information, 276
Right to Information Act, 2005, 275
   Disposal of request for information partly exempted, 279
   Exemption, 280
   Information not exempt from disclosure, 280
   Objectives, 275
   Penalties, 281
   Powers and functions of the Information Commissions, appeal and penalties, 278
   Processing of request, 279
   Public Information Officers and their role, 278

S

Scheme of testing and inspection for certification of disinfectant fluid, phenolic type, 288
  Control unit, 289
  Laboratory, 288
  Levels of control, 289
  Marketing, 288
  Packing, 289
  Production data, 290
  Quality control, 288
  Raw materials, 290
  Rejection, 290
  Replacement, 290
  Sample, 290
  Standard mark, 288
  Stop marking, 290
  Test records, 288
Shops and Establishment Act, 208
  Cleanliness, ventilation and lighting, 210
  Hours and timings for work, 209
  Inspection of establishments, 213
  Objectives, 208
  Offences and penalties, 213
  Service conditions, 210
  Work in establishments, 209
Standards of Weights and Measures Act, 1976, 235
Standards of Weights and Measures (Enforcement) Act, 1985, 235
State Drug Control Laboratories, 36
State Information Commission, 277
State Legal Metrology (Enforcement) Rules, 236
State Pharmacy Council, 17
  Constitution of, 17
  Functions of, 19

T

Technical education, 216
Technical institution, 216
Trademarks, 257
  Types of, 257

U

UN Single Convention on Narcotics Drugs 1961, 150

W

Wholesale of drugs, 95
  Categories of licence for, 95
  Conditions for grant of licence, 95
  Conditions of licence for drugs other than those specified in Schedules C, C1 and X, 95